Review of OPHTHALMOLOGY

Must for PG Entrance Examination

Seventh Edition

Ruchi Rai

MBBS, MS, DNB (Ophthalmology), MNAMS

PEEPEE PUBLISHERS AND DISTRIBUTORS (P) LTD.®

Review of Ophthalmology

Published by
Pawaninder P. Vij and Anupam Vij

Peepee Publishers and Distributors (P) Ltd.
Head Office: 160, Shakti Vihar, Pitam Pura
Delhi-110 034 (India)

Correspondence Address:

7/31, First Floor, Ansari Road, Daryaganj
New Delhi-110002 (India)

Ph: 41512412, 23246245, 9811156083

e-mail: peepee160@yahoo.co.in

e-mail: peepee160@gmail.com

www.peepeepub.com

First Edition: 2006
Seventh Edition: 2019

ISBN: 978-81-8445-267-9

Dedicated

To my dear mentor Dr Daisaku Ikeda
who taught me to live with a "Big Heart and a Big Smile".

"Perseverance is strength. Lets live with the spirit–Still I am Not Discouraged".

PREFACE TO THE FIRST EDITION

Trends are changing, with more and more number of questions being asked from ophthalmology each year in various entrance examinations. In addition, with advances in ophthalmology occurring at a frantic pace, it is becoming increasingly difficult for the students to keep abreast with the latest. In my pursuit to help students cope with this problem, this edition has been reformatted, and is now topic based while the previous one was examination based. Each chapter contains author notes along with the corresponding questions and the key. In every chapter, the notes have been revised extensively to incorporate recent advances and contain all the information related to the questions asked. The book contains the entire latest questions and these questions are included chapter-wise. This makes the learning for the students more easy and methodical.

Wish you all the best for a bright future.

Ruchi Rai
ruchiraidr@gmail.com

PREFACE TO THE SEVENTH EDITION

A very focussed and tailored study is required to crack the PG entrance exams.

This edition includes major changes, with two separate sections of image-based and recently asked questions being added chapter-wise.

With more illustrations and images, this coloured version of the book is a visual treat for the students.

All feedback and criticism is taken with utmost seriousness and is used as a source of continuous refinement. This is the reason for the huge success of the book.

Kindly send your feedbacks at **ruchiraidr@gmail.com**

"Keep Striving Till You Win"

Stay blessed !

Ruchi Rai

ruchiraidr@gmail.com

ACKNOWLEDGEMENTS

To my dear mentor who inspired me to keep striving harder and become a better version of myself.

To my dear parents for always being a strong pillar of support.

To my husband, Dr Ashish Rai, for always being by my side.

To my lovely angels Ananya and Namya, the blessings of my life.

To my dear sister Vijaya, who is the joy and pride of my life.

To my family for all the support.

To my wonderful friends for always being a source of encouragement and making my life whole.

To Dr. Sumer Sethi and the DAMS team for their support and a wonderful working environment.

To Mr. Pawaninder P. Vij and Mr. Anupam Vij, Directors, Peepee Publishers and Distributors (P) Ltd., New Delhi for his keen interest and sincere efforts in getting the book published.

Ruchi Rai
ruchiraidr@gmail.com

CONTENTS

1. Diseases of Lens ---------- 1

2. Glaucoma ---------- 33

3. Cornea ---------- 66

4. Conjunctiva ---------- 105

5. Sclera and Episclera ---------- 127

6. Uveitis ---------- 132

7. Orbit ---------- 162

8. Ocular Adenexae ---------- 201

9. Lacrimal Drainage System ---------- 215

10. Neurophthalmology ---------- 221

11. Fundus ---------- 258

12. Vitreous ---------- 313

13. Squint and Optics ---------- 317

14. Community Ophthalmology ---------- 365

15. Embryology ---------- 371

16. Recent Advances ---------- 374

Appendices ---------- 379

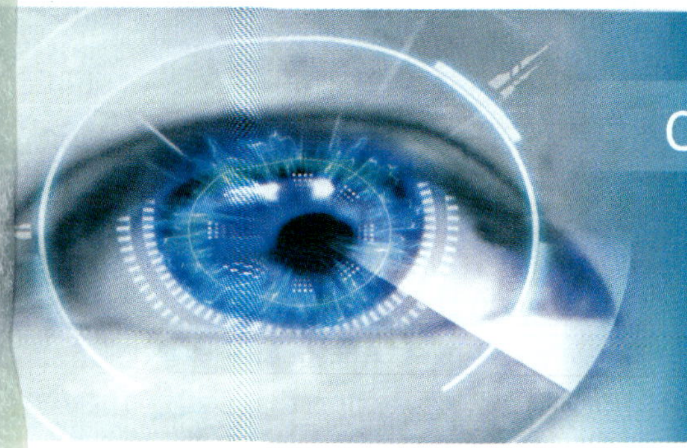

CHAPTER 1

Diseases of Lens

ANATOMY

- Lens is biconvex in shape.
- Diameter: 9–10 mm.
- Refractive index: 1.39.
- Total refractive power: 16 D–17 D.

Structure of Lens

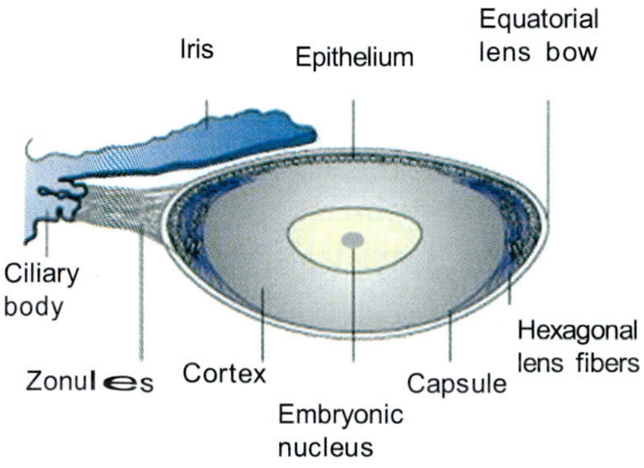

Fig. 1.1: Structure of lens

Lens constitutes of:

1. *Lens capsule:*
   - Lens capsule is a thin, transparent, hyaline collagenous membrane which surrounds the lens completely.
   - Lens capsule is highly elastic but does not have any elastic tissue.
   - It is secreted at embryonic stage as a basement membrane of lens epithelium **(Thickest basement membrane in the body)**.
   - It is thicker anteriorly than posteriorly and at the equator than the poles.

   Capsule is thinnest at the posterior pole.
2. *Anterior epithelium:* It constitutes single layer of epithelium cells. They are cuboidal at the centre and become columnar at the periphery.
3. *Lens fibres:* They are of two types:
   a. *Nucleus* (old lens fibres). It is further divided into: Embryonic (1–3 months gestation), Foetal, Infantile, Adult.
   b. *Cortex* (youngest lens fibres). Embryonic nucleus is the oldest fibres.
4. *Zonules of zinn:* They are the suspensory ligaments which support the nucleus.

PHYSIOLOGY

- 80% of glucose is metabolized anaerobically. This leads to formation of lactic acid in the lens which diffuses into the aqueous humour. Hence, absence of lens will lead to decreased lactic acid in the aqueous humour.

- Lens derives its nutrition from aqueous humour.
- Antioxidative system of the lens constitutes of Vitamin C, i.e., ascorbic acid, Vitamin E and glutathione. The detoxifying enzymes which are responsible to counteract the oxidative damage in the lens are catalase and superoxide dismutase. Cataract occurs due to the oxidative damage to the lens.
- Glutathione plays a central role in protecting the lens from oxidative damage. It is a tripeptide synthesized in the lens. Its levels are reduced in patients of cataract.
- Myoinositol is actively transported into the lens by sodium dependent carrier mediated mechanism. Its levels are markedly reduced in cataract. It is a precursor of membrane phosphoinositides which are involved in Na/Ka ATPase function. It also participates in ascorbic acid transport in the lens.

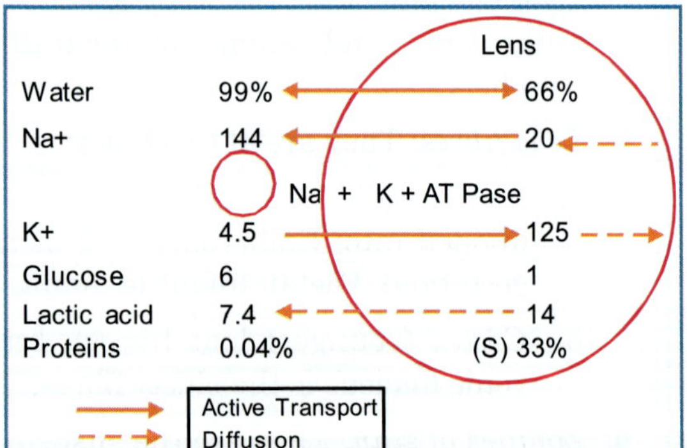

Fig. 1.2

Development of lens: Lens develops from lens vesicle which is derived from surface ectoderm.

Cataract

Definition: Any interference in the optical homogeneity of the lens is called cataract.

Classification

a. *Etiologically:* (1) Senile (2) Metabolic (3) Complicated (4) Traumatic (5) Radiational (6) Toxic (7) Electric (8) Skin diseases (9) Osseus diseases (10) Syndromes.

b. *According to maturity:* (1) Immature (2) Mature (3) Hypermature.

c. *Anatomically:* (1) Capsular cataract–Anterior and Posterior (2) Subcapsular cataract–Anterior and Posterior (3) Cortical cataract (4) Supranuclear cataract (5) Nuclear cataract (6) Polar cataract–Anterior and Posterior.

Most common cause of acquired cataract is senile cataract.

CONGENITAL AND DEVELOPMENTAL CATARACT

Etiology

a. *Heredity:* Usually dominant.

b. *Maternal factors:*
   1. Malnutrition.
   2. TORCHS infections, i.e., Toxoplasmosis, rubella, cytomegalovirus, Herpes and syphilis.
   3. Drug: Thalidomide, Corticosteroid.
   4. Radiation.

c. *Foetal or Infantile factor:*
   1. Anoxia.
   2. Metabolic:
      a. Galactosemia–Galactokinase deficiency.
      b. Neonatal hypoglycemia.
   3. *Congenital anomaly:* Lowe's syndrome, Myotonia dystrophica.
   4. Birth trauma.
   5. Malnutrition.

d. *Idiopathic.*

Types

a. *Cataracta centralis pulverulenta:*

1. Embryonic nuclear cataract.
2. Opacity has powdery appearance.
3. Does not affect vision.

b. *Zonular/lamellar:*

Most common type of congenital cataract causing decreased vision.

1. Involves the foetal nucleus.
2. Etiology may be:
   A. Genetic: Dominant inheritance.
   B. Environmental: (1) **Vitamin D deficiency,** (2) Rubella infection in 7th–8th week of gestation.
3. Usually bilateral.
4. Causes severe visual defect.
5. **Small linear opacities towards equator called Riders are characteristic of lamellar cataract.**

c. *Sutural cataract:* Along anterior and posterior sutures.

d. *Anterior polar cataract.*

e. *Posterior polar cataract.*

f. *Coronary cataract:* Occurs in adolescence, club shaped opacities peripheral in distribution.

g. *Punctate cataract:* Also called *Blue-dot cataract* or *Cataracta-punctate-cerulea*–Bluish dots in peripheral part of adolescent nucleus and deeper cortex are seen. It is the most common type of congenital cataract.

h. *Total congenital cataract.*

i. *Congenital membranous cataract:* It is due to total or partial absorption of congenital cataract.

CONGENITAL RUBELLA SYNDROME

It is characterized by the classical triad of–Cataract, Headache and Deafness.

MNEMONIC

CHD **(**Cataract, Headache and Deafness**)**

Ocular Features

1. Microphthalmos.
2. *Cataract:* Pearly nuclear or lamellar.
3. *Retinopathy:* Salt-pepper retinopathy at posterior pole. It is non progressive.
4. Glaucoma.
5. Optic nerve abnormalities.
6. Other complications:
   A. Pendular nystagmus and strabismus.
   B. Keratitis.
   C. Iritis and iris atrophy.
   D. Extreme refractive error.

   The most common type of cataract in rubella is–Nuclear Pearly.

ACQUIRED CATARACT

1. Senile Cataract

Etiology:

- Heredity.
- Dehydrational crisis in diarrhea and cholera.
- UV-Rays.
- Dietary deficiency of vitamin E,C,B and proteins.

It is broadly divided into:

- Nuclear.
- Cortical.

Nuclear Cataract:

It occurs due to following factors:

- Increased age-related nuclear sclerosis.
- Increase in insoluble proteins.
- Deposition of pigments like urochrome and melanin.

Sclerosis makes the lens hard and inelastic leading to shrunken lens with wrinkled capsule due to leakage of water. This causes inability to accommodate and progressive index myopia. It manifests as **"Second sight of old age".**

Maturation of Nuclear Cataract:

A. Immature cataract.

B. Mature cataract.

C. Hypermature nuclear sclerotic cataract.

Nuclear Cataract may be Tinted:

A. Amber.

B. Brown—Cataracta Brunescens.

C. Black—Cataracta Nigra.

D. Red—Cataracta Rubra.

Nuclear cataract causes Hamarlopia (Day Blindness).

Causes of Hamarlopia:

1. Central corneal opacities.
2. Central lenticular opacities.
3. Congenital absence of cones.

Cortical Cataract: Decreased levels of total protein, amino acids and potassium alongwith increased concentration of Na+, leads to hydration and coagulation of proteins causing cataract. It is of two types:

1. *Cuneiform:* It generally starts as wedge shaped radial spokes from periphery to center. Hence visual disturbances are comparatively at the late stage.
2. *Cupulliform:* These are posterior subcapsular opacities. This type of cataract lies right in the pathway of the axial rays, **at the nodal point of the eye** (Nodal point of eye is just behind the lens) and thus causes an early loss of visual acuity.

Maturation of Cortical Cataract:

1. Stage of Lamellar Separation.
2. Stage of Incipient Cataract.
3. Immature Senile Cataract (Intumescent Cataract—*It causes frequent change of presbyopic glasses).*
4. Mature Senile Cataract (Ripe Cataract).
5. Hypermature *Morgagnian Cataract.*

Causes of frequent change of presbyopic glasses are:

1. Early cataract (Intumescent cataract).
2. Late stage of primary open angle glaucoma.
3. Diabetes mellitus (Hyperglycemia causes myopic shift and hypoglycemia causes hypermetropic shift).

Note:

- **Intumescent cataract is a cause of Phacomorphic glaucoma.**
- **Morgagnian cataract is the most common form of senile cataract causing glaucoma.**
- **Most common complication of Morgagnian cataract is Phacolytic Glaucoma. Other complication possible is Phacoanaphylactic uveitis.**
- **Most common complication of hypermature nuclear sclerotic cataract is subluxation of lens.**

2. Metabolic Cataract

a. Diabetes Mellitus:

- Causes senile cataract at early age (i.e., presenile cataract).

- **Typical morphology is Snow-Flake Or Snow-Storm Cataract.**
- Increased glucose leads to sorbitol pathway (Due to saturation of other metabolic pathways like glycolysis and krebs cycle. *When enzyme hexokinase is saturated or inhibited, sorbitol pathway is the only pathway remaining for glucose metabolism.*
- This sorbitol accumulation in the lens (Due to Aldose Reductase pathway) leads to overhydration of lens causing cataract.

b. *Galactosaemia:*

- Deficiency of GPUT (Galactose-phosphouridyl transferase) causes **Oil Droplet Cataract.**
- Deficiency of Galactokinase causes lamellar cataract.

c. *Hypocalcaemia:* Due to decreased parathyroid activity, i.e., Hypoparathyroidism.

d. *Wilson's Disease:* Wilson's disease (Hepatolenticular degeneration) is a rare condition caused by deficiency of alpha$_2$—globulin, ceruplasmin. It is characterized by widespread deposition of copper in the tissues and becomes manifest in 3 ways:

1. Liver disease.
2. Neurological involvement of the basal ganglion.
3. Psychiatric features.

Ocular Features are:

1. *Sunflower Cataract:* This type of cataract also occurs in blunt trauma where it is also known as Rossete Cataract.
2. *K.F. Ring (Kayser-Fleischer Ring):* Golden brown discoloration of descements membrane is due to copper deposition and is pathognomic of Wilson's disease.

   Note: Fleischer's ring is iron deposition at the base of the cone in patients of keratoconus.

e. *Lowe's Syndrome (Oculocerebrorenal syndrome):* It is an inborn error of aminoacid metabolism.

Ocular Features:

1. Congenital cataract.
2. Microphakia.
3. Posterior lentiglobus/Posterior Lenticonus.
4. Glaucoma.

f. *Mannosidosis:* Deficiency of alpha-mannosidase leads to mannose rich oligosaccharides in tissues causing spoke like posterior capsular cataract.

g. *Fabry's Disease:*

- It is due to deficiency of alpha-Galactosidase.

Ocular Features:

1. Spoke like cataract—No impairment of vision.
2. Vortex Keratopathy.

3. Complicated Cataract

Clinical Features:

- It is posterior cortical or more commonly posterior subcapsular due to posterior segment disease.
- It is anterior cortical due to anterior segment disease.
- Most commonly it is **Posterior subcapsular.**
- Spreads axially.

- *Has Bread Crumb appearance.*
- **Polychromatic luster is the pathognomic feature of complicated cataract.**

Causes:

1. Inflammatory–Iridocyclitis, Parsplanitis, Choroiditis, Endophthalmitis, Corneal ulcer.
2. Degenerative–Retinitis pigmentosa, Best disease (It is dystrophy of RPE cells), Myopia.
3. Tumours.
4. Glaucoma–Primary and Secondary.
5. Retinal detachment.

Hypermetropia is not a degenerative disease hence complicated cataract does not occur in hypermetropia but occurs in myopia.

4. Toxic Cataract

Causes:

1. *Corticosteroids:* Typically discoid, posterior sub-capsular cataract which at a later stage involves anterior subcapsular region. Steroids both systemic and topical are cataractogenic.
2. *Phenothiazines:* Deposition of fine yellow brown granules under the anterior capsule in pupillary zone which develop into large stellate opacities and finally anterior polar cataract.
3. *Chloroquine:* (Not hydroxychloroquine) causes white, flaky posterior subcapsular cataract.
4. *Anticholinesterases:* Commonly causes anterior subcapsular cataract. Mainly due to long acting miotics like DFP, Ecothiophate, Demecarium bromide.
5. *Busulphan:* It is given for treatment of CML. It causes PSC, i.e., posterior subcapsular cataract.
6. *Amiodarone:* Anterior subcapsular cataract. Also causes vortex keratopathy.
7. *Cu, Fe, Au:* Gold is used for the treatment of rheumatoid arthritis and causes ASC.
   - **Most common ocular complication of steroid is–Glaucoma.** Occurrence of glaucoma is genetically monitored. Less common in short term steroid therapy or alternate day therapy.
   - **Oral steroids more commonly lead to cataract and topical steroids more commonly lead to glaucoma.**
   - Both phenothiazines (chlorpromazine) and chloroquine can cause cataract but phenothiazines are most commonly mentioned in relation to cataract formation.

5. Traumatic Cataract

Features of Blunt Trauma/ Concussion Injury:

1. *Rossette-shaped cataract:* It is also called sunflower cataract. It mainly involves posterior cortex first.
2. *Vossius ring:* It is the imprint of iris pigment on the anterior capsule of the lens, due to blunt trauma.
3. *Berlins edema:* It is also called Commotio Retinae. It is macular edema after blunt trauma and is morphologically described as "cherry-red spot".
4. *Angle-recession glaucoma:* Angle recession occurs due to tear in ciliary body after blunt trauma. Glaucoma is due to damage in trabecular network.

6. Radiational Cataract

- It occurs due to damage to lens by all types of radiations namely UV rays, Infrared rays, X-rays/Y-rays or neutrons.
- Infrared rays causes "Glass Blower's" or Glass worker's cataract.
- MRI has no radiation exposure as it is done by ultrasonic energy and not radiations.
- *Most common type of radiational cataract is Posterior subcapsular cataract.* They are punctate subcapsular opacities which mature rapidly.

7. Syndermatotic Cataract

These are cataracts which occur due to skin diseases.

Causes:

- Atopic dermatitis is the most common cause.
- Poikiloderma.
- Scleroderma.

8. Pre-Senile Cataract

These are cataracts which occur in young age.

Causes:

1. *Myotonic dystrophy:* Myotonic dystrophy or Dystrophia myotonica is a generalized dominantly inherited myopathy characterized by myotonia of peripheral muscles and muscle wasting.

   Ocular Features:

   1. *Pre-senile cataract*
      - **"Christmas-tree cataract"**—posterior subcapsular, stellate plaque.
      - Small iridescent, polychromatic crystals.
   2. *Ptosis*—Usually bilateral.
   3. *Pigmentary retinopathy*, i.e., salt and pepper fundus.
   4. *Pupillary changes*—Light-near dissociation.
   5. *Low intraocular—pressure.*

   Hence, we remember its ocular features as 5 Ps.

2. *Atopic dermatitis:* Stellate opacities mostly posterior.
3. *Diabetes mellitus:* It causes snowstorm or snowflake opacities.

SYNDROMES ASSOCIATED WITH CATARACT

A. Down's Syndrome

Ocular Features:

1. Shortened and slanted palpebral fissure.
2. Neonatal ectropion.
3. Lateral trichiasis and entropion.
4. Keratoconus.
5. Cataract.
6. *Brushfield spots are light coloured spots on iris.*

B. Others

- Werner's syndrome.
- Rothmund's syndrome.

CLINICAL FEATURES OF CATARACT

1. Misty vision with distortion of vision.
2. Loss of vision.
3. Coloured halos.

   Other causes of coloured halos are:

   - Mucopurulent conjunctivitis.
   - Acute congestive angle closure glaucoma.

Finchams Test: It helps to know the cause of halos whether it is due to cataract or glaucoma. A stenopic slit is passed in front of the eye which is seeing the halos, if the halos break then it is due to cataract and if not then it is due to glaucoma.

4. Black spots in front of eyes.
5. Glare.
6. Uniocular diplopia or polyopia seen in stage of intumescent cataract.

COMPLICATIONS OF LONG STANDING CATARACT

1. Uveitis.
2. Subluxation or dislocation of lens (In nuclear sclerotic cataract).
3. Glaucoma: Phacoanaphylactic/Phacomorphic/Phacolytic.

MANAGEMENT OF CATARACT

The first line of treatment in cataract is surgery.

Modalities of Treatment of Cataract

1. *ICCE (Intracapsular cataract extraction):* It constitutes removal of lens alongwith the capsule. The methods of ICCE are: 1. Cryoextraction 2. Forceps method (Arrugas forceps are used) 3. Irisophake 4. Wire Vectis 5. Indiansmith method (Also called tumbling method). **The best method is cryoextraction. Today the only indication of ICCE is subluxation of lens.**
2. *ECCE with PC IOL (Extracapsular cataract extraction):* It constitutes removal of lens leaving behind the posterior capsule on which artificial lens is implanted.
3. *Manual small incision cataract surgery:* This is sutureless small incision cataract surgery without using the phacoprobe.
4. *Phacoemulsification:* Cataract removal using phacoemulsification is achieved by ultrasonic fragmentation and aspiration of the lens material. The tip of the phacoemulsification hand piece is composed of a hollow (approximately 1 mm) titanium needle that transmits vibrations at a high speed (30,000 to 60,000 cycles/sec) to emulsify the cataract. These vibrations are transferred from piezoelectric or magnetostrictive crystals.
5. *Lensectomy with anterior vitrectomy:* Lens in toto with anterior vitreous is removed. This procedure is specially opted in children when ICCE is indicated. This is because in children there is strong adhesion between posterior surface of lens and anterior hyaloid face of vitreous and hence any pulling can cause retinal detachment.
6. *Mydriatics/optical iridectomy:* This procedure can be opted for congenital stationary cataracts but now it is more of a theoretical purpose and not opted for.
7. *ECCE with PC IOL with primary posterior capsulotomy:* Primary posterior capsulotomy is done in children as they are very prone to develop posterior capsular opacification after few days of surgery due to intense postoperative inflammations.

Discission and Needling done in congenital cataract are now obsolete procedures.

Preoperative evaluation of cataract surgery includes:

I. *General Examination for:*

- Diabetes mellitus.
- Hypertension.
- Cardiac problems.
- Obstructive lung disorders.

- Any potential source of infection in the body like—septic gums, urinary tract infection.

II. *Ocular Examination:*

A. *Retinal function test:*

1. Perception of light.
2. Projection of rays—Easy test to assess the function of peripheral retina.
3. Test for Marcus Gunn pupillary response.
4. Two light discrimination. } Macular function test
5. Maddox rod test. } Macular function test
6. Laser interferometry. } Macular function test
7. Stereoacuity.
8. Color perception—It indicates that optic nerve is relatively normal.
9. Entoptic visualization is also used to indicate retinal function but it is a subjective test where the patient perceives his own vasculature.
10. Indirect ophthalmoscopy.

B. *Objective tests* are indicated if some retinal pathology suspected.

i. ERG—Electroretinogram.
ii. EOG—Electrooculogram.
iii. VER—Visually-Evoked-Response.

C. *Search for local source of infection:*

- Conjunctivitis.
- Blepharitis.
- Meibomitis.
- Lacrimal sac infection—lacrimal syringing is done.

D. *Slit lamp examination of anterior segment of eye:*

- Presence of uveitis.
- State of endothelial cells.

E. *Intraocular pressure measurement.*

F. *Gonioscopy* is not done routinely. It is only when the IOP is found raised, we can do to assess the state of the angle.

SURGICAL TECHNIQUES

ECCE

(a) Limbal partial thickness incision is made from 10 o' clock to 2 o' clock.

(b) Anterior chamber is formed by viscoelastic through a small full thickness incision.

(c) Anterior capsulotomy is done (Can opener technique or Envelope technique).

(d) Partial thickness limbal incision is made full-thickness by corneal scissors.

(e) Hydrodissection and hydrodelineation is done.

(f) Nucleus is prolapsed.

(g) Cortical matter is aspirated.

(h) IOL is implanted.

(i) Incision is sutured by radial sutures.

BSS (i.e., Basal salt solution) with glutathione is the ideal irrigating fluid in cataract surgery as it resembles the aqueous humour most.

After cataract surgery, stitches are removed at 6 weeks post-operative, and refraction should be done after 2 weeks of the suture removal so that any change in corneal curvature due to the sutures (tight or loose) is stabilized. (But if in the question, 8 weeks is not an alternative, we will mark 6 weeks as the correct answer). This schedule is for conventional cataract surgery (with sutures). *In case of sutureless cataract surgery with phaco, refraction can be done after 1–2 weeks.*

Small Incision Cataract Surgery (SICS)

ECCE can also be done through self-sealing small incision, which does not need any sutures. This sutureless surgery can be either by phaco machine, which is called *Phaco-emulsification or manually called Non-phaco sutureless cataract surgery.*

1. Manual small incision cataract surgery:

Procedure:

(a) Triplanar scleral tunnel is made.

(b) Anterior chamber is formed by viscoelastic.

(c) Anterior capsulotomy is done (Preferably CCC, i.e., continues curvilinear capsulorrhexis or can opener).

(d) Hydrodissection and hydrodelineation is done.

(e) Nucleus is first prolapsed in the anterior chamber and then prolapsed out by viscoelastic called viscoexpression.

(f) Cortical matter is aspirated and IOL implanted. If we have to implant a nonfoldable lens then we need to extend our scleral incision.

(g) No sutures are required as it is a self-sealing incision.

2. Phacoemulsification:

Procedure:

(a) **Scleral tunnel with an external incision of 3 mm to 3.5 mm is made/ Corneal incision can also be made.**

(b) Circular curvilinear capsulorrhexis done.

(c) Hydrodissection and Hydrodelineation done and lens material emulsified and aspirated along with the cortical matters.

(d) Foldable IOL implanted.

Advantages:

1. Normal life activity regained faster.
2. Minimum post-operative astigmatism.

Note:

- Vitreous haemorrhage and RD occurs more commonly in ICCE due to vitreous traction. In ECCE since the posterior capsule (PC) is intact this complication is less common.
- Cystoid macular edema (CME) after cataract surgery (called *Irvine-Gass syndrome*) is attributed to both *vitreous traction* and *prostaglandins released* during inflammation. As there is an intact PC in ECCE hence again this complication is less common in ECCE.
- IOL implantation in diabetic patient should be done after PRP (pan-retinal photocoagulation). But if the patient has developed diabetic cataract then IOL implantation becomes a prerequisite for proper visualization of fundus and PRP.
- An uncontrolled glaucoma is a contra-indication for IOL implantation surgery. First the glaucoma has to be controlled as increased intraocular tension can lead to per-operative complications.
- Phacoemulsification is less preferred in black cataract, i.e., grade 4 or grade 5 nuclear cataract.

MANAGEMENT OF PEDIATRIC CATARACT

In both bilateral and unilateral cases, primary implantation is indicated as soon as the patient is fit for anesthesia, ideally between 2 and 3 months of age. The earlier the surgery is done, the better is the chance that deep amblyopia can be overcome as the visual reflexes develop by 5–6 months of age. Unilateral cases are particularly at a risk of developing deep amblyopia and hence dealt with more seriously.

Management can be divided according to two age groups:

1. Patients younger than 2 years.
2. Patients between 2–8 years.

Guidelines for the Choice of Intraocular Lens

1. *< 2 years old:*
   - Do biometry and undercorrect by 20%.

     OR
   - Use axial length measurements only.

Axial length	IOL diopteric power
17 mm	28 D
18 mm	27 D
19 mm	26 D
20 mm	24 D
21 mm	22 D

2. *Between 2 years to 8 years:* Do biometry and undercorrect by 10%.

The undercorrection of the IOL power is done to take into account the myopic shift of power as the child grows.

The total diameter of IOL in children should not exceed 12 mm.

IOLS

Materials:

- Commonly used material of IOL (Non-foldable) is PMMA (Polymethylmethacrylate).
- Materials for foldable IOLs are: Hydrogel, Silicon and Acrylic.

Types of Non-Foldable IOLs:

- AC-IOL-Kelman multiplex.
- Iris-supported lens–Worst's or Singh's iris claw lenses.
- PC-IOL–It is of two types J-loop or C-loop. C-loop is preferred. Best option for IOL implantation is posterior capsule as it is most physiological.

Biometry:

The process of calculating the power of intraocular IOL is known as biometry.

It is done by SRK formula:

SRK–I

$P = A - 2.5\,L - 0.9\,K$

A is a constant depending on the surgeon and the type of IOL.

L is the axial length and is measured by USG-A scan.

K is the keratometry reading (Average of K1 and K2) and is measured by Keratometer.

SRK-II: It is the corrected form of SRK-I, taking into account any unusual axial length of the eye (i.e., too long or too short).

Hence preferred choice is SRK-II.

COMPLICATIONS OF CATARACT SURGERY

Operative:

1. SR muscle laceration.
2. Excessive bleeding during conjunctival flap preparation.
3. Irregular incision.
4. Injury to cornea, DM-detachment.
5. Iris injury and iridodialysis.
6. Accidental rupture of lens capsule.
7. Vitreous loss.
8. Expulsive haemorrhage.

Early Post-Operative:

1. Hyphema.
2. Iritis and iris prolapse.

3. Striate keratopathy.
4. Flat anterior chamber.
5. Bacterial endophthalmitis: Painful.
6. Glaucoma due to retained viscoelastic.

Late Post-Operative:

(All are painless conditions)

1. CME.
2. RD.
3. Epithelial in-growth.
4. Fibrous down growth.
5. After cataract.

RD occurs more commonly in aphakes compared to pseudophakes. The patient will present as floaters and sudden loss of vision.

IOL-Related

1. *Corneal endothelial damage.*
2. *Uveitis:* Mainly with AC-IOLs and iris-claw lenses.
3. *Secondary glaucoma.*
4. *Anisocoria (difference in size of pupil):* Commonly when iris claw lenses are implanted. It can also occur in PC-IOL implantation when there is iris hook by the haptic.
5. *Cystoid macular edema:* Its incidence is specially more in iris-claw lenses or AC-IOLs when, there is no posterior capsule. CME after cataract surgery is known as "*Irvine–Gass Syndrome*".
6. *UGH syndrome:*
   - Uveitis/glaucoma/hyphema syndrome.
   - Occurs with rigid AC-IOLs.
7. *Malposition of IOLs:*

   It causes:

   a. Astigmatism, if IOL is tilted.

   b. Decentration of IOL leads to glare, halos, rings of light, uniocular diplopia.

   Types:

   a. *Sunset syndrome:* Inferior subluxation of IOL.

   b. *Sunrise syndrome:* Superior subluxation of IOL.

   c. *Lost lens syndrome:* Complete dislocation of IOL in the vitreous cavity.

   d. *Windshield wiper syndrome:* It denotes the movement of the superior haptic with the movement of the head. This occurs due to implantation of a very small lens in the ciliary sulcus.
8. *Toxic lens syndrome:* It indicates the uveal inflammation which occurs due to lens material or the ethylene gas used to sterilise the lens.

- **Most dreaded complication of cataract surgery is–Endophthalmitis. It may be early onset or late onset.**

  Early Onset:

  1. Staphylococcal epidermidis is the most common organism isolated from post-surgical endophthalmitis.
  2. Other organisms are: Staph aureus, Pseudomonas and Proteus.

  Late Onset:

  1. Propionobacterium acne.
  2. Fungal infection.

- **Most common late complication of cataract surgery is–After cataract or PCO.**

After Cataract

- It denotes opacification of posterior capsule after cataract surgery.
- It is also known as secondary cataract.
- It may present with various morphological forms namely–Elschnig's pearls, Soemmering's rings or just a diffuse opacification.

- *Treatment:*
  (a) Surgical capsulotomy by zeiglers knife.
  (b) Laser capsulotomy by Nd-Yag laser which is a photodisruptive or cutting laser.

DISPLACEMENT OF THE LENS

Subluxation is partial dislocation of lens.

Causes:

1. *Congenital*—(a) Simple ectopia lentis (Symmetrical and upwards) (b) Ectopia lentis et pupillae (slit shaped pupil displaced in opposite direction) (c) Ectopia lentis with systemic anomalies (Marfan's syndrome, Homocystinuria, Weil-Marchesani syndrome and Ehlers-Danlos syndrome).
2. *Traumatic*—Blunt trauma.
3. *Consecutive or Spontaneous*—Hypermature cataract, Buphthalmos, High myopia and Uveitis.

Marfan's Syndrome

1. Megalocornea and Cornea plana.
2. Angle anomaly leading to glaucoma. {M}
3. Upward/temporal ectopia lentis.
4. Difficulty in pupil dilatation.
5. Lattice degeneration and rhegmatogenous retinal detachment.

The most PROMINENT manifestation of Marfan's syndrome is Megalocornea.

The most COMMON manifestation of Marfan's syndrome is Ectopia lentis.

Weil-Marchesani Syndrome

1. Microspherophakia.
2. Pupillary block glaucoma.
3. Ectopia lentis in inferior and forward direction.

Homocystinuria: It is an inborn error of metabolism caused by deficiency of enzyme – Cystathione synthetase leading to increased level of homocysteine in plasma and urine. It is characterized by skeletal deformities similar to Marfan's syndrome and mental handicap.

Ocular Features:

1. Ectopia lentis in inferonasal direction.
2. Angle anomaly leading to glaucoma or pupil block glaucoma due to incarceration of lens in the pupil.
3. Loss of accommodation due to disintegration of zonules.

Ehlers-Danlos Syndrome

1. Blue sclera.
2. Ectopia lentis.

Congenital Anomalies of Lens

A. *Colobomas:*
   1. Mostly occurs inferiorly.
   2. May be associated with defect in iris and choroid.

B. *Congenital Ectopia Lentis.*

C. *Lenticonus:* It is the conical protrusion of the lens.

Anterior Lenticonus:

Anterior lenticonus occurs in Alport's Syndrome.

Alport's Syndrome (Familial haemorrhagic nephritis)

Systemic Features:

1. Renal failure.
2. Hearing loss.

Ocular Features:

1. Posterior polymorphous corneal dystrophy.

2. Juvenile arcus.
3. Pigment dispersion.
4. Anterior lenticonus.
5. Retinal pigmentary changes.

Posterior Lenticonus:

It occurs in Lowe's Syndrome–i.e., Oculo-cerebrorenal syndrome.

D. *Congenital cataract.*

E. *Lentiglobus:* It is a generalised hemispherical deformity of the lens. Posterior lentiglobus is seen in Lowe's syndrome.

F. *Microphakia:* Lens is small in size. It is seen in Lowe's syndrome.

G. *Microspherophakia:* Small and spherical lens. Occurs in:

1. Weil-Marchesani syndrome.
2. Hyperlysinaemia.

NEET DRILL

1. The equatorial diameter of the lens is 9–10 mm.
2. The equatorial diameter of the lens at birth is 6.5 mm.
3. Thickness of the lens, i.e., the AP diameter is 3.5 mm–5 mm.
4. Radius of curvature of the anterior surface is 10 mm.
5. Radius of curvature of the posterior surface is 6 mm.
6. Refractive index of the lens is 1.39.
7. Refractive power is 16 D–17 D.
8. Accommodative power of the lens at birth: 14–16 D at birth, 7–8 D at 25 years and 1–2 D at 50 years of age.
9. The pigments responsible for the color change in the process of development of cataract are urochrome and melanin.
10. Snowflake or snowstorm cataract is more common in type 1 diabetes.
11. Cataract in diabetes is due to sorbital accumulation in the lens and sorbital is very hyperosmotic.
12. Lens capsule is thinnest at posterior pole with the thickness of 4 microns.
13. Lens capsule is thickest at equatorial region and is 23 microns in thickness.
14. Suspensory ligament or zonules have a diameter of 0.35–1 microns.
15. Lens nucleus is divided as–embryonic nucleus–1-3 months of gestation/fetal nucleus–3 months–birth/infantile nucleus-birth–puberty/adult nucleus–in adult life.
16. Lens is 66% water and 33% protein.
17. Antioxidative system of lens constitutes–vitamin C, i.e., ascorbic acid, glutathione, myoinositol that helps in ascorbic acid carrier system and detoxifying enzymes like catalase and superoxide dismutase.
18. Respiratory coefficient of the lens is: 1.
19. Microwave radiations can also cause cataract, proved in animals and claimed that there is maximum probability for humans also. It occurs in due to rise in temperature.
20. Length of incision in phacoemulsification is 2.75–3.2 mm.
21. Frequency of the phacoprobe is 40 khz.
22. Most commonly used foldable IOL is acrylic.
23. MICS, i.e., minimal incision cataract surgery: incision is between 1.8 and 2.4 mm.
24. Phaconit: Incision length is 0.9 mm.
25. Father of phaco: Charles D Kelman.
26. Causes of ectopia lentis: Marfan's syndrome, homocystinuria, Weil-Marchesani, Ehlers-Danlos, sulphite oxidase deficiency, hyperlysenemia, Refsum's disease and Sturge-Weber syndrome.

27. Anterior lenticonus: Alport's syndrome, Waardenburg syndrome.
28. Posterior lenticonus: Lowe's syndrome.
29. Expulsive haemorrhage after cataract surgery occurs due to bleeding from the posterior ciliary arteries.
30. The size of opening of posterior capsulotomy done by NdYAG laser ranges from 2–3 mm to 5–6 mm.
31. The insoluble proteins raised in a cataractous lens are: HM3, HM4.
32. In nuclear cataract, it is HM4.
33. The genes responsible for congenital cataract: CRY, i.e., crystallines, Cx, i.e., connexins and MIP, i.e., Major Intrinsic Protein.
34. The most recent in cataract surgery is Femtolaser cataract surgery called LACS, i.e., laser assisted cataract surgery.
35. Femtolaser is an ultrafast laser, with pulse duration in femtosecond, i.e., 10^{-15}.
36. Minimum chance of after cataract is seen with Acrylic Hydrophobic IOLSs.

MULTIPLE CHOICE QUESTIONS

1. Transport of ascorbic acid to lens is done by:
A. Myoinositol B. Choline
C. Taurine D. Na/K ATPase

2. Which of the following does not handle the free radicals in the lens?
A. Vitamin A B. Vitamin E
C. Vitamin C D. Catalase

3. Typical bilateral inferior subluxation of lens is seen in:
A. Marfan's syndrome
B. Homocystinuria
C. Hyperinsulinemia
D. Ocular trauma

4. In which of the following uveitic conditions is it contraindicated to put intraocular lens after cataract extraction?
A. Fuch's heterochromic cyclitis
B. Juvenile rheumatoid arthritis
C. Psoriatic arthritis
D. Reiter's syndrome

5. A two-week old child presents with unilateral cataract, which of the following statement represent the best management advice?
A. The best age to operate him to get the best visual results is four weeks
B. The best age to operate him to get the best visual results is four months
C. The best age to operate him to get the best visual results is four years
D. The eye is already lost, only cosmetic correction is required

6. Which prominent ocular manifestation is associated with Marfan's syndrome?
A. Microcornea
B. Microspherophakia
C. Megalocornea
D. Ectopia lentis

7. A child has got a congenital cataract involving the visual axis, which was detected by the parents right at birth. This child should be operated:
A. Immediately
B. At 2 months of age
C. At 1 year of age when globe becomes normal sized
D. After 4 years when entire ocular and orbital growth become normal

8. Dislocation of lens is seen in all the following conditions except:

A. Congenital rubella

B. Weil-Marchesani syndrome

C. Marfan's syndrome

D. Homocystinuria

9. **After cataract surgery, glasses are prescribed after:**

A. 2 weeks B. 6 weeks

C. 12 weeks D. 20 weeks

10. **Sunflower cataract is caused by:**

A. Siderosis

B. Chalcosis

C. Lead intoxication

D. Silicosis

11. **Anterior lenticonus is found in:**

A. Lowe's syndrome

B. Willium syndrome

C. Alport's syndrome

D. Down's syndrome

12. **Vossius ring is seen on:**

A. Cornea

B. Anterior capsule of lens

C. Posterior capsule of lens

D. Iris

13. **Steroid-induced cataract is:**

A. Posterior subcapsular

B. Anterior subcapsular

C. Nuclear cataract

D. Cupulliform cataract

14. **Which of the following is the most important factor for prevention of endophthalmitis in cataract surgery?**

A. Preoperative preparation with povidone iodine

B. One week antibiotic therapy prior to surgery

C. Trimming of the eyelashes

D. Use of intravitreal antibiotics

15. **The crystalline lens derives its nutrition from:**

A. Blood vessels B. Connective tissue

C. Aqueous D. Zonules

16. **Which laser is used in the management of after cataracts?**

A. Argon B. Krypton

C. Nd-YAG D. Excimer

17. **A 55 years old patient complains of decreased distance vision. However now he does not require his near glasses for near work. The most likely cause is:**

A. Posterior subcapsular cataract

B. Nuclear sclerosis

C. Zonular cataract

D. Anterior subcapsular cataract

18. **A 56 years old patient presents after 3 days of cataract surgery with a history of increasing pain and diminution of vision after an initial improvement. The most likely cause would be:**

A. Endophthalmitis

B. After cataract

C. Central retinal vein occlusion

D. Retinal detachment

19. **Which morphological type of cataract is most visually handicapping?**

A. Cortical

B. Nuclear

C. Posterior subcapsular

D. Zonular

20. **The standard sutureless cataract surgery done with phacoemulsification and foldable IOL has an incision of:**

A. 1 mm–1.5 mm

B. 2–2.5 mm

C. 3–3.5 mm

D. 3.5–4.5 mm

21. Oldest component of lens of the eye is:

A. Anterior capsule

B. Posterior capsule

C. Nucleocortical junction

D. Nucleus

22. Ideal fluid for irrigation during ECCE is:

A. Normal saline to dextrose

B. Normal saline

C. Balanced salt solution

D. Balanced salt solution + glutathione

23. The most common complication of hypermature sclerotic cataract is:

A. Dislocation of the lens

B. Phacomorphic glaucoma

C. Uveitis

D. Neovascularization of retina

24. A 60 years old male patient operated for cataract 6 months back now complains of floaters and sudden loss of vision. The diagnosis is:

A. Vitreous haemorrhage

B. Retinal detachment

C. Central retinal artery occlusion

D. Cystoid macular edema

25. Most common senile cataract causing glaucoma is:

A. Incipient type

B. Nuclear type

C. Morgagnian hypermature

D. Sclerotic hypermature

26. A diabetic patient gets cataract because of accumulation of sorbitol in lens. The enzyme responsible for this is:

A. Glucokinase

B. NADPH+ dependent aldolase

C. Phosphofructoisomerase

D. Hexokinase

27. In Finchams test–there is breakup of halo and rejoining (patient present with coloured halo and giddiness). Diagnosis is:

A. Open angle glaucoma

B. Cataract

C. Mucopurulent conjunctivitis

D. Acute angle closure glaucoma

28. All are methods of intracapsular extraction of lens, except:

A. Phacoemulsification

B. Cryosurgery

C. Forceps delivery

D. Erisophake

29. Snow flake cataract is a pathognomic feature of:

A. Chalcosis

B. Diabetes mellitus

C. Wilson's disease

D. Trauma

30. Chalcosis is associated with:

A. Copper B. Zinc

C. Lead D. Gold

31. Polychromatic lusture is seen in:

A. Zonular cataract

B. Posterior subcapsular cataract

C. Nuclear cataract

D. Anterior subcapsular cataract

32. Cataract is seen in all, except:

A. Rheumatoid arthritis

B. Glucocorticoid administration

C. Galactosemia

D. Hypoparathyroidism

33. Sunflower cataract is seen in:
A. Injury
B. Laurence-Moon-Biedl syndrome
C. Wilson's disease
D. Galactosemia

34. Before IOL implantation the following are done for the estimation of refractory power of IOL:
A. Keratometry
B. Axial length
C. Lens thickness
D. Corneal thickness
E. Corneal diameter

35. Most common cause of cataract is:
A. Age related changes
B. Hereditary
C. Diabetes mellitus
D. Trauma induced
E. Myxoedema

36. Treatment of cataract in infant is:
A. Lensectomy
B. ICCE
C. Discission
D. ECCE
E. Phacoemulsification

37. Cataract is evaluated by:
A. Gonioscopy B. Tonometry
C. Stereoacuity D. Contrast
E. Colour vision

38. Modern IOL is made up of:
A. Acrylic acid B. PMMA
C. PML D. Glass
E. Silicon

39. Leaving the capsule behind in cataract surgery is advantageous because it:
A. Prevents cystoid macular edema
B. Decrease endothelial damage
C. Progressively improves vision
D. Decrease chance of retinal detachment
E. Decrease chance of endophthalmitis

40. Infective complication in cataract operation can be decreased by:
A. Antibiotic eye drops
B. Intracameral instillation of antibiotic at the end of the operation
C. Intraoperative antibiotics
D. Preoperative antibiotics
E. Postoperative oral antibiotics

41. Cataract is caused by all except:
A. Ultraviolet radiation
B. MRI
C. Infrared radiation
D. Microwave radiation
E. Ionizing radiation

42. Best site for IOL implantation:
A. Iris
B. Capsular bag
C. Anterior chamber
D. Sulcus

43. Common complication of IOLs are all except:
A. Corneal dystrophy
B. Glaucomas
C. Anisocoria
D. Macular edema

44. Rosette shape cataract is seen in:
A. Trauma B. Radiation
C. DM D. Iridocyclitis

45. Christmas tree cataract is seen in:
A. Down's syndrome
B. Rubella

C. Myotonic dystrophy

D. Diabetes

46. Good vision in dim light and clumsy in day lights, seen in:

A. Cortical cataract

B. Morgagnian cataract

C. Nuclear cataract

D. Steroid induced cataract

47. Most common type of cataract is:

A. Blue dot B. Zonular

C. Cupulliform D. Cuneiform

48. The complication of extracapsular extraction of lens is:

A. Cystoid macular oedema

B. Opacification of capsule

C. Iritis

D. Glaucoma

E. None of the above

49. Factor leading to raised intraocular pressure after cataract extraction:

A. Vitreous touch syndrome

B. Use of alpha chymotrypsin

C. Choroidal detachment

D. Epithelial ingrowths

E. Residual lens cortex

50. Lens develops from:

A. Surface ectoderm

B. Neuroectoderm

C. Visceral mesoderm

D. Paraxial mesoderm

51. Downward and nasal subluxation of lens is typically seen in:

A. Homocystinuria

B. Marfan's syndrome

C. Weil-Marchesani syndrome

D. Ehlers-Danlos syndrome

52. Congenital cataract is seen in:

A. Lowe's syndrome

B. Tyrosinemia

C. Maple syrup urine disease

D. Beckwith-Wiedemann's syndrome

53. Cataract can be caused by prolonged ingestion of which drug?

A. Phenothiazines

B. Methotrexate

C. Ethambutol

D. Chloroquine

54. Statement not true about rubella cataract is:

A. Pearly white

B. Bilateral

C. Stationary

D. Associated with subluxation

55. Cataract is caused by all except:

A. Systemic corticosteroids

B. Busulphan

C. Thioridazine

D. Metronidazole

56. Organism most commonly isolated from the vitreous following endophthalmitis developing 4 days after cataract surgery is:

A. Staph epidermidis

B. Bacillus subtilis

C. Pseudopyocyanea

D. Propionobacterium

57. All are risk factors for cataract except:

A. Diabetes mellitus

B. Hypertension

C. Smoking

D. Recurrent diarrhoea

58. After phacoemulsification, sutures applied are:

A. Continuous
B. Interrupted
C. No sutures needed
D. None of the above

59. Increased lactic acid in aqueous humour is found in:

A. Aphakia
B. Ectopia lentis
C. Traumatic dislocation of lens
D. Senile cataract

60. Earliest visual rehabilitation occurs with:

A. ICCE + IOL
B. ECCE + IOL
C. ICCE alone or laser
D. Phacoemulsification

61. Lens has a respiratory quotient of:

A. 1 B. 0.6
C. 0.7 D. 0.9

62. True about complicated cataract is all except:

A. Axial involvement
B. Sutural involvement
C. Polychromatic luster
D. Posterior subcapsular involvement

63. Hypermature cataract leads to:

A. Phacomorphic glaucoma
B. Phacotoxic glaucoma
C. Phacolytic glaucomas
D. None of the above

64. Scan used to calculate power of intraocular lens is:

A. A scan B. C scan
C. S scan D. None

65. Lens capsule is thinnest at:

A. Anterior pole B. Posterior pole
C. Equator D. Pupillary margin

66. Spontaneous absorption of the lenticular material is seen in:

A. Myotonic dystrophy
B. Hallerman Streif syndrome
C. Aniridia
D. Persistent hyperplastic primary vitreous

67. Anterior cortical cataract is caused by:

A. Perforating injury to eye
B. Radiation
C. Steroid
D. Senile

68. Traumatic dislocation of lens is diagnosed by:

A. Direct ophthalmoscopy
B. Indirect ophthalmoscopy
C. Distant direct ophthalmoscopy
D. Slit lamp examination

69. Constantly changing refractory error is seen in:

A. Traumatic cataract
B. Diabetic cataract
C. Morgagnian cataract
D. Intumescent cataract

70. What is the most important complication of anterior chamber lenses?

A. Glaucoma
B. Hyphema
C. Subluxation
D. Retinal detachment

71. The biochemistry of cataract formation is:

A. Hydration intumescence

B. Denaturation of lens proteins

C. Slow sclerosis

D. All of the above

72. Which is not associated with zonular cataract?

A. Diabetes

B. IUGR

C. Rickets

D. Dental abnormalities

73. Uniocular diplopia is seen in which stage of cataract?

A. Incipient B. Intumescent

C. Mature D. Hypermature

74. Modern criteria for cataract operation is:

A. Maturation of cataract

B. Loss of vision

C. Complications

D. All of the above

75. Vossius ring is seen in:

A. Chalcosis

B. Siderosis

C. Lens concussion

D. Pseudomonas infection

76. Most common complication of extracapsular cataract surgery is:

A. Retinal detachment

B. Opacification of posterior capsule

C. Vitreous haemorrhage

D. None

77. Zonular cataract is:

A. Bilateral

B. Stationary

C. Autosomal dominant

D. Associated with hypocalcemia

E. None of the above

78. The most common type of cataract in adults:

A. Nuclear cataract

B. Cortical cataract

C. Morgagnian cataract

D. Hypermature nuclear sclerotic cataract

79. Cataract is associated with:

A. Pseudomuscular hypertrophy

B. Myotonic dystrophy

C. SLE

D. Rheumatoid arthritis

E. All of the above

80. Which of the following is not correct about the cataract in cases of galactosemia?

A. It is most often central

B. It is zonular or lamellar

C. Involve the embryonal and foetal nuclei

D. Is polar

81. Equatorial diameter of the lens is:

A. 7 mm B. 9 mm

C. 8 mm D. 10 mm

82. Which continues to grow in a lifetime?

A. Cornea B. Lens

C. Iris D. Retina

83. All of the following lead to the formation of complicated cataract, except:

A. Pigmentary retinal dystrophy

B. Progressive hypermetropia

C. Progressive myopia

D. Iridocyclitis

84. Maximum refractive index in eye is of:

A. Cornea
B. Anterior capsule of lens
C. Posterior capsule of lens
D. Centroid of lens

85. Dislocation of the lens is seen in:

A. Retinoblastoma
B. Medulloblastoma
C. Neuroblastoma
D. None of these

86. Which is the most important complication of anterior chamber IOLs?

A. Glaucoma
B. Hyphema
C. Subluxation
D. Retinal detachment

87. A 55 years old patient complains of decreased distant vision. However, now he does not require his near glasses for near work. The most likely cause is:

A. Posterior subcapsular cataract
B. Zonular cataract
C. Nuclear sclerosis
D. Anterior subcapsular cataract

88. Complicated cataract is seen in:

A. Blunt trauma
B. Diabetes mellitus
C. Neovascular glaucoma
D. Myopic chorioretinitis

89. Ectopia lentis is not seen in:

A. Homocystinuria
B. Down's syndrome
C. Pseudoexfoliation
D. Marfan's syndrome

90. Christmas-Tree cataract is seen in:

A. Myotonic dystrophy
B. Irradiation cataract
C. Diabetes
D. Traumatic cataract

91. An elderly male on eye examination shows limbal scar, deep anterior chamber, iridodonesis, dark pupillary reflex, visual acuity 6/6 with 11D lens. Diagnose:

A. Aphakia
B. Pseudophakia
C. Hypermetropia
D. Posterior dislocation of lens

92. A patient presents with diplopia in one eye. On examination with oblique illumination– golden crescent and on axial illumination black/dark crescent is seen. Likely diagnosis would be:

A. Ectopia lentis
B. Lenticonus
C. Coloboma
D. Microspherophakia

93. A child presents bilateral white pupillary reflex, on slit lamp examination there is zone of opacity around fetal nucleus with some spoke of wheel like arrangement towards centre. Probable diagnosis would be:

A. Cataracta purvulenta
B. Lamellar cataract
C. Posterior pole cataract
D. Coronary cataract

94. Following 2 days of successful phaco-emulsification and IOL placement, a diabetic patient presents with redness, pain and grey white pupillary reflex.

Patient also shows hypopyon, retro-lental flare and posterior synechiae. Likely diagnosis is:

A. Post operative endophthalmitis
B. Post operative glaucoma
C. Post operative keratitis
D. Post operative cyclitis

95. Congenital cataract occurs due to abnormalities in protein formation in which of the following genes?

A. PAX6 B. SIX5
C. CryG D. PITX3

96. In a case of senile cataract, which of the following occurs?

A. Soluble protein increases, insoluble protein decreases
B. Soluble protein decreases, insoluble protein increases
C. Soluble protein increases, insoluble protein increases
D. Soluble protein equal to insoluble protein

97. Ascorbate and α-tocopherol are maintained in a reduced state in the lens by:

A. Glucose B. Glycoprotein
C. Glutathione D. Fatty acid

98. Chronic systemic steroid use causes:

A. Open angle glaucoma
B. Conjunctival and lid papillomatis
C. Uveitis
D. Cataract

99. What is to be done of congenital cataract involving visual axis?

A. Wait and watch
B. Operated when the baby reaches an appropriate age
C. Mydriatics are given
D. Immediately operate

100. Causes of ectopia lentis are all except:

A. Homocystinuria
B. Marfan's syndrome
C. Cogan-Reese syndrome
D. Sulphite oxidase deficiency

101. Lens contains which antigen?

A. Sequestered antigens
B. Cross antigens
C. Heterophile antigens
D. Isoantigens

102. Which type of lenticonus is more common in males?

A. Posterior
B. Anterior
C. Both are equally common
D. Inferior

103. Marfan's syndrome associated with all except:

A. Retinal detachment
B. Vitreous hemorrhage
C. Ectopia lentis
D. Roth spots

104. Thinnest part of lens is:

A. Anterior pole
B. Posterior pole
C. Posterior capsule
D. Apex

105. In a district hospital in India, an ophthalmologist is expected to perform which of the following surgeries most commonly?

A. Phacoemulsification
B. Dacryocystectomy
C. Bilamellar tarsal rotation
D. Trabeculectomy

106. Congenital cataract occurs due to abnormalities in protein formation in which of the following genes?

A. PAX6 B. SIX5

C. CRYGS3 D. PITX3

107. High molecular weight proteins in cataractous lens seen only in humans:

A. HM 1 and 2 B. HM 2 and 4

C. HM 3 and 4 D. HM 2 and 3

108. The frequency of pulse in laser assisted cataract surgery is:

A. 10^{-12} B. 10^{-15}

C. 10^{-20} D. 10^{-10}

ANSWER AND EXPLANATION

1.	a	Lens has a special carrier system for the ascorbic acid which is a major antioxidant in the lens. This carrier system is mediated by myoinositol.
2.	a	Lens has two major antioxidants, i.e., Vitamin C and Vitamin E. Also it has two detoxifying enzymes, i.e., catalase and superoxide dismutase.
3.	b	In homocystinuria, the subluxation is inferonasal whereas in Marfan's it is superotemporal. Hyperinsulinemia does not present with subluxation whereas in ocular trauma there is no specific direction.
4.	b	Inflammatory reaction in children is always severe, and if the child is already suffering from uveitis, IOL implantations can deteriorate the condition.
5.	a	Ideally the child has to be operated as soon as feasible, this is to prevent amblyopia (visual reflex formation occurs by 5–6 months). As no ideal age has been recommended, we will mark the answer with the shortest duration.
6.	c	Most prominent feature is Megalocornea and most common is Ectopia Lentis.
7.	a	We have to opt for the minimum duration mentioned hence we will mark the answer immediately.
8.	a	Congenital Rubella is characterized by nuclear pearly cataract, but there is no dislocation of the lens.
9.	b	After ECCE, we prescribe the glasses after 6 weeks whereas after SICS we can prescribe after 2 weeks.
10.	b	Chalcosis is copper alloy in the eye.
11.	c	Alport's syndrome is Familial Haemorrhagic Nephritis.
12.	b	Vossius ring is the iris pigments imprinted on the anterior capsule of the lens, in shape of pupil–due to blunt trauma.
13.	a	Steroid induced cataract are posterior subcapsular cataracts.
14.	a	Part preparation is the most critical factor to prevent infection during any surgery.
15.	c	Lens is avascular and hence derives its nutrition from aqueous humour.
16.	c	NdYAG is a photodisruptive laser and is used for both posterior capsulotomy and peripheral iridotomy.
17.	b	Nuclear sclerosis causes mild increase in the refractive index of the lens and hence the refractive power of the lens increases, leading to improvement in the near vision.
18.	a	Pain which is increasing alongwith D/V, particulary after only 3 days of

		cataract surgery strongly suggests endophthalmitis.
19.	c	PSC is near the nodal point of the eye and hence diminishes the vision most.
20.	c	The incision size in phacoemulsification is 2.75 mm–3.2 mm.
21.	d	Nucleus is the oldest part of the lens.
22.	d	BSS with glutathione resembles the aqueous most and hence the most ideal.
23.	a	Subluxation of the lens is the most common complication of Nuclear Sclerotic Hypermature cataract.
24.	b	Retinal detachment can be the most probable cause of floaters occurring after 6 months of surgery.
25.	c	Morgagnian cataract complicates into phacolytic glaucoma.
26.	b	The enzyme responsible for sorbitol pathway is Aldose Reductase.
27.	b	If the halos break it is due to cataract and if not it is due to angle closure glaucoma.
28.	a	Phacoemulsification is method of SICS.
29.	b	In diabetes we get snowflake or snowstorm cataract.
30.	a	Chalcosis is copper deposition whereas gold deposition is called Chrysiasis. Long-term intake of gold of more than 1000 mg (in patients of RA) leads to corneal deposits and anterior subcapsular cataract.
31.	b	Polychromatic luster is a pathognomic feature of complicated cataract which is most commonly posterior subcapsular.
32.	a	Rheumatoid arthritis causes thinning and melting of the peripheral cornea and scleritis called Scleromalacia perforans.
33.	c	Wilson's disease is characterized by copper deposition, it is characterized by sunflower cataract and KF ring.
34.	a,b	The process of calculating the refractive power of the IOL is called Biometry. It is calculated by applying the SRK formula.
35.	a	Most common cause of acquired cataract is senile cataract.
36.	a,d, e	ICCE is contraindicated in children, because there is a strong adhesion between the posterior capsule of the lens and the vitreous called hyaloidocapsular ligament (ICCE will cause traction on the vitreous due to this adhesion leading to retinal detachment). Dissicision is an obsolete procedure.
37.	a,b, c,e	A patient of cataract is evaluated under all the above headings before being treated.
38.	a,b, e	Non foldable IOLs are made up of PMMA whereas foldable IOLs are made up of three materials, i.e., Acrylic, Silicon and Hydrogel.
39.	a,d, e	Posterior segment complications are least if posterior capsule is retained.
40.	a,d	Intraoperative and intracameral antibiotic injections are not given routinely. Role of oral postoperative antibiotics is controversial and many surgeons do not prescribe it.
41.	b	Radiational cataracts occur due to electromagnetic radiations.
42.	b	In-the-bag implantation is most physiological with least complications.

43. a Corneal dystrophies are idiopathic spontaneous changes with no inflammatory component.

44. a Rossete shaped cataract occurs in blunt trauma.

45. c Myotonic dystrophy presents as ptosis, Christmas tree cataract, pupillary changes and pigmentary retinopathy.

46. c In the day time pupil is constricted and hence nuclear cataract will diminish the vision in the day time.

47. a Most common type of congenital cataract is blue dot.

48. a,b,c,d All the above mentioned complications can occur after ECCE. CME is particularly common if there is posterior capsular tear.

49. a,b,d Choroidal detachment occurs due to hypotony. Rest all other can cause increased IOP.

50. a Area of the surface ectoderm overlying the optic vesicle thickens to form the lens placode which later converts into lens vesicle which separates from the surface ectoderm.

51. a Inferonasal–Homocystinuria, Superotemporal–Marfan's syndrome, Inferior and forward–Weil-Marchesani.

52. a Lowe's syndrome is inborn error of aminoacid metabolism and causes metabolic cataract.

53. a Toxic cataract can occur due to following drugs—Steroids, Phenothiazines, Long acting miotics, Amiodarone, Busulphan and Gold.

54. d Rubella does not present with subluxation of lens.

55. d Metronidazole does not cause cataract.

56. a Most common cause of endophthalmitis is staphylococcus epidermidis.

57. b Hypertension is the least documented risk factor among the other options mentioned. Recurrent diarrhoea causes dehydrational crisis which is said to cause cataract.

58. c Phacoemulsification is a sutureless surgery.

59. d Primary metabolism of lens is anaerobic and leads to lactic acid formation. In all other three options lens is not present in its place.

60. d Phacoemulsification—Main advantages of this surgery are negligible post operative astigmatism and early rehabilitation.

61. a RQ is the ratio of CO_2/O_2. In lens it is 1 which indicates that carbohydrates are the main source of energy in lens.

62. b Sutures of the lens are involved in sutural cataract.

63. c Phacomorphic glaucoma occurs in intumescent cataract whereas Phacotoxic glaucoma occurs in trauma and Phacolytic glaucoma occurs in Morgagnian cataract.

64. a USG A-scan measures the axial length whereas USG–B scan is used to examine the posterior segment of the eye.

65. b Lens capsule is thinnest at the posterior pole with the thickness of 0.4 mm.

66. b Other features of Hallermann-Strief syndrome are: microphthalmos,

macular pigment changes and Coats' disease.

67. a Radiational and steroid induced cataract are most commonly posterior subcapsular. Traumatic cataracts are most commonly posterior cortical.

68. d Slit lamp examination is the choice of method to diagnose a dislocated lens.

69. d Causes of frequent changes of presbyopic glasses are: Early cataract (i.e., intumescent cataract), late stage of primary open angle glaucoma and diabetes (It is not diabetic cataract but diabetes).

70. a AC lenses can complicate as glaucoma, uveitis and corneal decompensation.

71. d Hydration leads to cortical cataract whereas sclerosis leads to nuclear cataract.

72. a Zonular cataracts are associated with vitamin D deficiency.

73. b Most common cause of uniocular diplopia is subluxation of lens. Other causes are intumescent cataract and polycoria.

74. b Decreased visual acuity is the major criteria considered to operate cataract.

75. c Vossius ring is a feature of concussion injury located in the anterior capsule of the lens.

76. b After cataract is the most common long term complication of cataract surgery.

77. a,b, c,d Most common type of congenital cataract causing diminution of vision is Zonular cataract.

78. b Nuclear cataracts are more common than cortical cataract.

79. b Myotonic dystrophy and Atopic dermatitis are causes of presenile cataract.

80. d If Galactosemia occurs due to GPUT (Galactose phospho uridyl–transferase), it causes Oil Droplet cataract whereas if it occurs due to Galactokinase deficiency, it causes lamellar cataract.

81. b Diametre of the lens is 9–10 mm less than 9 mm is called Microphakia.

82. b Lens fibres grow throughout life.

83. b One of the causes of complicated cataract is retinal pathologies. Retinal degenerations and other fundal changes is a feature of pathological myopia but not of hypermetropia.

84. d Refractive index is maximum at the centre of the lens where the nucleus is hard compared to the cortex.

85. a Endophytic retinoblastoma (which grows towards the vitreous) may lead to dislocation of the lens.

86. a Other complications are corneal decompensation and uveitis.

87. c Nuclear sclerosis causes increased refractive index leading to lenticular myopia. This is called "second sight of old age".

88. d Pathological myopia may complicate as PSC and early onset of nuclear sclerosis. These patients are also predisposed to develop POAG.

89. b In pseudoexfoliation syndrome, the suspensory ligaments are weak and hence there are chances of subluxation.

90. a Christmas tree cataract is a presenile cataract in patients of myotonic dystrophy.

91. a An aphakic eye has a deep anterior chamber and there is iridodonesis, i.e., trembling of the iris due to loss

of support by the lens. Also since his vision is corrected by the high convex lens, diagnosis is aphakia.

92. a The above features are typical of ectopia lentis. Other features are:
 1. Iridodonesis.
 2. Fluctuating anterior chamber depth.
 3. Phacodonesis.
 4. Herniation of vitreous in the anterior chamber leading to pupillary block glaucoma.
 5. Monocular diplopia.
 6. Uveitis if the lens is displaced posteriorly.

93. b The description of the opacities is in favor of lamellar cataract and these spoke of wheel like arrangement is a typical description of Riders, these are the characteristic feature of lamellar cataract.

94. a A diabetic patient with the following signs and symptoms, just after two days of surgery–most favourable diagnosis is endophthalmitis. The most strong points in favor is the grey white reflex. Though the incidence of infection in phaco is less, but as the patient is diabetic and hence always a possibility.

95. c Mutation in distinct genes which encode the main cytoplasmic proteins of human lens has been associated with cataract.
 1. Genes encoding crystalline: CRYA, CRYB, CRYG.
 2. Lens specific connexins: Cx43, Cx46, Cx50.
 3. MIP major intrinsic protein or Aquaporin.

96. b Insoluble proteins are albuminoids and souble proteins are crystallines. Cataract occurs due to decrease in soluble proteins and increase in insoluble proteins.

97. c Glutathione plays a central role in protecting the lens from oxidative damage.

98. d Systemic steroids most commonly cause cataract which is posterior subcapsular cataract whereas topical steroids most commonly leads to open angle glaucoma.

99. d Congenital cataract should be operated immediately to prevent amblyopia. This is because foveal reflex formation completes within 5–6 months of age.

100. c Cogan Reese syndrome is an irido-corneoendothelial syndrome causing secondary glaucoma.

101. a It is sequestered in the lens capsule and whenever there is leakage of the protein outside the capsule, it causes immune reaction.

102. b Anterior lenticonus.

103. d Roths spot is flame shaped haemorrhage with a white pale centre which is soft exudate.

104. b Thinnest part is capsule at the posterior pole. It is 4 microns.

105. a If the question would have SICS as one of the options, then it would have been the answer as this is the most common surgery performed in a district hospital and hence an ophthalmologist should be able to perform the same. Here the best option is A.

106. c **Gamma-S-crystallin gene (CRYGS) mutation causes dominant progressive cortical cataract in humans.** Other genes that are responsible for congenital cataract are:

1. Cx: Connexins.
2. MIP: Major intrinsic protein.

107. c High molecular weight proteins are seen in the lens. HM1 HM2 HM3 HM4.

HM1, HM2 are soluble type.

HM3, HM4 are insoluble type seen in cataractous lens.

HM4, occurs exclusively in nuclear cataract.

108. b Femtosecond laser is a focussed infrared laser, with a wavelength of 1053 nm that uses ultrafast pulses with duration of 100 fs (100 into 10 to power of –15 seconds) it is a solid state Nd Glass laser which operates on the principle of **photo-ionisation**.

RECENTLY ADDED QUESTIONS

1. **A 55-year-old man complaints of glare in eye while driving his car in the night, his best corrected vision 6/12. What is the most probable diagnosis?**
   A. ARMD
   B. Post capsular opacification lens
   C. Corneal degeneration
   D. Diabetic retinopathy

2. **Dislocation is not seen in: (PGI)**
   A. Marfan's syndrome
   B. Myotonic dystrophy
   C. Sulphite oxidase deficiency
   D. Homocystinuria
   E. Diabetes mellitus

ANSWERS OF RECENTLY ADDED QUESTIONS

1. b Posterior capsular opacification or After cataract is the most common long-term complication of cataract surgery. The above history of glare at night with dimunition of vision is most suggestive of PCO compared to other options.

2. b,e Myotonic dystrophy and diabetes mellitus cause cataract but not ectopia lentis.

Common causes of lens dislocation/ ectopia lentis include:

- Marfan syndrome.
- Ehlers-Danlos syndrome.
- Sulphite oxidase deficiency.
- Homocystinuria.
- Weil-Marchesani syndrome.
- Stickler syndrome.
- Hyperlysinemia.

IMAGE-BASED QUESTIONS

1. **The diagnosis is:**

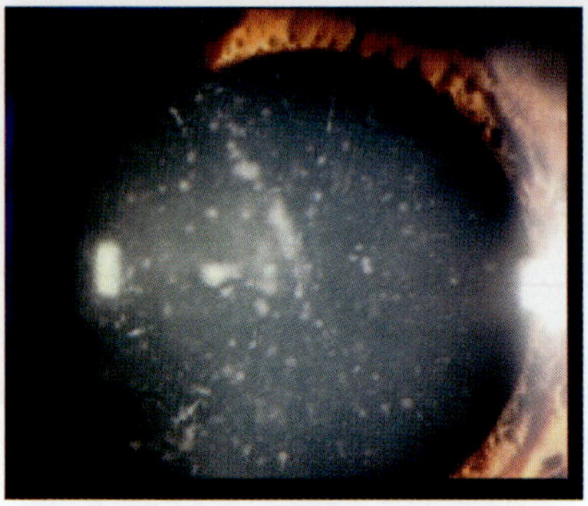

A. Snowflake cataract
B. Sunflower cataract
C. Radial spokes
D. Posterior subcapsular cataract

2. **The diagnosis is:**

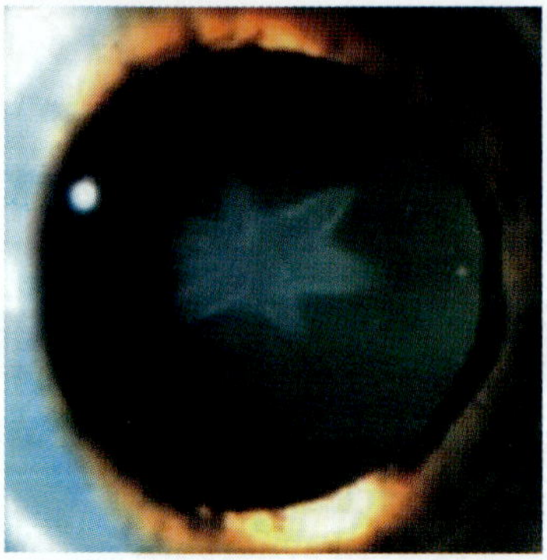

A. Blunt trauma B. Electric cataract
C. Chalcosis D. Rubella

3. **The diagnosis is:**

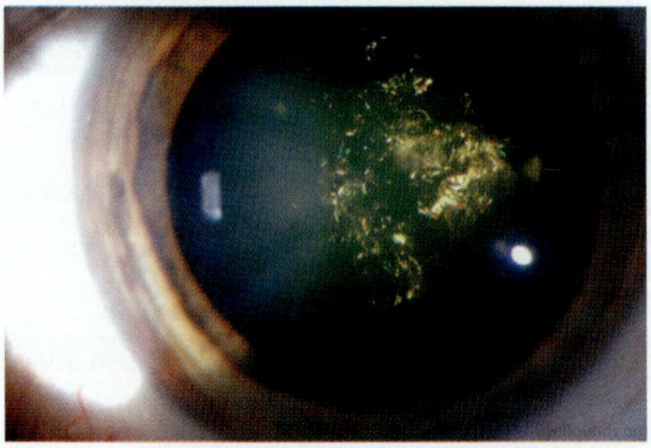

A. Nuclear pearly cataract
B. Christmas tree cataract
C. Glaucomaflecken
D. Anterior subcapsular cataract

4. **The diagnosis is:**

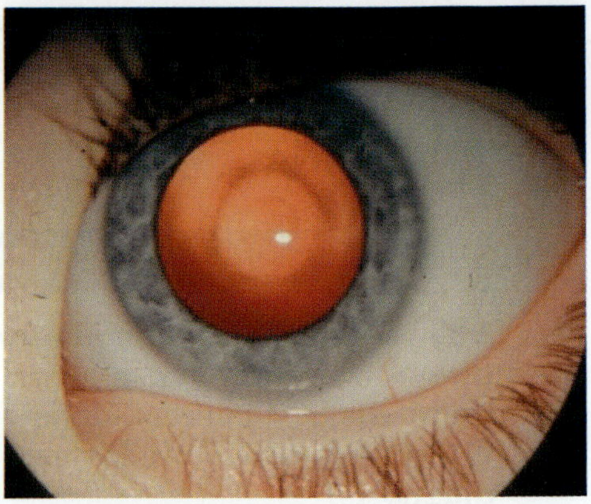

A. Vossius ring
B. Oil globule reflex
C. Oil droplet reflex
D. Oil droplet cataract

5. **The diagnosis is:**

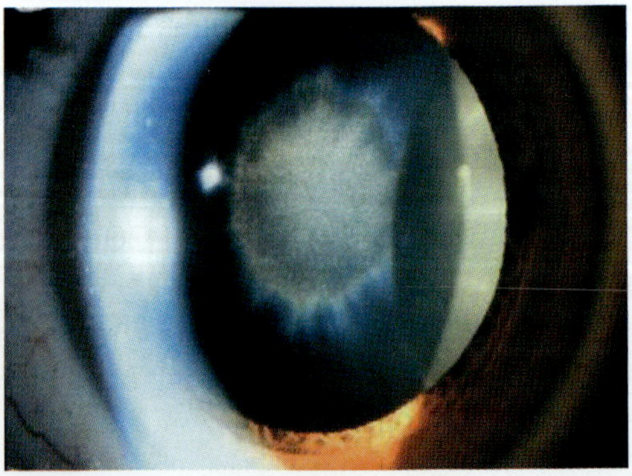

A. Chalcosis
B. Trauma
C. Rubella
D. Posterior polar cataract

6. **Most common cause of the image given below is:**

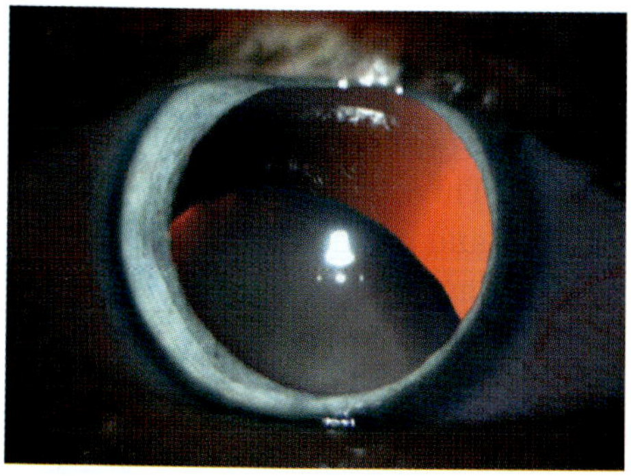

A. Trauma
B. Marfan's Syndrome
C. Homocystinuria
D. Ehlers-Danlos

7. **The procedure given below is done by:**

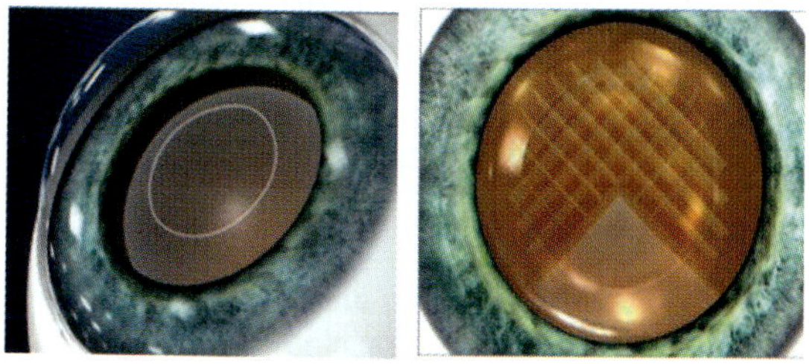

A. Photodisruptive lasers
B. Photocoagulative lasers
C. Photoablative lasers
D. Excimer lasers

8. **Choice of treatment for the condition given below:**

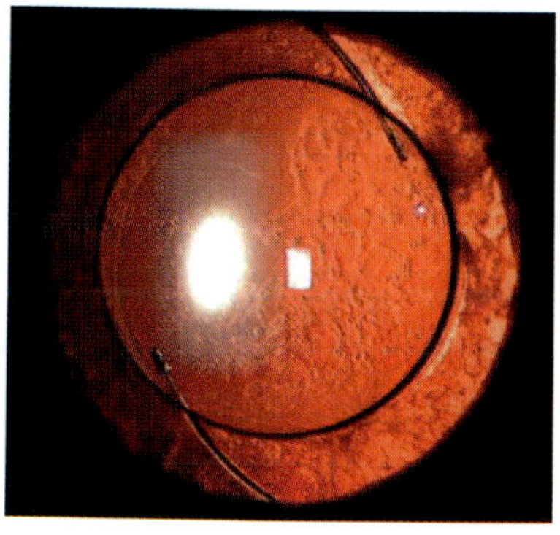

A. Excimer
B. Femtolaser
C. Nd YAG
D. Diode

9. **The most common complication of the image given below:**

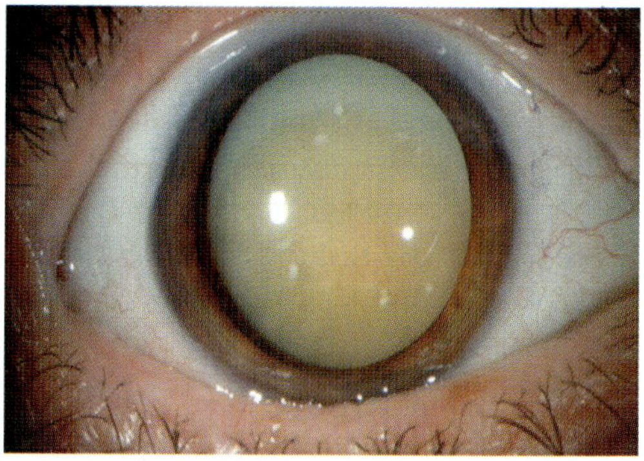

A. Phacotoxic glaucoma
B. Phacolytic glaucoma
C. Phacoanaphylactic glaucoma
D. Phacomorphic glaucoma

10. **The incision length for procedure given below is:**

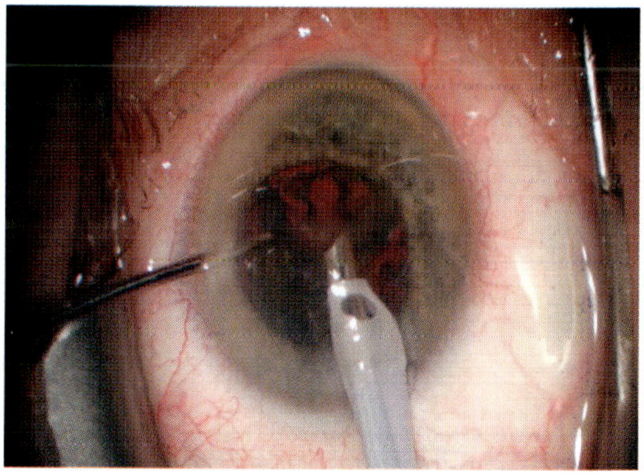

A. 2.75 – 3.2 mm
B. 5.0 – 5.5 mm
C. 1.8 – 2.4 mm
D. 3.0 – 3.5 mm

ANSWERS OF IMAGE-BASED QUESTIONS

1. a It is a feature of diabetes and more common in type 1 diabetes.
2. a It is a rossette shaped cataract, characteristic of blunt trauma. It involves posterior cortex.
3. b It is Christmas tree cataract. It is a feature of myotonic dystrophy.
4. d It is oil droplet cataract and is a feature of galactosemia.
5. a This is sunflower cataract and is a feature of chalcosis.
6. a It is subluxation of lens, most commonly caused by trauma.
7. a It is a femtolaser cataract surgery which is a photodisruptive laser with a wavelength of 1052 nm.
8. c The above is a slide of after cataract and its choice of treatment is Nd YAG laser posterior capsulotomy.
9. b The above is a slide of morgagnian cataract and hence the most common complication is phacolytic glaucoma.
10. a The above slide is of phacoemulsification with the incision length of 2.75–3.2 mm.

GUIDANCE

In all things, patience is the key to victory. Those who cannot endure cannot hope to win. Ultimate triumph belongs to those who can forbear.

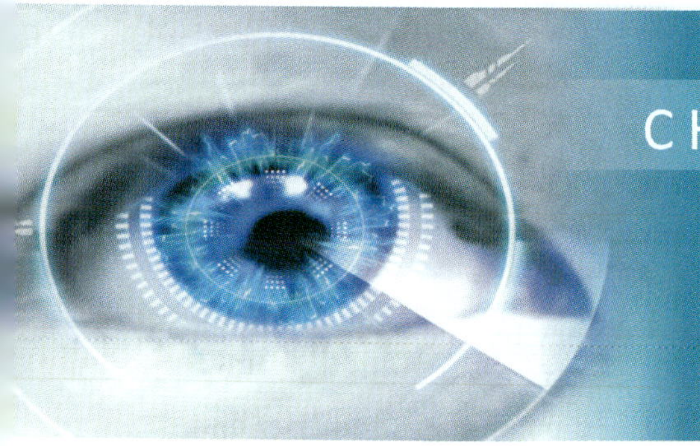

CHAPTER 2

Glaucoma

DEFINITION

Glaucoma is a multifactorial optic neuropathy in which there is characteristic loss of optic nerve fibre. **The most common cause of glaucoma is primary open angle glaucoma accounting for more than 90% of all cases.** It is the second leading cause of irreversible blindness (1.8% of Indian population).

Pathogenesis: Glaucoma involves loss of retinal ganglion cells. This ganglion cell death occurs by apoptosis.

Factors which are responsible are:

1. Lack of trophic factors.
2. Autoimmune reactions.
3. Increased concentration of nitrous oxide.
4. Increased concentration of glutamate.

Genetics: 20 genetic loci are there for occurrence of primary open angle glaucoma. 11 are designated from GLC1A to GLC1K. GLC1A is for myocillin and GLC1E is for optineurin [on chromosome 10 (p15–p14)].

CLASSIFICATION

a. Angle Closure Glaucoma

1. *With pupillary block:*

   Primary: Acute, subacute and chronic.

   Secondary: Lens induced, miotic induced, synechiae.

2. *Without pupillary block:*

   Primary: Plateau iris.

   Secondary: Anterior pulling mechanism, Posterior pushing mechanism.

b. Open Angle Glaucoma

A. Primary open angle glaucoma.

B. Normal tension glaucoma.

C. Secondary open angle glaucoma.

c. Combined Mechanism Glaucoma.

d. Developmental Glaucoma.

A. Primary congenital glaucoma.

B. Glaucoma associated with congenital anomalies/syndrome.

AQUEOUS HUMOUR

1. Normal rate of formation of aqueous is 2.3 uL/min (about 1% of the anterior-chamber volume/min).
2. Total volume of aqueous humour is 0.31 ml—0.25 ml in anterior chamber and about 0.06 ml in the posterior chamber.
3. Refractive index of aqueous is 1.33.
4. Osmotic pressure: It is slightly hyperosmotic to plasma by 3–5 mOsm/L.
5. pH of aqueous: pH = 7.2.

6. **Aqueous is produced by the non pigmented epithelial cells of ciliary process by secretion (90% of aqueous). Other processes like ultrafiltration and diffusion also take part.**
7. Aqueous humour provides nutrition to both the avascular structures of eye, i.e., lens and cornea.
8. Protein content of aqueous is less than 1% of plasma as blood aqueous barrier is impermeable to large molecular weight plasma proteins. Small molecular weight proteins like globulin can cross the barrier hence its concentration in aqueous humor is more than albumin.
9. **The normal intraocular pressure in the eye is between 10 mm Hg to 21 mm Hg and mean pressure is 16 ± 2.5 mm Hg.**
10. The intraocular pressure refers to the pressure exerted by intraocular contents on the coats of the eyeball.
11. **Normal IOP is pulsatile**, reflecting its vascular origin and the effects of blood flow on internal ocular structures.
12. **Diurnal variation in IOP:** IOP fluctuates cyclically throughout the day. The pressure is highest in early morning and lowest in late evening. **The mean amplitude of daily fluctuation is usually less than 5 mm Hg in normal individuals. A diurnal variation in IOP of more than 8 mm Hg is considered pathognomic of glaucoma.**

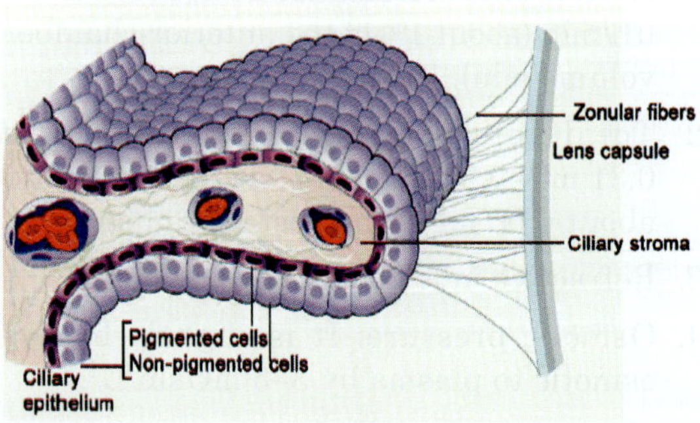

Fig. 2.1

Biochemical Composition of Aqueous Humour

1. *Water:* It constitutes 99.9% of aqueous humour.
2. *Colloid contents:*
   a. *Proteins:*
      - Very less compared to plasma, i.e., 5–15 mg/100 ml.
      - In plasma–6–7 gm/100 ml.

   b. *Amino acids:*
      Aqueous/plasma ratio—varies from 0.08 to 3.14. Hence, there is active transport of amino acids.
3. *Non-colloidal constituents:* These are dissolved solids which give a clear solution.
   a. Concentration of ascorbate, pyruvate and lactate are much higher in aqueous humour than in plasma.
   b. Concentration of urea and glucose are much less in aqueous humour compared to plasma.

Control of Aqueous Formation

1. Vasopressin causes increase in active transport of Na^+ ions leading to increase in aqueous formation.
2. Adenylcyclase decreases aqueous formation.
3. Carbonic anhydrase inhibitors decrease aqueous formation.

Drainage of Aqueous Humour

1. **Conventional Outflow** (90% of total outflow):

   Ciliary processes→Aqueous in posterior chamber→Anterior chamber→Trabecular meshwork (Uveal, Corneoscleral, Juxta-canalicular)→Schlemns canal (Through formation of giant vacuoles)→Collector channels→Episcleral veins.

   Juxtacanalicular (Endothelial) meshwork is responsible for maximum

resistance to aqueous outflow compared to other parts of the trabecular meshwork.

2. **Uveoscleral outflow** (10% of total outflow):

   Ciliary processes→Aqueous in posterior chamber→Ciliary body→Suprachoroid space→Venous circulation of ciliary body, choroid and sclera.

DEVELOPMENTAL GLAUCOMA

Primary Congenital Glaucoma (Inheritance—AR): It can be divided into three types: (1) True congenital glaucoma (2) Infantile glaucoma (Before 3 years of age) (3) Juvenile glaucoma (3–16 years).

Buphthalmos or enlargement of eyeball occurs within three years of age as the sclera is elastic due to low scleral rigidity.

Pathogenesis:

1. *Developmental anomaly of angle of anterior chamber, i.e., Flat iris insertion or Concave iris insertion.*
2. *Trabeculodysgenesis:* Trabecular meshwork is not formed properly.

Clinical Features:

1. *Photophobia, blepharospasm, lacrimation and eye-rubbing.*
2. *Corneal signs:*
   a. Corneal edema.
   b. Corneal enlargement (>13 mm).
   c. Haab's Striae-break in DM (Descements memb).
3. *Buphthalmos:*
   a. Blue and thin sclera.
   b. Iridodonesis.
   c. Deep AC.
   d. Anteroposteriorly flat lens; which may subluxate.
4. *Cupping of disc:*

   Enlarged C:D ratio may be either due to neuronal loss or enlargement of scleral canal.
5. *IOP:* Raised but neither marked nor acute.

Differential Diagnosis:

a. *Cloudy cornea:*
   1. Birth trauma.
   2. Intrauterine rubella.
   3. Metabolic disorders–Mucopolysaccharidosis, lipidosis and cystinosis.

b. *Large cornea:*
   1. Megalocornea.
   2. Very high myopia.

c. *Lacrimation:* Non-patent NLD.

d. *Secondary causes of glaucoma:*
   1. Retinoblastoma.
   2. Juvenile Xanthogranuloma.
   3. Persistent hyperplastic primary vitreous.
   4. ROP: Retinopathy of prematurity.

Treatment:

a. *Goniotomy:* It is the treatment of choice of congenital glaucoma.

b. *Trabeculotomy:* It denotes cutting opening of Schlemm's canal.

c. Combined trabeculotomy and trabeculectomy.

GLAUCOMA ASSOCIATED WITH CONGENITAL ANOMALIES

A. With Iridocorneal dysgenesis

a. *Axenfeld's anomaly:*

   C/F:

   1. *Posterior embryotoxon:* It is prominent schwalbe line displaced anteriorly.

2. Iris strands attached to the posterior embryotoxon.

b. *Reiger's anomaly:*

C/F:

1. Posterior embryotoxon.
2. *Iris anomalies:* Stromal hypoplasia, Pseudopolycoria (Full-thickness holes), Corectopia (Displacement of pupil) and Ectropion uveae.

c. *Reiger's syndrome:* It constitutes all the features of Reiger's anomaly alongwith hypodontia, microdontia and facial abnormalities.

d. *Peter's anomaly:*

1. Corneal opacity with iris adhesions to its margin.
2. Keratolenticular adhesions.

B. With Aniridia: It is a rare bilateral condition. Its features vary from total absence to relative mild hypoplasia.

C/F:

1. Absence of iris or hypoplasia of iris.
2. *Corneal lesions:* Microcornea, sclerocornea, corneal opacity, limbal dermoids and keratocorneal adhesions.
3. *Lenticular opacity:* Cataract, subluxation of lens, absence of lens, and persistent pupillary membrane.
4. *Posterior segment:* Hypoplasia of fovea hypoplastic disc and choroidal coloboma.
5. Glaucoma.

It can be divided into four phenotypes:

1. *With normal vision:* Inheritance is autosomal dominant.
2. *With poor vision, due to foveal hypoplasia:* Inheritance is autosomal dominant.
3. *With Wilms' tumour of the kidney also known as nephroblastoma:* These cases occur sporadically but are associated with deletion of short arm of chromosome 11.
4. *With mental retardation:* Inheritance is autosomal recessive.

C. Associated with Ectopialentis syndromes: Marfan's syndrome, Weil-Marchesani syndrome and homocystinuria.

SECONDARY CONGENITAL GLAUCOMA

A. *Congenital ectropion uveae:* It is a rare anomaly showing iris pigments on the anterior surface of iris. The pupil is round and reacting. Glaucoma occurs due to associated angle anomaly.

B. *Nanophthalmos:* It is a rare disorder characterized by hypermetropia with very short axial length. Glaucoma develops due to progressive narrowing of angle.

C. *Naevus of ota:* It is also known as oculodermal melanosis. It is charac-terized by conjunctival subepithelial melanosis alongwith dermal melanosis. Some of the patients have associated glaucoma (which could be due to similar changes in the trabecular meshwork).

D. *Lowe's syndrome:* It is characterized by:

1. Microphakia.
2. Cataract.
3. Posterior lenticonus or posterior lentiglobus.
4. Glaucoma.

E. *Phacomatosis:*

1. *Sturge-Weber syndrome:* It consti-tutes a triad of angioma of face, ipsilateral angioma of meninges and brain and

glaucoma (It occurs due to increased episcleral pressure or angle anomaly).

2. *Von-Recklinghausen's diseases:* Glaucoma occurs due to associated angle anomaly.

PRIMARY OPEN ANGLE GLAUCOMA (POAG)

Predisposing Risk Factors:

1. Heredity, i.e., positive family history.
2. Age (above 40)–Common in elderly.
3. Myopes–More common.
4. Diabetics–More common.
5. Hypertension–More common.
6. Cigarette smoking.
7. Thyrotoxicosis.

Pathogenesis: Thickening and sclerosis of trabeculae and absence of giant vacuoles in the cells lining schlemn canal leads to obstruction of outflow of aqueous humour.

Clinical Features:

1. Mild headache, eyeache.
2. Difficulty in reading and close work.
3. Frequent change of presbyopic glasses.
4. Delayed dark adaptation.

Signs:

1. IOP changes.
2. Optic disc changes.
3. Visual field defect.

A. IOP Changes:

1. Exaggeration of normal diurnal variation (>8 mm Hg).
2. Increase in IOP.

Variants:

a. *Normal Tension Glaucoma:* In this condition, the intraocular tension is normal but there is damage to the optic nerve leading to both disc changes and field defects.

b. *Ocular Hypertension:* Here, the intraocular tension is more than the normal but the disc is normal and there are no field defects.

B. Fundus Changes:

Disc Pattern Changes:

1. C:D>0.3.
2. C:D asymmetry > 0.1–0.2 between two eyes.

   Cupping always starts in a vertical direction as the arcuate fibres from the temporal retina exit from optic disc at superior and inferior location. Horizontal cupping occurs last. *First vertical dimension is important, then oblique and lastly horizontal.*
3. Neuroretinal rim thinning/notching.
4. Visibility of openings of lamina cribosa called **"Laminar-dot-sign"**. It is a feature of advanced stage of glaucoma due to deepening of the cup.
5. **Cavernous optic atrophy**–It is also known as **"Schnables' atrophy"**.

Features:

1. Atrophy of nerve fibres.
2. No glial cell proliferation.
3. Mucoid degeneration of glial cells leading to formation of lacunae or clear pools.

Occurs in:

1. Glaucoma.
2. Methyl alcohol poisoning.
3. High myopia.

C. Vascular Signs:

1. Flame shaped haemorrhage at inferior quadrant of the optic disc.

2. Nasal shifting of vessels.
3. *Bayonetting sign:* It denotes double bending of vessels.
4. Tortuosity of retinal vessels in advanced stage.

D. Peripapillary Changes:

1. Wedge-shaped and slit-shaped defects in retinal nerve fibre layer.
2. Diffuse loss of striations.

E. Visual Field Defects:

Early Defects:

1. Central or paracentral scotoma at Bjerrums area: (Bjerrums area corresponds to the arcuate fibres which are first affected in glaucoma). **It is the earliest field defect in primary open angle glaucoma.**
2. Siedel scotoma: When central or paracentral scotoma joins with the blind spot, it is known as Siedel scotoma.
3. Baring of blind spot: Earliest sign is localized constriction of central field to very small test objects (1/2000) so that instead of skirting the 30° isopter concentrically, the field becomes deformed curving inwards to exclude the blind spot called **"BARING OF BLIND SPOT"**, i.e., isopter contraction, but this sign is not pathognomic of early glaucoma and also can be manipulated by change in illumination or size of pupil. Hence, the earliest sign is scotoma (initially relative) in the same isopter as blind spot and generally above it (Bjerrums area).
4. Isolated paracentral nasal scotoma.
5. Roenne's nasal step.

Late Defects:

1. Arcuate scotoma.
2. Double arcuate or ring scotoma.
3. Total field loss except small island of central and temporal vision.

PRIMARY ANGLE CLOSURE GLAUCOMA (PACG)

Predisposing Risk Factors:

1. Hypermetropic eyes with shallow anterior chamber.
2. Iris-Lens diaphragm placed anteriorly.
3. Narrow angle of anterior chamber.
4. Plateau iris configuration.
5. Age–More common in 5th decade.
6. Sex–Females are more prone.
7. Personality–Nervous individuals.
8. Season–Peak in rainy season.
9. Family history–Positive.

Clinical Features:

Stages of PACG:

1. Latent Glaucoma (Prodromal Phase)

1. Shallow AC.
2. Convex shaped iris—lens diaphragm.
3. Normal IOP.
4. Narrow angle capable of closure.

2. Intermittent Glaucoma (Stage of Constant Instability)

1. Rapid partial closure and re-opening of the angle (Angle is narrow in only one part).
2. *Clinical Features:*
   - Transient blurring of vision.
   - Halos around light.
   - Eye ache and frontal headache.
3. *On Examination* (during attack)
   - Corneal epithelial edema.
   - Semi-dilated pupil.
   - Eye not congested.

In between attacks eye is perfectly normal. Although angle is narrow.

3. **Acute Congestive Angle—Closure Glaucoma**
   1. Sudden and severe elevation of IOP due to total closure of angle.
   2. *Clinical Features:*

      Rapid impairment of vision with periocular pain, may be accompanied with nausea and vomiting.
   3. *On Examination:*
      - Ciliary congestion.
      - Severely elevated IOP (upto 60 mm Hg).
      - Corneal edema.
      - Shallow AC.
      - Closed angle.
      - Vertically dilated and fixed pupil (Pathognomic feature of acute angle closure glaucoma).
4. **Chronic Closed Angle Glaucoma**

   All features of open angle glaucoma, i.e., increased intraocular pressure, fundus changes and field defects but the angle is closed.
5. **Absolute glaucoma:** It is an end stage.
   1. *Clinical Features:*
      - Eye is painful, irritable and completely blind.
      - Slight ciliary flush around cornea.
      - "Caput medusae"—In long-standing cases few prominent and enlarged blood vessels seen around cornea are caput medusae.
      - Cornea initially clear but **corneal sensation is decreased.**
   2. *Late Features of Absolute Glaucoma:*
      1. Bullous keratopathy.
      2. Filamentary keratitis.
      3. Shallow AC.
      4. Iris atrophy.
      5. Pupil dilated and fixed.
      6. Optic disc—Glaucomatous optic atrophy.
      7. High IOP—Eyeball stony hard.

Stages in Natural History

1. *Primary angle-closure suspect (PACS):* Gonioscopy shows posterior meshwork ITC (Iridotrabecular contact) in three or more quadrants but no PAS (Peripheral anterior synechiae).
   - Normal IOP, optic disc and visual field.
2. *Primary angle-closure (PAC):* Gonioscopy shows three or more quadrants of ITC with raised IOP and/or PAS, or excessive pigment smudging on the TM.
   - Normal optic disc and field.
3. *Primary angle-closure glaucoma (PACG):* Gonioscopy shows ITC in three or more quadrants.
   - Optic neuropathy.

Medical Treatment of Acute Congestive Stage of PACG

1. Intravenous mannitol or glycerol or acetazolamide.
2. Oral acetazolamide, if the patient is not vomiting.
3. Pilocarpine eye drops: It is given every two minutes till the pupil constricts.
4. Injectable analgesics like pethidine.
5. Topical beta blockers: It can be given alongwith pilocarpine.

   Acetazolamide is given first and simultaneously pilocarpine is instilled as there is severe iris ischemia due to very high intraocular pressure hence it will not react to pilocarpine alone.

Laser Iridotomy

- **This is the definitive treatment of angle closure glaucoma.**
- In patients of acute angle closure glaucomas, fellow eye is given prophylactic treatment to prevent the advent of angle closure in the other eye. **There is no role of prophylactic treatment in open angle glaucoma.**
- Laser iridotomy is done by Nd: YAG laser which is a photodisruptive (cutting) laser.
- If laser is not available, can go for surgical iridectomy.

Trabeculectomy: It is opted as a last resort in the management of ACG when the patient is not responding to other means of treatment or if peripheral anterior synechiae is formed in greater than 2/3rd of the angle.

Treatment Modalities in Absolute Glaucoma

1. The choice of treatment is cyclotherapy either by Cryo or Laser (Nd: YAG in free thermal mode).

   Cyclophotocoagulation

   It is used in treatment of absolute glaucoma to destroy the ciliary processes. The laser used is Nd:YAG in free-running or thermal mode.

   Cyclocryotherapy

   It can also be done instead of laser therapy. Cryotherapy destroys the ciliary processes by freeze and thaw method, hence aqueous humour is not formed leading to decrease in the IOP thus relieving pain.
2. Retrobulbar injection of absolute alchohol. But in this modality the disadvantage is that it has to repeated at regular intervals.
3. Evisceration.

SECONDARY GLAUCOMAS

1. Lens-Induced Glaucoma

A. *Phacomorphic Glaucoma:* It denotes glaucoma due to alteration in morphology of lens.

   1. Intumescent lens.
   2. Microspherophakia is generally associated with anterior subluxation or dislocation of lens.

B. *Phacolytic Glaucoma:* It occurs due to leakage of proteins from the wrinkled capsule of hypermature morgagnian cataract which block the trabecular meshwork leading to glaucoma.

C. *Lens Particle Glaucoma or Phacotoxic Glaucoma:* It occurs due to rupture of lens capsule (due to trauma), leading to release of lot of lens particles causing clogging of trabecular meshwork hence causing glaucoma.

D. *Glaucoma Associated with Phacogenic Uveitis:* It denotes to the uveitis occurring due to leaked lens proteins and contributing to the development of glaucoma.

E. *Glaucoma Associated with Phacoanaphylaxis:* It denotes to the anaphylactic reaction, causing accumulation of macrophages, which engulf the lens protein and block the trabecular meshwork leading to glaucoma.

2. Inflammatory Glaucoma

- It is glaucoma occurring due to uveitis.
- It is broadly divided into three types:
  1. ACG with pupillary block.
  2. ACG without pupillary block.
  3. *OAG:* **It is also known as POSNER-SCHLOSSMAN SYNDROME or Glaucomatocyclitic crisis or Hypertensive uveitis.**

In this condition, the primary pathology is uveitis. However, the patient presents with very few KPs and the rise in intraocular pressure is upto 26 mm Hg. Hence, sometimes if misdiagnosed as angle closure glaucoma, pilocarpine is given which further aggravates the condition. **The most diagnostic is the pupil which if constricted, it is uveitis and not glaucoma.**

3. Pigmentary Glaucoma

- It is secondary open angle glaucoma.
- Pigments are dispersed from the pigment epithelial layer of the iris, due to rubbing against the suspensory ligament leading to accumulation of pigments in the trabecular meshwork causing glaucoma.
- Other features: (a) Pigments at the back of cornea called Krukenberg spindles. (b) Pigmented line anterior to the schwalbe's line called **sampolesi's line.**

4. Pseudo-Exfoliative Glaucoma "Glaucoma Capsulare"

- It is due to deposition of grey dandruff-like material in the trabecular meshwork, which is exfoliated from the basement membranes of the structures of the eye.
- Treatment is on lines of POAG.

5. NVG–Neovascular Glaucoma

- Glaucoma due to encroachment of neovascular tissue at the angle of anterior chamber. This occurs due to neovascularisation of iris called rubeosis iridis.
- It occurs in hypoxic conditions of retina like: Diabetic retinopathy, Central retinal vein occlusion, Eales' disease, Sickle cell retinopathy etc.
- Initially it is an open angle glaucoma and later leads to closed angle due to contraction of the fibrous tissue.
- **Treatment modalities:**
  - (a) **Pan retinal photocoagulation is the treatment of choice of NVG.**
  - (b) Antiglaucoma drugs.
  - (c) Trabeculectomy with aqueous drainage implants.
  - (d) Enucleation or Eviceration

6. Glaucoma Associated With Intra-ocular Tumours

Intraocular tumours raise the IOP hence leading to glaucoma.

7. Steroid-Induced Glaucoma

It occurs due to deposition of mucopolysaccharides in the trabecular meshwork.

Steroid-induced Complications in Eye

It generally occurs with long-acting steroids like Dexamethasone, Betamethasone.

1. **Glaucoma:** It is the most common complication of steroids. It is more common with topical steroids compared to oral steroids.
2. **Cataract (Posterior subcapsular):** It is more common with oral steroids.
3. Increased incidence of infections.
4. Corneal ulceration.
5. Myopathy leading to ptosis.

8. Traumatic Glaucoma

Glaucoma after trauma occurs due to following factors:

a. *Angle-Recession (cleavage) glaucoma:* It occurs due to blunt injury which causes tear in the ciliary body leading to recession of the angle. Glaucoma occurs due to associated damage to the trabecular meshwork.

b. *Inflammatory glaucoma:* Uveitis secondary to trauma can lead to glaucoma.

c. Due to intraocular haemorrhage.

d. *Lens-induced glaucoma:* Trauma can lead to subluxation of lens leading to glaucoma.

9. Ciliary-Block-Glaucoma (Malignant Glaucoma)

- It occurs as a complication of any intraocular procedure.

Clinical Features:

1. Persistent flat anterior chamber following any intraocular operation.
2. Markedly raised IOP, in early postoperative period.
3. Negative Siedel's test, indicating no leakage from anterior chamber.
4. Unresponsiveness or even aggravation by miotics.
5. It may be phakic, aphakic or pseudophakic.

Mechanism:

a. Ciliolenticular block (ciliary processes press against equator of lens).

OR

b. Ciliovitreal block (ciliary processes press against anterior hyaloid face of vitreous)

↓

Aqueous humour is diverted posteriorly and collects as aqueous pockets in the vitreous

↓

Raised IOP

↓

Anterior chamber becomes flat

Management:

- *Medical:*
  a. 1% Atropine drops or ointment to dilate ciliary ring and break the block. Since mydriatic is used to treat this condition it is also known as INVERSE GLAUCOMA.
  b. Timolol maleate eye drops and oral acetazolamide to decrease the aqueous formation.
  c. I/V mannitol to shrink the vitreous.
- *Laser:* Disruption of anterior hyaloid face by Nd: YAG through patent iridectomy opening.
- *Surgical:* Pars plana vitrectomy.

10. With Intraocular Haemorrhage

A. After Hyphema:

1. *Red cell glaucoma:* It occurs when RBCs block the trabecular meshwork.
2. *Haemolytic glaucoma:* It occurs when macrophages laden with RBC's block the trabecular meshwork.
3. *Hemosiderotic glaucoma:* It occurs when iron from phagocytosed haemoglobin block the trabecular meshwork.

B. After Vitreous Haemorrhage:

Ghost cell glaucoma: In vitreous haemorrhage, RBC's get transformed into ghost cells. When these ghost cells block the trabecular meshwork it leads to glaucoma.

11. Glaucoma Associated With Irido-Corneal Endothelial Syndromes

It typically affects young to middle aged women. It constitutes the following three overlapping disorders:

A. Progressive iris atrophy.

B. Chandler's syndrome.

C. Cogan-Reese syndrome (Iris naevus).

Pathogenesis: It is a proliferative endotheliopathy where the endothelial cells (*which normally do not proliferate*) starts proliferating and migrating across the angle and onto the surface of iris. 50% of such cases present with glaucoma.

Clinical Features:

1. Corectopia, i.e., eccentric pupil.
2. Pseudopolycoria, i.e, supernumerary false pupil.
3. Iris atrophy of varying severity.
4. Corneal edema due to endothelial decompensation.
5. PAS on gonioscopy.
6. Glaucoma.

Specific Features:

1. *Progressive Iris Atrophy:* It is characterized by stromal atrophy and hole formation in the iris.
2. *Cogan-Rheese Syndrome:* It is characterized by diffuse naevus or pedunculated nodules on the iris. Iris atrophy is absent in 50% of cases.
3. *Chandler's Syndrome:* It is characterized by severe corneal changes leading to corneal edema. Patient complains of blurred vision and halos. Glaucoma is less severe.

Treatment: Medical therapy is ineffective. Trabeculectomy with aqueous drainage implants is required.

INVESTIGATIONS FOR GLAUCOMA

A. Provocative Tests

For PACG

1. *Mydriatic test:* Rise in IOP of > 8 mm Hg after instillation of tropicamide is suggestive of angle closure glaucoma.
2. *Dark room test:* Patient is made to sit in the dark room for 60–90 min. If >8 mm Hg rise in IOP occurs then the test is positive.
3. *Prone test:* Patient is made to lie prone for 60–90 minutes. If >8 mm Hg rise in IOP occurs then the test is positive.
4. *Dark room prone test:* In this test the patient is made to lie flat in a dark room, any rise of pressure >8 mm Hg indicates that the patient will develop angle closure glaucoma.
5. *Phenylephrine-Pilocarpine test:* 10% phenylephrine and 2% pilocarpine – causes middilated pupil and maximum pupillary block. Any rise of IOP of more than 8 mm Hg is suggestive of glaucoma.

For POAG

1. *Water drinking test:* The patient is asked to come empty stomach and an IOP reading is taken and then the patient is made to drink 1 litre of water. IOP readings are taken every 15 minutes for one hour. Any difference between the initial and the final reading of > 8 mm Hg, indicates a positive test.
2. *Venous congestion test:* The patient lies on his back, jugular veins in the neck are compressed by the cuff of sphygomomanometer, inflated to pressure of 50 mm Hg for 1min. Increase in IOP by 9–10 mm Hg after the test indicates positive test.

B. Measurement of IOP

It is known as tonometry. Tonometry is of two types:

(a) *Indentation tonometry:* Schiotz tonometre.

(b) *Applanation tonometry:* Goldmann, Perkins, Draeger, Mackay–Marg, Pulsair, Tonopen and Maklakow.

- The non contact type of applanation tonometres are Pulsair and Air puff tonometre.
- *Tonography:* It is used to measure the **facility of aqueous outflow**. In this procedure, continuous recording of intraocular pressure is done for 4 minutes by electronic schiotz tonometre. This method is more for research purpose and not done commonly in clinical practice. Normal value is: 0.22 to 0.28 µl/min/mm Hg.
- **Applanation tonometry is more reliable than indentation tonometry as its readings are not affected by the scleral rigidity.**

Ocular or Scleral Rigidity:

It is the expression of stretchability of eye in response to increase in IOP. Small increase in intraocular volume at a low pressure causes small increase in IOP whereas at high pressure will lead to much large increase in IOP.

Co-efficient of scleral rigidity is donated by **"E"** value which normally is–0.0215. It is calculated by **"Friedenwald Nomogram"**.

Factors Affecting Ocular Rigidity:

1. *Refractive errors:* Scleral rigidity is higher in hypermetropia whereas lower in myopia.
2. *Elevated IOP:* Scleral rigidity decreases if IOP increases.
3. *Drugs:* Miotics reduce scleral rigidity.
4. *Surgery:* Scleral rigidity is reduced following RD surgery.

High ocular rigidity will cause a falsely high IOP and a low ocular rigidity will lead to falsely low IOP.

C. Gonioscopy

Bimicroscopic examination of A-C angle is known as Gonioscopy.

It is of two types:

1. *Indirect:* In this procedure the angle is examined by reflected light, e.g., Goldmann, Zeis.
2. *Direct:* The angle is examined by direct light, e.g., Keoppe lens, direct surgical goniolenses like Barkan, Medical Workshop, Thorpe and Swan-Jacob goniolenses etc.

The following are three main purposes of gonioscopy:

1. Identification of abnormal angle structures.
2. Estimation of width of the chamber angle.
3. Visualization of the angle during procedures such as Argon laser trabeculoplasty and goniotomy.

Indentation gonioscopy helps to differentiate appositional closure and synechial closure.

Indentification of Angle Structures on Gonioscopy

(From Anterior to Posterior)

Schwalbe's line→Corneal Wedge→ Trabeculum→Schlemm's canal→Scleral spur→Ciliary body→Angle Recess→Iris processes.

D. Visual Field Testing (Perimetry)

It is broadly divided into two main types:

1. *Kinetic perimetry:* Peripheral field is measured by Lister's perimeter and central field is measured by Bjerrum's screen or Tangent screen.
2. *Static perimetry:* It is also known as Automated perimetry. It is done by Octopus or Humphery field analyzer.

Goldmann Perimeter: Both static and kinetic perimetry is possible with this perimeter.

Campimetry: Central visual field evaluation (Central 30°) is known as campimetry.

E. Evaluation of Optic Nerve Head (ONH)

It can be done by:

1. **Direct Ophthalmoscopy.**
2. **Slit-Lamp Fundoscopy:** It is a more preferred method as the examiner can have a binocular view in contrast to direct ophthalmoscopy where the examiner is using only one eye.
3. **Monophotography and Stereophotography of ONH.**
4. **Confocal scanning laser topography and nerve fibre layer analyser.**

F. Slit Lamp Fundoscopy

It is possible by two types of lenses:

1. *Contact lenses:* Goldmann, Rodenstock.
2. *Non-contact:* It is further divided into
   (a) Concave lenses: Hruby lens (-58.6D)
   (b) Convex lenses: +60D, +78D or +90D.

Investigations in Children

Following procedures are done under GA:

1. Tonometry.
2. Corneal diameter measurement.
3. Gonioscopy (Koeppe).
4. Ophthalmoscopy.
5. Axial length measurement.

Treatment of Glaucoma

Three modalities of treatment are:

1. Medical therapy.
2. Laser therapy.
3. Surgical treatment.

Antiglaucoma Drugs

Topical:

A. Beta Blockers:

Timolol, Levobunolol, Betaxolol (Beta1 selective), Carteolol, Metipranolol.

Mechanism of action: It decreases the formation of aqueous humour.

Side Effects:

1. Bronchospasm due to non-selective blockers.
2. Bradycardia and hypotension, more common in elderly patients, due to beta-1 blockade.
3. Corneal punctate epithelial erosions.
4. Occasional allergies.
5. Delayed recovery from hypoglycemia specially in patients of IDDM.
6. Timolol causes nasolacrimal duct.

B. Adrenergic Agonists:

1. *Non-Selective:* Epinephrine, Dipivefrine.
2. *Alpha-2 Selective:* Brimonidine, Apraclonidine.

Mechanism of Action: It has dual action:

(a) It decreases the formation of aqueous humour.

(b) It increases the drainage of aqueous humour.

Brimonidine has a dual action, it is an alpha agonist and also a **neuroprotective drug.**

Side Effects:

1. Blepharoconjunctivitis.
2. Stinging sensation.

3. Rebound conjunctival injection.
4. *Naso-lacrimal duct obstruction* may rarely occur with long term use.
5. *Pigmented conjunctival adrenochrome* deposits are common in long-term use; although they are innocuous.
6. *Mydriasis:* It is usually innocuous but may precipitate angle–closure glaucoma.
7. *Cystoid macular edema:* It may be precipitated or aggravated in *aphakic eyes*, particularly when 2% adrenaline is used hence it is contraindicated in aphakic glaucoma.

C. Miotics:

Pilocarpine:

Mechanism of action:

a. In angle closure glaucoma, it causes constriction of pupil and hence opens the angle.
b. It increases the conventional/trabecular meshwork.

Side Effects:

1. *Miosis:*
   A. Problem in presence of axial lens opacities.
   B. Generalised constriction of visual field and apparent increase in size of visual field defects.
2. *Spasm of accommodation:* It causes myopic shift and frontal headache, hence it is not indicated in young patients. **Pilocarpine should be avoided in patients with myopia.**
3. *Retinal detachment:* It is a rare complication.
4. *Increased capillary permeability leading to disruption of the blood aqueous barrier:* **Hence, it is contraindicated in patients of uveitis as it will aggravate inflammation and due to constriction of pupil there is more chances of developing posterior synechiae.**
5. Shallow anterior chamber.
6. Iritis/Iris cyst.
7. Cataract.
8. Rarely punctal stenosis.

D. Prostaglandin Analogues ($PG\ F_2$ alpha agonist):

Latanoprost, Isopropyl Unoprostone, Bimatoprost, Travoprost.

Mechanism of action:

It acts by increasing the uveoscleral outflow.

Dose of latanoprost is 0.005% once a day.

Side Effects:

A. *Ocular:*
   - Conjunctival hyperaemia, burning, stinging, tearing and pain.
   - Increased pigmentation.

B. *Systemic:* Headache, back, muscle and joint pain.

E. Topical Carbonic-Anhydrase Inhibitor:

Dorzalamide, Brinzolamide.

Mechanism of action: It decreases the formation of aqueous humour.

It is contraindicated in sulfa allergy.

Systemic:

A. *Carbonic Anhydrase Inhibitors:* Acetazolamide, Dichlorphenamide, Methazolamide.

B. *Hyperosmotic Agents:* Mannitol, Glycerol, Isosorbide.

Note:

- Both pilocarpine and latanoprost should never be used in patients of uveitis.
- In hypertensive uveitis, most useful drug is dipivefrine as hypertensive uveitis is primarily a uveitic condition leading to open angle glaucoma, hence as dipivefrine will dilate the pupil as well as decrease the IOP it is a preferred option.

NEWER ANTIGLAUCOMA AGENTS

Brimonidine, Prostaglandin analogues and topical CA inhibitor, i.e., Dorzalamide are the newer antiglaucoma drugs. Other drugs which are under study are:

a. *Calcium Channel Blockers (CCB):* It is specially useful in normal tension glaucoma, as it has neuroprotective effect (by increasing the optic nerve blood flow).

b. Gene therapy.

c. Neuroprotective drugs.

Laser Therapy

1. *Argon Laser Trabeculoplasty:* It is a modality of treatment of OAG, when the patient does not respond, to medicines. Laser burns are given at the junction of pigmented and non-pigmented parts of trabecular meshwork.
2. *Nd-YAG Laser Iridotomy:* It is done for treating ACG.
3. *Nd-YAG* in free thermal mode is used for **cyclophotocoagulation in absolute glaucoma, to destroy the ciliary processes.** This cyclotherapy can also be done by cryo.

Surgical Treatment

1. **Goniotomy:** It is the choice of treatment of congenital glaucoma.

   Procedure: In this procedure circumferential incision is made in the trabecular meshwork. It can only be done if the cornea is clear.

2. **Trabeculotomy:** It denotes the cutting opening of Schlemm's canal. It is generally done in combination with trabeculectomy.

   Procedure: In this procedure the trabeculotome is inserted in the Schlemm's canal and rotated into the anterior chamber.

3. **Trabeculectomy:** It is the choice of treatment of acquired glaucoma, if the patient does not respond to other conservative modes of treatment.

   Procedure: In this procedure, fistula is formed between the anterior chamber and subtenon's space allowing free flow of the aqueous humour. The fistula is protected by superficial scleral flap.

Anti-Metabolites in Trabeculec-tomy: They are used in cases in which, there is high risk of fibrosis leading to closure of the fistula. These are:

a. 5-Fluorouracil (5-FU).

b. Mitomycin C (MMC).

Artificial Filtering Shunts: They are used in cases where conventional filtering procedure has failed or likely to fail. These are plastic devices which create a communication between the anterior chamber and subtenon's space.

Few commonly used shunts are:

a. Krupin-Denver valve.

b. Molteno implant.

c. Schoket implant.

d. *American Glaucoma Valve (AGV)/ Ahmed Glaucoma Valve:* This is the latest implant and is valved. It prevents hypotony due to excessive filtering as the valve closes when pressure reaches 10 mm Hg.

NEET DRILL

1. Rate of formation of aqueous humour is 2–2.5 microlitres/minute: Amounting to around 2.3 mircrolitres/min.
2. Number of ciliary processes is: 70–75.
3. Each ciliary process is 2 mm long and 0.5 mm in thickness.
4. Total volume of aqueous is: 0.31 ml:0.25 ml in anterior chamber and 0.06 ml in posterior chamber.
5. Refractive index of aqueous is: 1.33.
6. pH of the aqueous is: 7.2.
7. Aqueous is hyperosmotic to plasma by 3–5 mosmol/liter.
8. Normal IOP is: 10–21 mm Hg with mean of 16 +/- 2.5 mm Hg.
9. Maximum amount of the aqueous is formed by secretion.
10. 99.9% of aqueous is water.
11. 90% of the aqueous outflow is conventional outflow.
12. The most common type of glaucoma is primary open angle glaucoma.
13. It is the most common cause of irreversible blindness in the world.
14. There are 20 genetic loci for occurrence of POAG including myocillin and optineurin on chromosome no. 10.
15. Tonography measures the facility of aqueous outflow. The normal value is 0.22–0.28 microlitres/min/mm Hg.
16. Coefficient of scleral rigidity is denoted by E which normally is 0.0215.
17. Angle of anterior chamber:
    a. 0°: Closed (no angle structures are visible).
    b. 10°: Very narrow (only Schwalbe's line).
    c. 20°: Moderately narrow (Schwalbe's line and trabecular meshwork).
    d. 20–35°: Open angle (Schwalbe's line, trabecular meshwork and sclera spur).
    e. 35–45°: Wide open (Schwalbe's line, trabecular meshwork, scleral spur and ciliary body band).
18. Steroid induced glaucoma is open angle glaucoma.
19. Trabecular meshwork is derived from neural crest.
20. Antiglaucoma causing iris pigmentation is latanoprost.
21. Antiglaucoma causing conjunctival pigmentation is adrenaline.
22. Antiglaucoma contraindicated in infants is Brimonidine.
23. Tonometre more reliable than Goldmann is Pascals Dyanamic Contour Tonometre.
24. Tonometre used for self measurement is Rebound Tonometre.
25. Diaton Tonometre is used over closed lids.
26. Antiglaucoma which causes hypertrichosis: Prostaglandins analogues.
27. Antiglaucoma which causes lid retraction: Apraclonidine.

MULTIPLE CHOICE QUESTIONS

1. Which of the following antiglaucoma medications can cause drowsiness?

A. Latanoprost
B. Timolol
C. Brimonidine
D. Dorzalamide

2. Latanoprost used topically in glaucoma primarily acts by:

A. Decreasing aqueous humour formation
B. Increasing uveoscleral outflow
C. Releasing pupillary block
D. Increasing trabecular outflow

3. Which of the following drugs is not used topically for the treatment of open angle glaucoma?

A. Latanoprost B. Brimonidine
C. Acetazolamide D. Dorzolamide

4. Tonography helps you to determine:

A. The facility of outflow of aqueous
B. Diurnal variation
C. The levels of intraocular pressure at different times
D. None of the above

5. Kusumlata presents with acute painful red eye and mild dilated vertically oval pupil. Most likely diagnosis is:

A. Acute retrobulbar neuritis
B. Acute angle closure glaucoma
C. Acute anterior uveitis
D. Severe keratoconjunctivitis

6. You have been referred a middle-aged patient to rule out open angle glaucoma. Which of the following findings will help in the diagnosis?

A. Cupping of the disc
B. Depth of anterior chamber
C. Visual acuity and refractive error
D. Angle of the anterior chamber

7. In a case of hypertensive uveitis, most useful drug to reduce intra-ocular pressure is:

A. Pilocarpine B. Latanoprost
C. Physostigmine D. Dipivefrine

8. A patient having glaucoma develops blepharoconjunctivitis after instilling some antiglaucoma drug. Which of the following drug can be responsible for it?

A. Timolol B. Latanoprost
C. Dipivefrine D. Pilocarpine

9. Treatment of choice in acute congestive glaucoma:

A. Pilocarpine B. Laser iridotomy
C. Timolol D. Trabeculoplasty

10. Secondary glaucoma is seen in all except:

A. Intraocular lens implantation
B. Epidemic dropsy
C. CRVO
D. Interstitial keratitis

11. Most common complication of topical steroid is:

A. Glaucoma B. Cataract
C. Ptosis D. Iritis

12. Iridocorneal endothelial syndrome is associated with:

A. Progressive atrophy of iris stroma
B. Bilateral symmetrical stromal edema of iris and cornea
C. Deposition of collagen in descements membrane
D. Deposition of glycosaminoglycans in the descements membrane

13. Painless sudden visual loss is seen in all except:

A. CRAO
B. Retinal detachment
C. Vitreous haemorrhage
D. Angle closure glaucoma

14. The conversion of CO_2 and H_2O into carbonic acid during the formation of aqueous humour is catalysed by which one of the following enzymes?

A. Carboxylase
B. Carbamylase
C. Carbonic anhydrase
D. Carbonic deoxygenase

15. Which of the following drugs is contraindicated in a patient with history of sulpha allergy presenting with an acute attack of angle closure glaucoma?

A. Glycerol B. Acetazolamide

C. Mannitol D. Latanoprost

16. A 55 years old female comes to the eye casualty with history of severe eye pain, redness and diminution of vision. On examination the visual acuity is 6/60, there is circumcorneal congestion, corneal oedema and a shallow anterior chamber. Which of the following is the best drug of choice?

A. Atropine ointment

B. I.V. mannitol

C. Ciprofloxacin eye drops

D. Betamethasone eye drops

17. In which of the following condition, aniridia and hemihypertrophy are most likely present?

A. Neuroblastoma

B. Wilms' tumour

C. Non-Hodgkin's lymphoma

D. Germ cell tumour

18. All of the following conditions are contraindicated or likely to worsen in a case of primary open angle glaucoma when treated with timolol maleate 0.5% eye drops, except:

A. Hypertension

B. Hypercholesterolemia

C. Depression

D. Bronchial asthma

19. A male patient with a history of hypermature cataract presents with a 2-day history of ciliary congestion, photophobia, blurring of vision and on examination has a deep anterior chamber in the right eye. The left eye is normal. The diagnosis is:

A. Phacomorphic glaucoma

B. Phacolytic glaucoma

C. Phacotoxic glaucoma

D. Phacoanaphylactic uveitis

20. A 30-day-old neonate was presented with a history of photophobia and excessive lacrimation. On examination, both the lacrimal duct systems are normal, but there was a large cornea and corneal haziness. The diagnosis is:

A. Megalocornea

B. Keratoconus

C. Congenital glaucoma

D. Hunter's syndrome

21. All the following anatomical changes will predispose to primary angle closure glaucoma, except:

A. Small cornea

B. Flat cornea

C. Anterior chamber shallow

D. Short axial length of eyeball

22. A patient complains of evening halos and occasional headache for some months. On examination anterior chamber of both the eyes are shallow and the intraocular pressure is normal. This condition represents what stage of glaucoma?

A. Constant instability

B. Prodrome

C. Absolute

D. Acute

23. In a patient predisposed to glaucoma, the drug contraindicated is:

A. Pilocarpine B. Atropine

C. Echothiophate D. Timolol

24. A lady with chronic simple glaucoma with bronchial asthma took anti-glaucoma drug which exaggerated her asthma. The likely drug is:

A. Timolol B. Brimonidine

C. Pilocarpine D. Latanoprost

25. All are side effects of pilocarpine, except:

A. Shallow anterior chamber

B. Folliculosis

C. Posterior synechiae

D. Punctal stenosis

26. Epinephrine is used in all, except:

A. Aphakic glaucoma

B. Open angle glaucoma

C. Secondary glaucoma

D. Neovascular glaucoma

27. Earliest field defect in primary open angle glaucoma is:

A. Seidel's scotoma

B. Arcuate scotoma

C. Nasal spur

D. Scotoma in Bjerrum field

28. Which examination is of least value in open angle glaucoma?

A. Tonometry

B. Perimetry

C. Indirect ophthalmoscopy

D. Direct ophthalmoscopy

29. Pilocarpine is not used in young adults as it causes:

A. Retinal detachment

B. Myopia

C. Iris cysts

D. Shallow anterior chamber

30. True about acute angle closure glaucoma:

A. Pupil vertically oval

B. Increased IOP

C. AC deep

D. AC shallow

E. Painful eye

31. True about buphthalmos:

A. Large cornea

B. Haab's stria

C. Shallow AC

D. Glaucoma

E. Medical treatment helps

32. Buphthalmos is associated with:

A. Epiphora

B. Shallow anterior chamber

C. Megalocornea

D. Surgery is used for treatment

E. KF ring is pathognomic

33. Which of the following causes least increase in IOP?

A. Fluorometholone

B. Triamcinolone

C. Dexamethasone

D. Hydrocortisone

34. In angle closure glaucoma, treatment given to the fellow eye is:

A. Pilocarpine eye drops

B. Atropine

C. LASER iridotomy

D. Trabeculoplasty

E. Physostigmine eye drops

35. Regarding aqueous humor, which of these are correct?

A. It is secreted at rate of 2.3 ml/min

B. Secreted by ciliary processes

C. Provides nutrition

D. Normal pressure is 5–15 mm Hg

36. Haab's striae are seen in:
A. Angle closure glaucoma
B. Infantile glaucoma
C. Stargardt's disease
D. Disciform keratitis

37. Malignant glaucoma is seen in:
A. Malignancy
B. After surgery for cataract or glaucoma
C. Trauma
D. Thrombosis

38. A 30 years old woman with sudden right-sided painful red eye associated with nausea, vomiting and headache. The diagnosis is:
A. Acute congestive glaucoma
B. Endophthalmitis
C. Eales' disease
D. Trachoma

39. Which should not be used in raised IOT associated with uveitis?
A. Timolol B. Pilocarpine
C. Atropine D. Acetazolamide

40. Coloured halos is seen in all except:
A. Open angle glaucoma
B. Closed angle glaucoma
C. Cataract
D. Any of the above

41. In buphthalmos, seen are all except:
A. Subluxated lens
B. Large cornea
C. Small cornea
D. Big eyeball

42. In buphthalmos, lens is:
A. Anteroposteriorly flat
B. Small
C. Large
D. None of the above

43. Treatment of malignant glaucoma is:
A. Topical atropine
B. Topical pilocarpine
C. IV mannitol
D. Vitreous aspiration

44. Treatment of primary open angle glaucoma:
A. Timolol maleate
B. Atropine
C. Acetazolamide
D. Prostaglandin analogue

45. The canal of Schlemm possesses the following anatomic characteristics:
A. Contains red cells
B. Contains aqueous
C. Lined by endothelium
D. Contains partitions resembling the dural venous sinuses

46. In a patient of bronchial asthma with open angle glaucoma, drug of choice is:
A. Pilocarpine drops
B. Timolol drops
C. Ipratropium bromide drops
D. Betaxolol drops

47. Normal intraocular tension is:
A. 0–10 mm Hg
B. 10–20 mm Hg
C. 20–30 mm H_2O
D. 100–120 cm H_2O

48. Applanation tonometry is more useful than indentation tonometry:
A. In cases where corneal ulcer is present
B. It eliminates the factor of scleral rigidity
C. It accurately measures tension in uncooperative patient
D. None of the above

49. Increased intraocular tension is seen in all except:

A. Epidemic dropsy
B. Branch vein occlusion
C. Malignant melanoma
D. Pthisis bulbi

50. Drug useful in open angle glaucoma with uncorrected myopia is:

A. 2% Pilocarpine
B. 0.5% Timolol
C. 10% Phenylephrine
D. None of the above

51. Pathognomic of open angle glaucoma is:

A. Pulsation of retinal arterioles
B. Arcuate scotoma
C. Enlargement of blind spot
D. Spiral field defect

52. Coloured halos in acute congestive glaucoma is due to:

A. Raised IOP B. Corneal edema
C. Raised ICT D. Mydriasis

53. Not given in glaucoma:

A. Beta blocker B. Cyclopentolate
C. Ecothiophate D. Urea

54. Glaucoma causes:

A. Secondary optic atrophy
B. Cavernous optic atrophy
C. Pressure optic atrophy
D. No optic atrophy

55. Campimetry measures:

A. Field of vision
B. Acuity of vision
C. Colour vision
D. Includes all

56. All are changes in chronic glaucoma except:

A. Cupping of disc
B. Cavernous optic atrophy
C. Scotomas of various types
D. Synechiae

57. Aqueous as compared to plasma has all more, except:

A. Higher glutathione
B. Higher pH
C. Higher ascorbate
D. Higher lactate

58. Following are important in production and release of aqueous except:

A. Pigmented epithelium
B. Ultrafiltration and diffusion
C. Adenylcyclase
D. Carbonic anhydrase

59. Acute congestive glaucoma all are present except:

A. Ciliary congestion
B. Shallow anterior chamber
C. Edematous cornea
D. Miosis

60. Phacomorphic glaucoma is an example of:

A. Primary open angle glaucoma
B. Secondary open angle glaucoma
C. Primary angle closure glaucoma
D. Secondary angle closure glaucoma

61. Shallow anterior chamber is seen in all except:

A. Old age
B. Steroid-induced glaucoma
C. Hypermetropia
D. Angle closure glaucoma

62. Ratio of incidence of open angle to closed angle glaucoma is:

A. 1 : 1 B. 2 : 1
C. 3 : 1 D. 4 : 1

63. Gonioscopy is used to study:
A. Anterior chamber
B. Posterior chamber
C. Angle of anterior chamber
D. Retina

64. Secondary glaucoma following corneal perforation is due to:
A. Anterior synechiae formation
B. Peripheral synechiae
C. Intraocular haemorrhage
D. Angle disruption

65. 100-day glaucoma is seen in:
A. Central retinal artery occlusion
B. Central retinal vein occlusion
C. Neovascular glaucoma
D. Steroid induced glaucoma

66. The most reliable provocative test for angle closure glaucoma:
A. Homatropine-mydriatic test
B. Mydriatic-Miotic test
C. Water drinking test
D. Dark room test

67. The technique of goniotomy includes all except:
A. Anterior chamber air injection
B. Use of contact lens
C. Dilatation of the pupil
D. Diamox preoperatively
E. Insertion of knife posterior to the descements membrane

68. Argon laser trabeculoplasty is used in:
A. Closed angle glaucoma
B. Primary open glaucoma
C. Neovascular glaucoma
D. Aphakic glaucoma

69. Pain in the eye, while sitting in cinema is due to:
A. Prodromal angle closure glaucoma
B. Intermittent angle closure glaucoma
C. Acute congestive angle closure glaucoma
D. Chronic angle closure glaucoma

70. The following antiglaucoma drug decreases the uveoscleral outflow:
A. Latanoprost B. Timolol
C. Pilocarpine D. Acetazolamide

71. Photophobia in an infant could be due to:
A. Buphthalmos
B. Congenital cataract
C. NLD obstruction
D. None of the above

72. Following trabeculectomy, all these changes occur except:
A. Haemorrhage
B. Malignant glaucoma
C. Shallow anterior chamber
D. Choroidal degeneration

73. Schwalbe's line corresponds to:
A. Corneal endothelium
B. Descements membrane
C. Schlemm's canal
D. Ciliary body

74. Normally the cup disc ratio is:
A. Below 0.5 B. Below 1.0
C. Below 1.5 D. Below 0.1

75. A patient came to the casuality with acute bronchial asthma after treatment for glaucoma. The probable drug may be:

A. Timolol B. Betaxolol
C. Latoprost D. Anticholinesterase

76. Secondary glaucoma following corneal perforation is due to:

A. Anterior synechiae formation
B. Peripheral synechiae
C. Intraocular haemorrhage
D. Angle disruption

77. Shallow anterior chamber is seen in all except:

A. Old age
B. Steroid induced cataract
C. Hypermetropia
D. Angle closure glaucoma

78. Laser iridotomy is done in:

A. Open angle glaucoma
B. Posterior capsular opacification
C. Angle closure glaucoma
D. Acute iridocyclitis

79. Field defects in open angle glaucoma is best charted with:

A. Listers perimeter
B. Goldmann perimeter
C. Humphrey perimeter
D. Bjerrum screen

80. Laser iridotomy is done by:

A. Argon laser B. Nd:YAG
C. Xenon D. None

81. Angle of anterior chamber is visualized by:

A. Slit lamp examination
B. Ophthalmoscope
C. A scan
D. CT scan

82. A 40 years old lady presented with a history of seeing coloured halos in the evening. On examination her intraocular pressure was normal. The diagnosis is:

A. Prodromal stage of acute congestive glaucoma
B. Acute attack of acute congestive glaucoma
C. Incipient stage of chronic congestive glaucoma
D. Incipient cataract

83. Acquired nasolacrimal duct obstruction is a side effect of therapy of which of the following medications?

A. Timolol B. Brimonidine
C. Dorzolamide D. Pilocarpine

84. Which of the following is a variable range tonometer?

A. Mackay-Marg tonometer
B. Draeger's tonometer
C. Barraquer tonometer
D. Rebound tonometer

85. Which of the following can be used for self tonometry?

A. Dynamic contour tonometer
B. Draeger tonometer
C. Rebound tonometer
D. Perkin's tonometer

86. Which diagnostic procedure is not done in a dilated pupil?

A. Gonioscopy
B. Laser inferometry
C. Fundus examination
D. Electroretinography

87. Laser trabeculoplasty is done for:

A. Chronic angle closure glaucoma
B. Neovascular glaucoma
C. Pseudoexfoliative glaucoma
D. Uveitic glaucoma

88. **A middle aged female presents with history of coloured halos and severe ocular pain that aggravates in dark room and lying in prone position. The examining physician should avoid which of the following drugs in her?**
A. Pilocarpine B. Acetazolamide
C. Homatropine D. Timolol maleate

89. **Cells affected in glaucomatous optic neuropathy are:**
A. Amacrine cells B. Bipolar cells
C. Ganglion cells D. Rods and cones

90. **Which of the following pairs of drugs is correctly matched with its mechanism of action?**
A. Pilocarpine – increased uveoscleral outflow
B. Latanoprost – carbonic anhydrase inhibitor
C. Brimonidine – decreased aqueous formation
D. Betaxolol – increased trabecular outflow

91. **Which of the following drugs acts on trabecular meshwork and affects the aqueous outflow?**
A. Timolol B. Pilocarpine
C. Brimonidine D. Brinzolamide

92. **Express glaucoma implant is made up of:**
A. Silicone B. Titanium
C. Gold D. Stainless steel

93. **In acute angle closure glaucoma all are seen except:**
A. Cupping of disc
B. Bayonetting sign
C. Snow banking
D. Oval cup

94. **Which of the following can be used for self tonometry?**
A. Dynamic contour tonometer
B. Diaton tonometer
C. Rebound tonometer
D. Perkin's tonometer

95. **Which diagnostic procedure is not done in a dilated pupil?**
A. Gonioscopy
B. Laser inferometry
C. Fundus examination
D. Electroretinography

96. **A young male presents with painless diminution of vision with an intraocular pressure of 60 mm Hg. Which of the following is the most likely diagnosis?**
A. Acute angle closure glaucoma
B. Acute anterior uveitis
C. Chronic papilledema
D. Glaucomatocyclitic crisis

97. **Laser trabeculoplasty is done for:**
A. Chronic angle closure glaucoma
B. Neovascular glaucoma
C. Pseudoexfoliative glaucoma
D. Uveitic glaucoma

98. **Which of the following topical agents cause heterochromia iridis?**
A. Latanoprost B. Prednisolone
C. Timolol D. Olopatadine

99. **Which of the following drugs acting on dilator pupillae has an action analogous to that of pilocarpine on sphincter pupillae?**
A. Timolol B. Phenylephrine
C. Neostigmine D. Tropicamide

100. Variable range tonometre is:

A. Draeger

B. Mac Kay Marg

C. Barraquer

D. Rebound

101. Well-known weight of the rabbit for ophthalmic drug testing is:

A. 0.5 kg to 1.0 kg

B. 1.5 kg to 3.0 kg

C. 3.5 kg to 4.5 kg

D. 5.0 kg to 6.0 kg

ANSWER AND EXPLANATION

1.	c	Brimonidine causes drowsiness and is also a neuroprotective drug.
2.	b	Prostaglandin analogues increase the uveoscleral outflow whereas pilocarpine decreases it.
3.	c	Acetazolamide is a systemic CA inhibitor, not topical.
4.	a	Tonography measures the "facility of aqueous outflow". It is done by electronic schiotz.
5.	b	Red eye with vertically oval dilated pupil–diagnosis is angle closure glaucoma.
6.	a	Increased C:D ratio, i.e., cupping is a pathognomic feature of glaucoma.
7.	d	Hypertensive uveitis means that uveitis which leads to increase in the IOP. Pilocarpine and Prostaglandin analogues are contraindicated in uveitis. Dipivefrine being an alpha agonist also dilates the pupil and helps in treatment of uveitis.
8.	c	Alpha agonists are known to cause blepharoconjunctivitis.
9.	a	In acute congestive stage we cannot do laser treatment; hence the choice of treatment is pilocarpine.
10.	d	Glaucoma is more common in AC-IOL implantation. In CRVO we get neovascular glaucoma called 100-day glaucoma. In epidemic dropsy we get hypersecretory glaucoma.
11.	a	Most common complication of topical steroids is glaucoma.
12.	a	ICE syndrome is a group of disorder where the endothelium cells become proliferative. It is one of the causes of secondary glaucoma. The disease has three forms–Progressive iris atrophy, Cogan-Reese syndrome and Chandler's syndrome.
13.	d	Angle closure glaucoma is a painful condition not painless.
14.	c	Carbonic anhydrase enzyme is responsible for formation of the aqueous humour.
15.	b	Acetazolamide is a sulphonamide and is contraindicated in patients with sulpha allergy.
16.	b	The history suggests that the patient is suffering from angle closure glaucoma.
17.	b	Wilms' tumour or Nephroblastoma is associated with Aniridia.
18.	a	All are complications of beta–blockers except hypertension. Hypertension is a complication of alpha agonists.
19.	b	Hypermature cataract complicates to phacolytic glaucoma.
20.	c	A neonate presenting with watering and photophobia with hazy cornea, the most probable diagnosis is congenital glaucoma.

21.	b	Flat cornea is not a risk factor of angle closure glaucoma.
22.	a	Patient is asymptomatic in prodromal stage of angle closure glaucoma.
23.	b	Dilatation of pupil can close the angle.
24.	a	Beta blockers aggravate asthma.
25.	d	Among all punctal stenosis is the least common complication of pilocarpine. Punctal stenosis occurs most commonly due to physostigmine, i.e., Eserine.
26.	a	An important side effect of Epinephrine is cystoid macular edema; hence it should be avoided in aphakics.
27.	d	The first damage in glaucoma occurs in Arcuate fibres. The area corresponding to these fibres is called Bjerrums area; hence the first field defect is central and paracentral scotoma in the Bjerrums area.
28.	c	Magnification of indirect ophthalmoscope is only 5 times, hence the details of the disc is not visible nicely.
29.	b	Pilocarpine causes miosis which leads to accommodation spasm hence the myopic shift.
30.	a,b, d,e	Angle closure is mostly associated with shallow AC.
31.	a,b, d	Buphthalmos is enlargement of the eyeball and hence is associated with enlarged cornea. Treatment of buphthalmos is Goniotomy.
32.	d	In buphthalmos, there is lacrimation (increased production of the tear) whereas Epiphora occurs in the cases where lacrimal drainage system is blocked. Large cornea in buphthalmos is a differential diagnosis of Megalocornea.
33.	a	Fluoromethalones affect the IOP least.
34.	c	Laser iridotomy should always be done prophylactically in the other eye also.
35.	b,d	Rate of formation of aqueous humour is 2.3 μl/min. Normal pressure is 10–21 mm Hg.
36.	b	Break in the descement's membrane due to overstretching of the cornea in patients of buphthalmos is called Haab's striae.
37.	b	Malignant glaucoma, also called Ciliary-block glaucoma occurs after any intraocular surgery. In this condition aqueous starts collecting in the vitreous cavity.
38.	a	A middle-aged female with history of painful red eye, associated with nausea and vomiting – most probable diagnosis is angle closure glaucoma.
39.	b	Pilocarpine aggravates inflammation and is not given in patients suffering from uveitis.
40.	a	Open angle glaucoma is an insidious condition and hence acute rise of pressure is not seen therefore no corneal edema (which is a cause of coloured halos in angle closure glaucoma).
41.	c	In buphthalmos, stretching of the cornea leads to large cornea.
42.	a	Enlargement of the eyeball leads to stretching of the lens, hence it becomes flat. In the later stage, stretching can break the zonules leading to subluxation of the lens.
43.	a,c, d	Malignant glaucoma is treated by a mydriatic, i.e., Atropine, hence, it is also known as INVERSE glaucoma.

44. a,c,d Atropine is not an antiglaucoma drug, and has no affect on formation or drainage of the aqueous humour.

45. b,c,d It is an endothelium lined oval channel present circumferentially in the sclera sulcus. Endothelium of the inner wall are irregular and contains giant vacuoles whereas in the outer wall the endothelial cells are smooth and contain the openings of the collector channels.

46. d Betaxolol is a selective α-blocker, and can be used in asthmatic patients.

47. b Normal IOP is 10–21 mm Hg.

48. b Scleral rigidity can affect the IOP readings if measured by indentation, i.e., schiotz tonometre, whereas it has no affect in applanation readings.

49. d Pthisis bulbi is shrinkage of eyeball and will lead to decreased IOP.

50. b Pilocarpine causes myopic shift due to increased accommodation.

51. b OAG presents as arcuate scotoma. Enlargement of blind spot is a feature of papilloedema.

52. b Coloured halos are due to corneal edema which is an epithelial edema occurring due to ACUTE rise of IOP.

53. b Cyclopentolate is not an anti-glaucoma drug. It is a mydriatic with cycloplegic.

54. b In cavernous optic atrophy, along-with the damage of the nerve fibres, the glial tissue also degenerates (due to lack of blood supply) leading to formation of large caverns or lacunae.

55. a Central field charting is known as Campimetry.

56. d Synechiae are adhesions and are feature of uveitis.

57. b pH of aqueous humour: 7.2. It is acidic compared to plasma.

58. a Aqueous is formed from the non-pigmented epithelium of the ciliary processes.

59. d Pupil is vertically oval middilated in acute angle closure glaucoma.

60. d Phacomorphic glaucoma causes pupillary block leading to angle closure glaucoma.

61. b Steroid induced glaucoma is open angle glaucoma. AC depth is normal.

62. d 90% of glaucomas are open angle glaucomas. Hence the actual ratio will be 9:1.

63. c Gonioscopy is a bimicroscopic examination of the angle of the anterior chamber.

64. a Corneal perforation is sealed by the iris, leading to anterior synechiae, which can cause angle closure.

65. b NVG in central retinal vein occlusion is called 100-day glaucoma.

66. b Combination of miotic and mydriatic mid-dilates the pupil, and angle closure is maximum in a mid-dilated pupil. Hence it is most reliable.

67. c Goniotomy is done in a constricted pupil.

68. b Laser trabeculoplasty is opted in open angle glaucoma, if the patient does not respond with the medical therapy.

69. b It indicates the stage of constant instability.

70. c Pilocarpine decreases the uveoscleral outflow whereas prostaglandin analogues increase the flow.

71. a Congenital cataract and NLD obstruction never presents as photophobia.

72. d Choroidal detachment can be a complication of trabeculectomy due to hypotony, but not choroidal degenerations.

73. b Schwalbe's line is the anterior most structure seen in gonioscopy.

74. a Normal value of C:D is ≤ 0.3.

75. a Betaxolol is a selective beta blocker and can be given in asthmatics.

76. a Corneal perforation is sealed by the iris (leucoma adherens) and the anterior synechiae so formed can cause decreased aqueous drainage.

77. b Steroid induced glaucoma is open angle glaucoma.

78. c Laser iridotomy helps to treat a pupillary block.

79. c The choice of perimetry is automated perimetry.

80. b Argon is a photocoagulative laser used in the retina. Nd-YAG is a cutting laser.

81. a Patient is examined on the slit lamp through the gonioscope.

82. d Ideally it should be stage of constant instability, which is the second stage of angle closure glaucoma.

83. a Recent researches have shown that patients on long term topical timolol for treatment of glaucoma have a much higher incidence of NLD obstruction.

Pilocarpine may lead to punctal occlusion. Another drug known to cause punctal occlusion is physostigmine.

84. b All the above are applanation tonometers. Draegers is almost similar to Goldmann tonometer and is very reliable for a wide range of IOPs. Mac-Kay Marg and Rebound tonometers are less reliable for extremes of IOP.

Barraquer tonometers are used peroperatively in LASIK and Vitreretinal surgeries. Barraquer tonometer is based on the Maklaykov's principle of applanation tonometry where the force applied to the cornea is constant and the amount of the area applanated varies.

85. c The rebound technology is based on the rebound measuring principle, in which a very light-weight probe is used to make a momentary contact with the cornea. In the rebound technology, motion parameters of the probe are recorded during the measurement. Deceleration and the contact time of the probe change as a function of IOP. In simple terms, the higher the IOP, the faster the probe decelerates and the shorter the contact time.

86. a It's a bimicroscopic examination of the angle of anterior chamber, hence pupil should be constricted.

87. c Laser trabeculoplasty is done for open angle glaucoma in patients who are not responding to medical treatment.

88. c The history suggests that the patient is prone to angle closure glaucoma and hence mydriatics should be contraindicated.

89. c Optic nerve fibres are the axons of ganglion cells, and glaucoma is the damage of these nerve fibres.

90. c Pilocarpine increases the trabecular outflow.

Latanoprost increases the uveoscleral outflow.

Betaxolol decreases the aqueous formation.

Brimonidine has a dual action; it decreases formation and increases the uveoscleral outflow.

91. b Timolol and brinzolamide decrease the aqueous production, whereas brimonidine increases the uveoscleral outflow.

92. d The Ex-Press implant — This biocompatible device is almost 3 mm long with an external diameter of approximately 400 microns. It is a non valved, MRI compatible, stainless steel device with a 50 micron lumen. It has an external disc at one end and a spur like extension on the other to prevent extrusion. This implant is not put under the conjunctiva but it is implanted under the scleral flap. This has totally avoided the complication of extrusion and hypotony.

93. c Snow banking is the inflammatory exudate on pars plan and is pathognomic feature of pars planitis.

94. c
- The current gold standard for the measurement of intraocular pressure is the Goldmann applanation tonometer.
- Dynamic contour tonometer is also called Pascals tonometer. Its reading is independent of central corneal thickness and is considered more accurate than even Goldmann.

95. a Gonioscopy is a bimicroscopic examination of the angle of anterior chamber.

96. d **Glaucomatocyclitic Crisis:**
- Recurrent glaucomatocyclitic crisis, or Posner-Schlossman Syndrome (PSS), is a rare clinical entity associated with **acute uniocular elevation of intraocular pressure with minimal evidence of anterior segment inflammation.**
- It is reported to occur in 0.5% of all cases of uveitis.

Treatment includes management of increased pressure with antiglaucoma therapy, alongwith management of uveitis.

97. c **Laser trabeculoplasty** is typically performed with Argon or frequency-doubled neodymium: yttrium-aluminium-garnet (Nd:YAG) laser. It is indicated in open angle glaucoma.

The indications can be:
- Primary open angle glaucoma.
- Pigmentary glaucoma (secondary open angle glaucoma).
- **Pseudoexfoliation glaucoma (secondary open angle glaucoma).**

98. a Latanoprost causes iris pigmentation in the eye, hence leading to difference of iris colour.

99. b Phenylephrine will contract dilator pupillae which is arranged radially similarly to pilocarpine on sphincter pupillae which is circular.

100. a All are variable range except barraquer. But most reliable among the options is Draeger, so let's mark that.

101. b For ophthalmic drug testing the recommended weight is 1.5 to 3.0 kg.

RECENTLY ADDED QUESTIONS

1. A 2-year-old child is brought by the parents with complaints of enlarged eyes and photophobia. Examination finding is as below. Most probable diagnosis is:

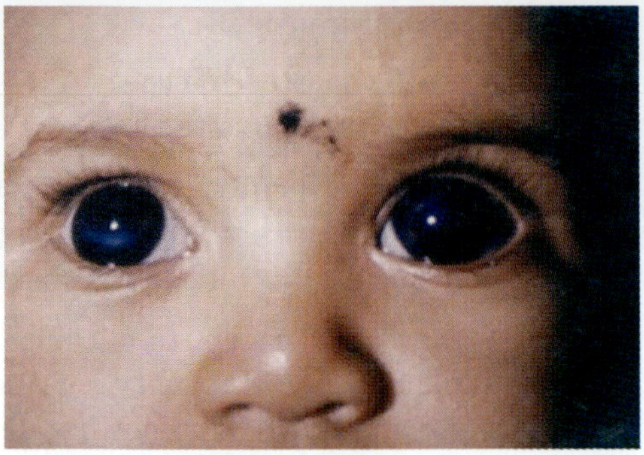

A. Congenital glaucoma
B. Retinoblastoma
C. Congenital endothelial dystrophy
D. Megalocornea

2. 100 days glaucoma is caused due to:

A. Central retinal vein occlusion
B. Phacolysis
C. Neovascularization in diabetes
D. Retinal detachment

3. Identify the test shown below:

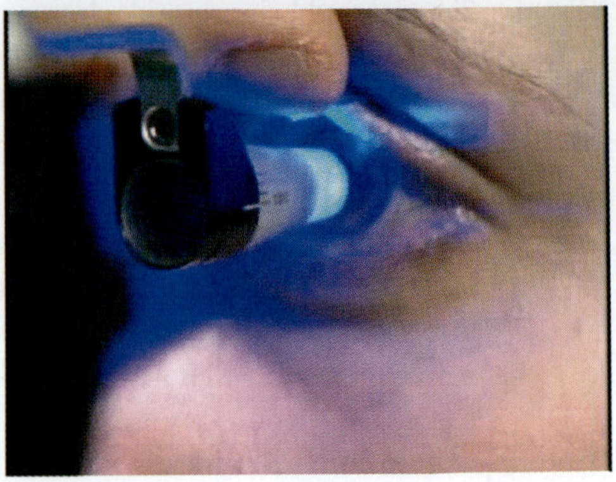

A. Tonometry
B. Laser interferometry
C. Pachymetry
D. Refractometer

4. First visual field defect in glaucoma:

A. Nasal B. Temporal
C. Superior D. Inferior

ANSWERS OF RECENTLY ADDED QUESTIONS

1. a 2 years child with photophobia and enlarged eye, most probably diagnosis is congenital glaucoma.

In retinoblastoma, patient presents with leukocoria. In megalocornea, it is corneal diameter of more than 13 mm, but no photophobia or enlargement of eye.

2. a 100 days glaucoma is neovascular glaucoma after central retinal vein occlusion typically seen to occur after 100 days, hence we call it 100 days glaucoma.

3. a Picture shows measurement of intraocular pressure (Tonometry) with Goldmann tonometer.

Goldmann tonometer: Considered gold standard.

The prism applanates the cornea in an area of 3.06 mm diameter.

It consists of double prism mounted on slit lamp.

Based on Imbert Fick's principle:

$P = F/A$

P = pressure inside the sphere

F = force necessary to flatten the area

A = area of flattening.

4. a The nerve fibres damaged FIRST are the temporal fibres (Arcuate fibres) hence the first field defect is nasal.

IMAGE-BASED QUESTIONS

1. Which tonometre is being used?

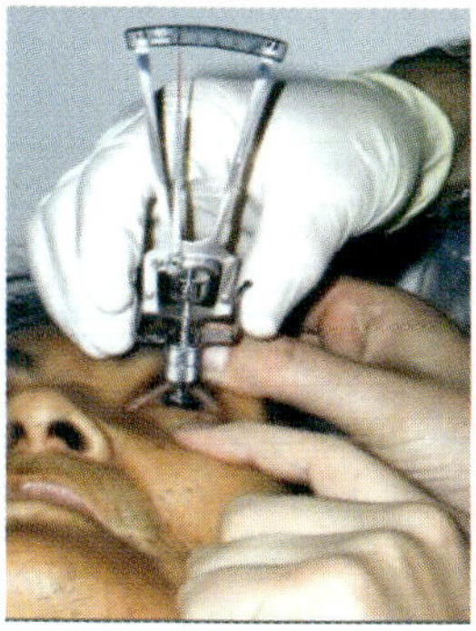

A. Schiotz tonometre
B. Goldmann tonometre
C. Tonopen
D. Mac Kay marg

2. The investigation is:

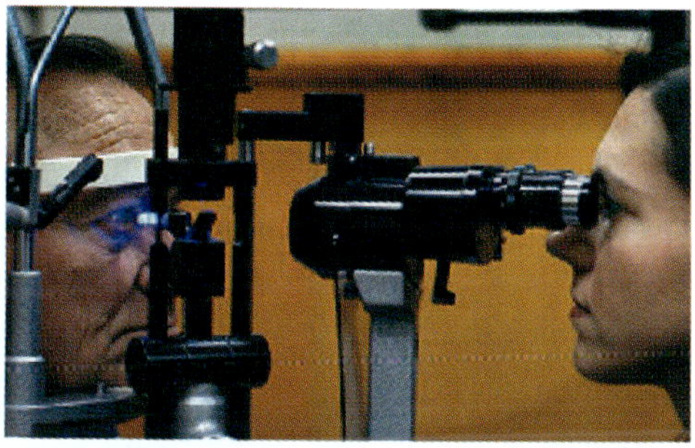

A. Pachymetry
B. Keratometry
C. Tonometry
D. Specular microscopy

3. The diagnosis is:

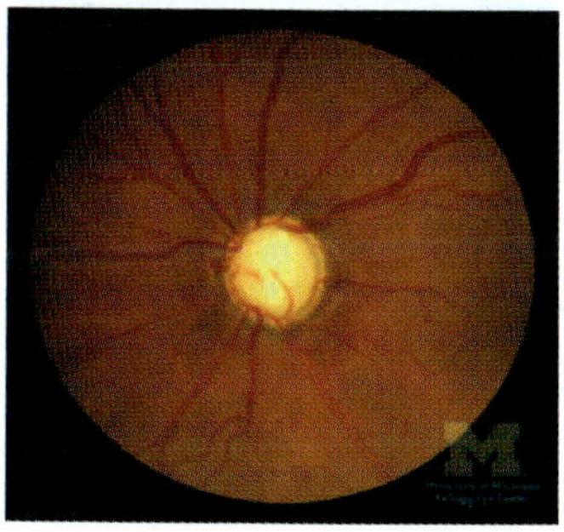

A. Primary optic atrophy
B. Secondary optic atrophy
C. Consequitive optic atrophy
D. Glaucomatous optic atrophy

4. The instrument is useful for:

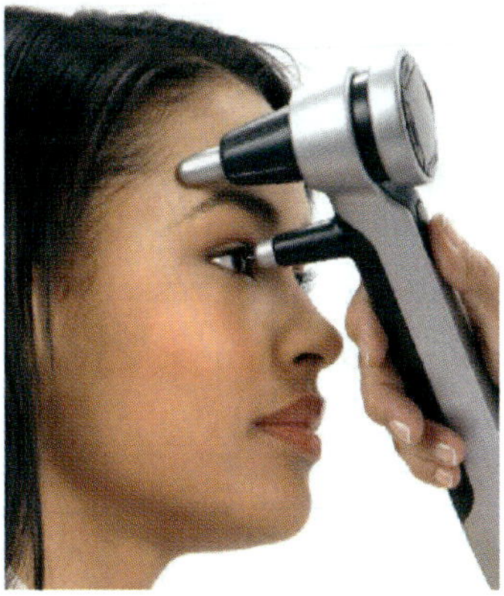

A. Measure IOP in scarred and irregular cornea
B. Measure IOP in infants
C. Self measurement of IOP
D. Measure IOP in thin cornea

5. The diagnosis is:

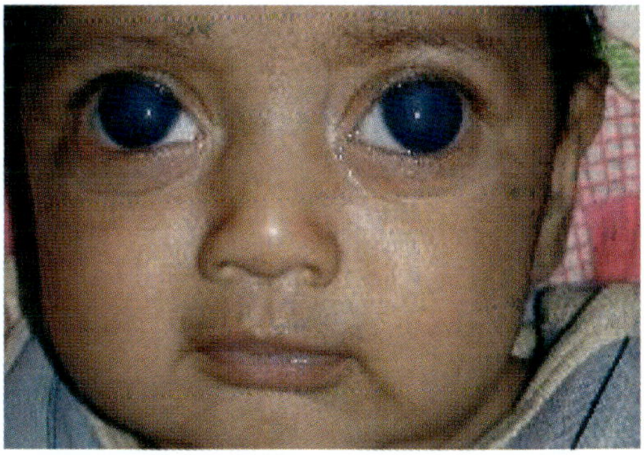

A. Congenital cataract
B. Congenital glaucoma
C. Congenital dacryocystitis
D. Megalocornea

6. The diagnosis is:

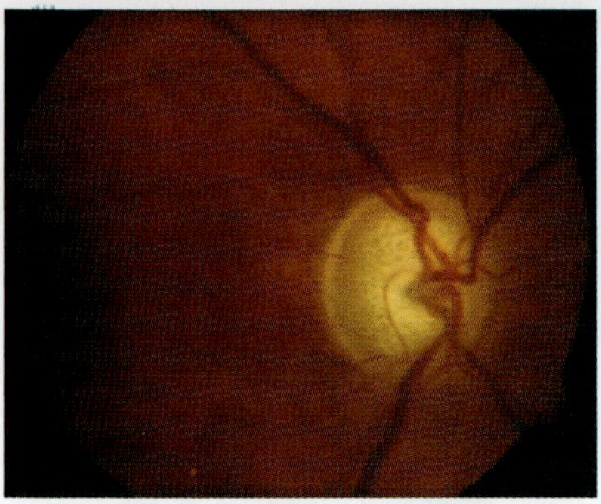

A. Laminar dot sign

B. Nasal shifting of vessels

C. Bayonetting sign

D. All of the above

7. The following is used for:

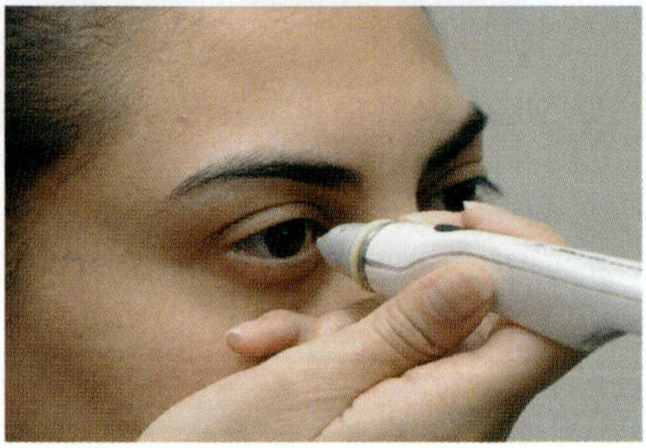

A. Infants B. Adults

C. Corneal opacities D. All of the above

8. The diagnosis is:

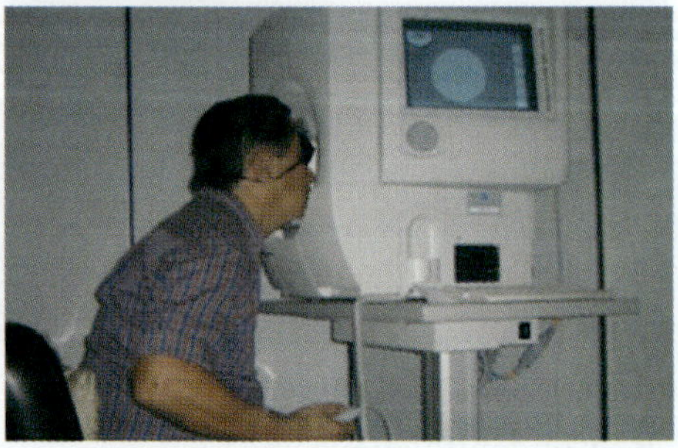

A. Auto refractometre

B. Automated perimetry

C. Goldmann perimeter

D. Kinetic perimetry

9. The following investigation is:

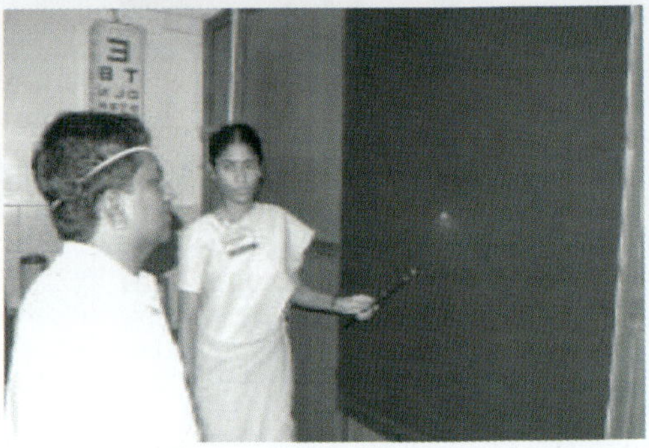

A. Listers perimetry

B. Goldmann perimetre

C. Bjerrums screen

D. None of the above

10. The diagnosis is:

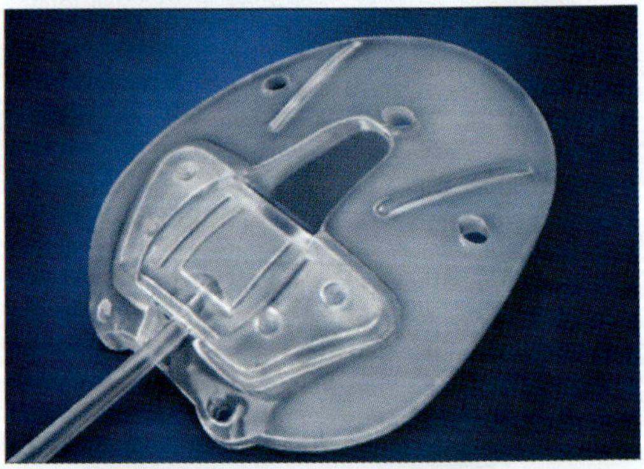

A. Express implant

B. Ahmed glaucoma valve

C. Molteno implant

D. Krupin Denver implant

ANSWERS OF IMAGE-BASED QUESTIONS

1. a It is a schiotz tonometre, where reading depends on the scleral rigidity of the patient.
2. c It is a Goldmann tonometre which is considered most reliable and is the gold standard for tonometry.
3. d The slide shows cupping of disc with bayonetting sign. Hence this is glaucomatous optic atrophy.
4. c This is rebound tonometre for self measurement of IOP.
5. b The slide shows buphthalmos with large cornea and corneal edema.
6. d Above slide shows glaucomatous changes with 0.8 cupping, nasal shifting of vessels, double bending of vessels (bayonetting sign) and visible openings of lamina cribosa (laminar dot sign).
7. d This is tonopen used in irregular and scarred corneas and also choice of tonometre for children.
8. b The slide shows automated perimetry which is most reliable method of perimetry.
9. c This is bjerrums screen for central field charting through kinetic perimetry.
10. b Ahmed glaucoma valve is most commonly used aqueous drainage implant made up of silicone.

GUIDANCE

Strength is the source of happiness. We mustn't shy away from life's challenges. We mustn't be defeated. Refusing to be defeated equals victory.

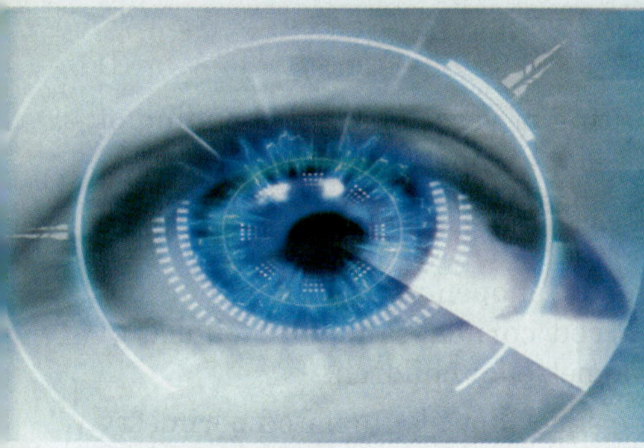

CHAPTER 3

Cornea

ANATOMY

It is a transparent, avascular structure, forming 1/6th of the outer fibrous coat of eyeball.

- **Refractive power** 43–45 D.
- **Refractive index** 1.37.
- **Structure**–It consists of five distinct layers; from anterior to posterior:

a. **Epithelium**

Corneal epithelium is 50μ to 90μ thick and consists of 5–6 layers of cells. It comprised:

1. **Basal layer:** It is the deepest layer and consists of tall columnar, polygonal shaped cells arranged in a palisade like manner on a basement membrane.
2. **The Wing cells:** It forms 2–3 layers of the polyhedral shaped cells.
3. **The flattened cells:** It constitutes two most superficial cell layers. The anterior cell wall of most superficial cells has many microvilli (0.5μ in height) which play an important role in tear film stability.

b. **Bowman's membrane.**

c. **Substantia propria or stroma.**

d. **Descements membrane.**

e. **Endothelium.**

There is a 6th layer in the cornea called Dua's layer. It is the tough layer between stroma and Descements membrane.

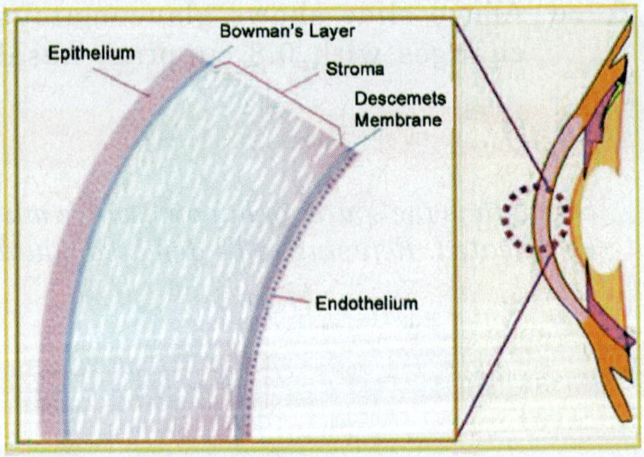

Fig. 3.1

PHYSIOLOGY

Cornea

- It acts as a refracting medium owing to it transparency.
- Transparency of cornea is maintained by:
  1. Regular arrangement of corneal lamellae.
  2. Avascularity of the cornea.
  3. Dehydrated state of the cornea.
- Cornea derives its nutrition mainly solutes (glucose and others) by simple diffusion or

active transport through aqueous humour and by diffusion from perilimbal capillaries.

- It derives oxygen from air through tear film. This is an active process undertaken by the epithelium. Hence, in contact lens use, the oxygen supply is interfered. **Since the nutrition to the cornea is through aqueous humour, hence it is the glucose utilization (through aerobic metabolism) which is affected on using contact lenses and not the glucose supply.**
- **The most metabolically active layer of cornea is endothelium**. Endothelium cells have Na+/K+ ATPase pump which extrudes out water from the cornea maintaining it in a dehydrated state. Hence, endothelial cell dysfunction if severe will cause corneal edema (stromal) followed by epithelial corneal edema leading to formation of fluid-filled bullae at the superficial layer of epithelium called Bullous Keratopathy, and the state of the cornea is termed as **decompensated cornea.** Decompensated cornea denotes that the endothelial loss cannot be compensated.
- **Most common cause of bullous keratopathy is post operative.**
- **Layer of the cornea involved in bullous keratopathy is epithelium.**
- The ionic exchange across the endothelium is inhibited by the **activation of the anaerobic glycolysis**. This is because the anaerobic metabolism leads to metabolic acidosis which inhibits the endothelial function.

INVESTIGATIONS RELATED TO CORNEA

1. **Pachymetry:** It measures the corneal thickness.
2. **Specular microscopy:** It photographs corneal endothelium and delineates various cellular characteristics like, size, shape, density and distribution.
3. **Keratometry:** It is used for the measurement of the radius of curvature of the anterior corneal surface.

   Principle: Keratometres utilize the reflective properties of the cornea to measure the radius of curvature of the anterior corneal surface. The anterior corneal surface acts as a convex mirror. An object of known size and position is then projected onto the cornea. The size of the image so formed is measured. The relationship between the object and image size is then used and from object distance and object size, *the radius of corneal curvature is calculated as—object distance × image size/object size.*

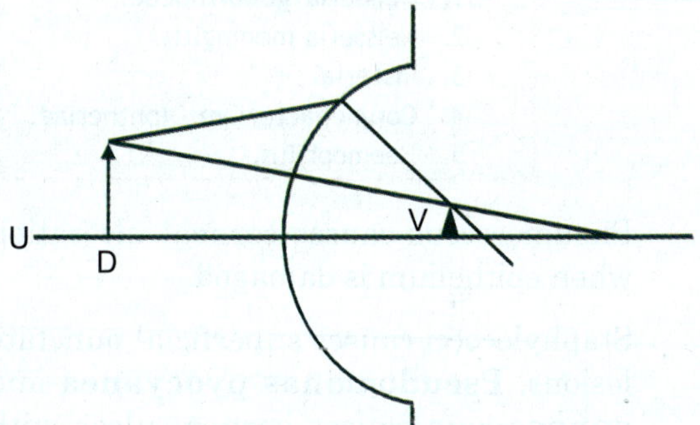

Fig. 3.2: Principle of keratometry

4. **Keratoscopy:** It denotes a qualitative assessment of the corneal shape. The three main types are:
   a. Hand-held placido's disc.
   b. Photokeratoscopes.
   c. Computer-assisted photokeratoscopes.
5. **Laboratory investigations:**
   a. Scrapings.
   b. Corneal biopsy.
6. **UBM (Ultrasound bimicroscopy):** It helps to measure the depth of the anterior chamber.

7. **Aesthesiometre:** It is an instrument to measure corneal sensation.

BACTERIAL KERATITIS

Etiological agents are Staphylococcus aureus, Streptococcus pneumoniae, Pseudomonas, Enterobacteriaceae, Pneumococcus, Klebsiella, Proteus, N gonorrhoeae, C diptheriae, N meningitidis.

Organisms which can penetrate intact cornea are:

MNEMONIC

NN-LDH

1. **N**eisseria gonorrhoeae.
2. **N**eisseria meningitis.
3. **L**isteria.
4. Corynebacterium **D**iphtheriae.
5. **H**aemophilus.

- Pneumococcus causes corneal ulceration when epithelium is damaged.
- Staphylococci causes superficial punctate lesions. **Pseudomonas pyocyanea** and **gonococcus** causes corneal ulcer with hypopyon whereas *proteus vulgaris causes simple corneal ulcer.*

Clinical Features:

a. Photophobia.
b. Pain.
c. Blepharospasm.
d. Ciliary congestion.
e. Corneal ulcer with or without stromal suppuration.
f. *Corneal rings:* It is seen in gram-negative infection due to infiltrates in stroma in response to endotoxins.
g. *Hypopyon:* **If present it is always sterile.**

Types of Corneal Ulcer

1. **Localised corneal ulcer:** It is generally described in four stages namely Infiltration, Active ulceration, Regression and Cicratisation.
2. **Corneal ulcer with perforation:** Deepening of ulcerative process reaching the descements membrane, leading to formation of descematocoele. Descematocoele later perforates. This site is further sealed by the iris causing **leucoma adherens.**
3. **Sloughing corneal ulcer:** It occurs due to very virulent organism. It causes sloughing of the whole cornea leaving a narrow rim at the margin, leading to total prolapse of iris with exudates and fibrosis known as **Pseudocornea formation**. It may further complicate into **Anterior Staphyloma**.

Pneumococcus

- Pneumococcus causes a characteristic **"hypopyon corneal ulcer"** known as **Ulcus Serpens.**
- It is named so because the ulcer has tendency to creep over the cornea in a serpiginous fashion.
- Typical ulcus serpens is a greyish white or yellowish disc near the center of the cornea.
- One edge of ulcer shows more dense infiltration along which the ulcer spreads. The other side of the ulcer may be showing simultaneous cicatrization.
- It is associated with virulent iridocyclitis.

Investigations

1. *Staining:* Gram stain and Geimsa stain.
2. *Culture:* Blood Agar.

Treatment of Bacterial Keratitis

1. *Topical Antibiotics:* It is given according to culture and sensitivity report or broad spectrum antibiotics are preferred.
2. *Fortified topical antibiotics:* It is given if the patient does not respond to the usual treatment.
   Gentamycin–15 mg/ml.
   Cephazoline–50 mg/ml.
3. Sub-conjunctival antibiotic injections may be needed.
4. Oral antibiotics are given in severe cases. Ciprofloxacin has excellent intraocular penetration.
5. *Topical cycloplegics:* It is given if there is an associated uveitis.
6. Systemic analgesics and anti-inflammatory.
7. Vitamin C, B, A.

- **Topical steroids are contra-indicated in ulcer except if of allergic origin.**
- **In any case of infection, purulent or mucopurulent never pad the eyes or close the lids by tarssoraphy, as it aggravates the condition.**

Treatment of a Non-Healing Ulcer

1. **Debridement:** It removes necrotic tissue from the ulcer and hence helps the epithelium to grow.
2. **Chemical cauterization:** This is done by trichloroacetic acid.
3. **Impending perforation:**
   a. *Tissue adhesive cynoacrylate glue:* They are used in the area of impending corneal perforation.
   b. *Conjunctival flapping:* The ulcer area is covered with conjunctiva to prevent any damage of the growing epithelium due to movement of lids.
   c. *Bandage contact lenses:* They are soft contact lenses with very high water content used for therapeutic purpose.
   d. Decreasing of IOP with anti-glaucoma drugs.
   e. Penetrating Keratoplasty (PK), if nothing works.

Complications of Corneal Ulcer

1. Descematocoele formation.
2. Perforation can lead to (a) Prolapse of iris (b) Subluxation of lens (c) Anterior capsular cataract (d) Purulent uveitis (e) Corneal fistula (f) Intraocular haemorrhage.
3. Toxic iridocyclitis.
4. Secondary scarring.

Corneal Opacity

Depending on the density, corneal opacity is graded as:

A. **Nebula:** Nebular corneal opacity is a faint opacity which results due to superficial scars involving Bowman's layer and superficial stroma.

B. **Macula:** It's a semi-dense opacity produced when scarring involves about half the corneal stroma.

C. **Leucoma** (also called **leucoma simplex**): It's a dense white opacity which results due to scarring of more than half of the stroma.

Treatment

1. **Optical iridectomy** is performed in the quadrant where the cornea is clearest and is determined by placing stenopic slit in the quadrant and finding the improvement of vision.
2. **Tatooing:** It is aimed in coloring the corneal opacity to obtain cosmetical

correction. This is done by Gold to color brown and Platinum to color black.

Procedure: Epithelium is debrided in the area of opacity and then gold or platinum is applied, and finally the area is washed with hydrazine hydrate to fix it.The eye is bandaged for one day, which helps the epithelium to grow.

3. **Keratoplasty, i.e., PK.**

Nebula produces maximum discomfort to the patient due to blurred image owing to irregular astigmatism (due to diffraction of light); than the leucoma.

VIRAL KERATITIS

Viral infection is associated with decreased corneal sensation.

Other causes of decrease/loss of corneal sensation are:

1. Leprosy.
2. Inflammations
   a. Stromal edema.
   b. Vascularized scar.
   c. Exposure keratitis.
   d. Congestive glaucoma.
3. Trauma due to constant wearing of contact lens.
4. Corneal dystrophies (stromal) like lattice, granular, macular.
5. Diabetes mellitus.
6. Skin lesions like psoriasis.

HERPES SIMPLEX VIRUS (HSV) KERATITIS

Clinical Features:

1. Blepharoconjunctivitis (self limited; occurs in primary ocular infection).
2. Keratitis:

A. Epithelial Disease

a. ***Dendritic ulcer:*** **It is a pathognomic feature of HSV infection.** The ulcer is linear in shape with knobbed ends. **Steroids are contraindicated in dendritic ulcer** as it will lead to geographical ulcer and later corneal perforation.

b. ***Geographical ulcer:*** It is amoeboid in shape. It is associated with stromal infiltrate.

B. Stromal Necrotic Keratitis: It occurs due to direct viral invasion and destruction of corneal stroma. Stroma has chessy, necrotic appearance with associated uveitis.

C. Disciform Keratitis: It refers to endothelitis involving the centre of the cornea. It is characterized by edema of the central cornea due to endothelial dysfunction.

D. Trophic Keratitis: It is also called **Metaherpetic keratitis**. Trophic ulcers are not due to active viral disease but due to denervation and drug toxicity.

Investigations:

1. **PCR, i.e., Polymerase chain reaction:** It detects even minute quantities of HSV viral DNA in tissue samples and hence is the most reliable method.
2. **Giemsa stain:** Giemsa stained smears of corneal scraping might reveal mononuclear cells, polymorphonuclear cells, multinucleated giant epithelial cells, and eosinophilic lipschutz inclusion bodies in cell nuclei. These bodies are best seen with papanicolaou's stain.
3. **Viral Culture:** A definitive diagnosis can be made by viral culture, if active virus is

present. Viral culture medium are of three types:

1. Organ culture.
2. Explant culture.
3. Cell Culture: It is the most common method.

   Some cell cultures in common use are:

   A. *Primary cell cultures:*
      1. Rhesus monkey kidney cell culture.
      2. Human amnion cell culture.
   B. *Diploid cell strains.*
   C. *Continuous cell lines:*
      1. HeLa.
      2. HEP-2.
      3. McCoy.

4. **Rose bengal staining:** Rose Bengal stains dead epithelial cell, debris and mucus. In typical herpetic dendritic ulcer, the base of ulcer stains with fluorescein and the margins (containing virus laden cells) with Rose Bengal.
5. **ELISA:** ELISA identifies viral antigens, whether or not live virus is present. HSV antigen can also be identified by direct immunofluorescence but this technique is less sensitive than ELISA test or Tissue Culture.

Treatment

Antiviral Drugs:

1. *Acycloguanasine also known as Acyclovir:* It is given as 3% ointment given five times a day.
2. *Trifluorothymidine (1% Drops):* It is more toxic to corneal epithelium and conjunctiva compared to acyclovir.
3. *Adenine arabinoside (3% Ointment):* It is given in rare circumstances when there is resistance to Acyclovir and Trifluorothymidine.
4. *Idoxuridine:* It is seldom used due to emergence of resistant strain and toxicity.
5. *Bromovinyl deoxyuridine (1% ointment):* It is a new promising antiviral, as potent as Trifluorothymidine.

Steroids are contraindicated in dendritic ulcer. Steroids are sometimes given (under antiviral cover) in disciform keratitis caused by HSV but not in dendritic ulcers or stromal keratitis.

HERPES ZOSTER OPHTHALMICUS (HZO)

It is more common in immunocompromised patients. It is a predicator of Leukemia, HIV, Lymphoma, disseminated TB and metastasis.

Hutchison's rule/sign: It says that if the tip of the nose is involved by the skin lesions then the eye will be involved. Skin lesion at the tip of nose indicates the involvement of nasociliary nerve.

Clinical Features:

Clinically HZO can be divided into the following three phases:

A. Acute phase
B. Chronic phase
C. Relapsing phase.

Acute Phase

It occurs within first 4 weeks and may totally resolve.

Clinical Features:

1. Fever, malaise and headache.
2. Neuralgia.
3. *Cutaneous lesions:*

i. The rash may involve one or all three branches of the ophthalmic nerve.
   (a) Frontal
   (b) Lacrimal
   (c) Nasociliary.
ii. Maculopapular rash→pustular→burst to form crusting ulcers.

4. *Ocular lesions:*

A. External lesions:

a. *Conjunctivitis:* It is always associated with vesicle on the lid margin.
b. Episcleritis.
c. Scleritis.

B. Corneal lesions:

1. ***Punctate epithelial keratitis:*** It consists of swollen epithelial cells containing replicating virus. It may be associated with filamentary keratitis.
2. ***Microdendritic ulcer:*** Unlike dendritic ulcers of HSV, they are peripheral, broader and more plaque like, with no central ulceration. They are more of stellate shape. They are also called **pseudodendrites.**
3. ***Nummular keratitis:*** It involves the stroma. These are multiple fine granular deposits (beneath Bowman's membrane) surrounded by stromal haze.
4. ***Disciform keratitis:*** It refers to endothelitis involving the centre of the cornea and manifests as edema of the central cornea.

C. Anterior uveitis.

D. Acute retinal necrosis.

E. Neurological complications:

1. **Cranial nerve palsies**—III nerve is most commonly involved.
2. Optic neuritis.
3. Encephalitis.
4. Contralateral hemiplegia.

Chronic Phase

Cutaneous Lesions:

- Typical punched out scars with varying degree of hyperpigmentation and hypopigmentation.
- Complications due to skin lesions include:
  a. Ptosis.
  b. Loss of lashes.
  c. Ectropion.
  d. Entropion.
  e. Lid notching.

Ocular Lesions:

1. **Mucus secreting conjunctivitis:** It consists of lipid filled granulomata under the tarsal conjunctiva.
2. Scleritis.
3. Nummular keratitis.
4. Disciform keratitis.
5. Neurotrophic and Exposure keratitis.
6. Mucus plaque keratitis.

Relapsing Phase

Recurrent lesions may reappear as long as 10 years after the acute lesions, commonly due to sudden withdrawal or reduction of topical corticosteroids.

Clinical Features:

1. Episcleritis, scleritis.
2. Iritis.
3. Glaucoma.
4. Keratitis: Nummular, Disciform and Mucus plaque keratitis.

Post Herpetic Neuralgia

- Affects about 7% of patients.
- Pain may be constant or intermittently severe.
- Pain is worse at night and aggravated by touch and heat.

Treatment:

A. Treatment of skin lesions:

The aim is, rapid healing of skin without the formation of massive crusts; as crusts cause scarring of nerves and post herpetic neuralgia.

1. *Systemic therapy:* Acyclovir (Zovirax)—800 mg tab 5 times/day.
2. *Topical therapy:* 3 times/day till all crust disappears.
   a. *Antiviral creams:* Acyclovir, Idoxuridine.
   b. *Steroid:* Antibiotic ointment like Neocortef ointment or Terracortil spray.

B. Treatment of ocular lesions:

1. *Indolent Episcleritis and Scleritis:* Oral flurbiprofen 100 mg thrice a day.
2. Antiviral therapy both oral and topical. Oral acyclovir is given 800 mg 5 times/day. Topical therapy is same as in HSV infection. In cases of severe inflammation topical steroids can be given but under antiviral cover.
3. Lateral tarsorrhaphy for neuroparalytic ulcer.
4. *Keratoplasty:* If dense scarring.

C. Treatment of post-herpetic neuralgia:

1. Systemic steroids inhibit development of post herpetic neuralgia.
2. Cimetidine – It reduces pain and pruritus due to histamine block.
3. Amitryptiline.
4. Carbamazipine—800 mg BD. It's an antiepileptic.
5. Dividing the sensory root of fifth nerve fibres.
6. Injection of absolute alcohol.

FUNGAL KERATITIS (KERATOMYCOSIS)

- Most common fungi (in India) to cause corneal ulcer is **Aspergillus fumigatus.**
- Most common fungi to cause lid infections are **Candida and Dermatophytes.**
- **Keratomycosis generally occurs after trauma to the eye by vegetable or organic matter.**

Clinical Features:

Patient is less symptomatic compared to the severity of disease, i.e., **signs are more than symptoms**.

Signs and Symptoms

1. Watering, photophobia, redness, pain, mild discharge.
2. Creamy stromal infilterates.
3. *Fungal ulcer:* The ulcer is dry and rough with feathery and hyphate margins.
4. Wessely ring, around central lesion, due to immune reaction.
5. *Satellite lesions in periphery:* Peripheral small ulcers apart from the main lesion. (It is also seen in acanthamoeba infections but more commonly seen in fungal infections).
6. **Unsterile hypopyon.**

Investigations

1. Smear examination

a. KOH wet preparation.

b. Gomori's methamine silver stain.

2. **Culture media**
   a. Saborauds glucose agar.
   b. Czapek-dox medium.
   c. Liquid brain-heart infusion broth.
3. **Serological tests.**

Treatment

Antifungal Drugs:

The most effective antifungal drug in India is Natamycin.

a. *Topical:* Fluconazole (0.2%), Nystatin eye ointment.
b. *Oral:* Fluconazole, Iatraconazole.
c. Atropine may be needed as an adjuvant due to associated uveitis.

Interestitial Keratitis: It is an inflammation of the corneal stroma with no primary involvement of epithelium or endothelium.

Causes

1. **Congenital Syphilis:** Deep vascularisation leads to bleeding in stroma and known as **Salmon patch.**
2. Tuberculosis.
3. **Cogan's syndrome:** Interestitial keratitis associated with deafness.
4. Leprosy.
5. Sarcoidosis.

ACANTHAMOEBA KERATITIS

- **Acanthamoeba does not depend upon a human host for the completion of its life-cycle.**
- Acanthamoebae are ubiquitous free-living protozoans found in air, soil and fresh or brackish waters. They exist in both active (trophozoite) and dormant (cystic) forms. The cystic form is highly resilient and able to survive under hostile environmental conditions.
- To a large extent, humans are resistant to its infection. Keratitis due to acanthamoeba occurs more due to prior corneal abrasion (e.g., in soft contact lens users) or in immunocompromised patients.
- Contact lens wearers who use distilled water to clean their lenses are at increased risk of acanthamoeba keratitis.

Clinical Features:

1. Blurred vision and pain which is characteristically severe and disproportionate to the extent of ocular involvement. The pain is disproportionately large because of the perineural invasion by the organism.
2. Multifocal patchy anterior stromal infilterates which gradually enlarge and coalesce to form a partial or complete, central or paracentral non suppurative ring.
3. Pseudodendrites.
4. Satellite lesions.
5. Hypopyon.
6. Stromal thinning and descematocele.

Investigations

A. Smear examination: Calcoflour White, Lactophenol Blue, F-CON-A (Fluorescein Conjugated Concavalin-A).

B. Culture medium: Non-nutrient agar with E. coli.

Treatment

Suggested Antimicrobials include:

1. **Cationic antiseptics:** Inhibit membrane function.
   a. Polyhexamethylene biguanide (PHMB).
   b. Chlorhexidine.

2. **Aromatic amidines:** Inhibit DNA synthesis.
   a. Propamidine isethionate.
   b. Pentamidine isethionate.
3. **Aminoglycosides:** Inhibit protein synthesis.
   a. Neomycin.
   b. Paromycin.
4. **Imidazoles:** Destabilize cell walls.
   a. Clotrimazoles.
   b. Fluconazole.
   c. Ketoconazole.
   d. Miconazole.

For synergistic approach, initial approach is chlorhexidine or PHMB with neomycin or propamidine isethionate.

KERATOCONUS

It is a hereditary disease characterized by non inflammatory, usually bilateral ectasia of the cornea giving it a conical shape with resultant irregular myopic astigmatism.

Classification

Morphologically:

a. Nipple cone (5 mm).
b. Oval cone (5–6 mm) displaced infero-temporally.
c. Globus cone (> 6 mm), may involve over 75% of cornea.

Clinical Features:

1. Impaired vision, due to progressing myopia and astigmatism.
2. **Retinoscopy: Irregular scissors reflex.**
3. **Keratometry:** Irregular astigmatism.
4. **Photokeratoscopy (Placido's disc):** Irregularity.
5. **Slit–Lamp Bimicroscopy:**
   a. **Vogt's striae:** Stress lines parallel to steep axis of cornea.
   b. **Prominent corneal nerves:** In keratoconus the visible corneal nerve is due to thin cornea. In condition like Herpes simplex, leprosy and neuro-fibromatosis the visibility of nerves is due to enlargement of nerves.
   c. Reduced corneal sensation.
   d. **Hurricane keratopathy:** Whorl pattern of SPK (Superficial Punctate Keratitis) due to effect of contact lens.
6. **Applanation tonometry:** Pulsating mires.
7. **Munson's sign:** V-shaped deformity of lower lid in down-gaze.
8. **Fleischer's ring:** Brown line encircling base of cone due to deposition of iron.
9. **Acute hydrops:** Sudden hydration of corneal stroma due to rupture of descements membrane.

Investigations: Corneal topographic picture is diagnostic.

Treatment

1. **Astigmatic spectacles:** It is effective in only initial stages of the disease.
2. **Rigid contact lens:** Soft contact lenses are of no use as it takes the shape of the irregular cornea. RGPs (rigid gas permeable) lenses replace the irregular surface of the cornea with its regular contour and hence helps to improve the vision.
3. **Penetrating keratoplasty:** In the later stage of the disease the contact lenses also become ineffective and the last resort is PK. The prognosis of PK in keratoconus is very good as it is a non inflammatory pathology.

KERATOGLOBUS

- It is an extremely rare disease and starts at birth.

- It is characterized by bilateral thinning and protrusion of the entire cornea, which is of normal size.
- Cornea is susceptible to rupture due to extreme thinness.
- It is associated with:
  a. Lebers congenital amaurosis.
  b. Blue sclera.

CORNEAL TRANSPLANTATION OR KERATOPLASTY

- It is the replacement of diseased cornea by a graft of homologous tissue.
- Donor cornea is obtained from cadaveric eye as soon as possible **(preferably within 6 hours but may be extended to 12 hours).**
- It is of two types:
  1. Penetrating Keratoplasty.
  2. Lamellar Keratoplasty.

Methods of Corneal Preservation

A. Short-term Storage:

In sterile moist chamber.

- It is stored at 4°C.
- It can be stored for 48 hours, but after 48 hours there is endothelial degeneration due to depletion of nutrient.

B. Intermediate-term Storage:

1. In McCarey-Kaufman medium (MK Medium)
   - Original formulation of MK medium consists of:
     a. Tc^{199}.
     b. 5% Dextran.
     c. Bicarbonate buffer.
     d. Penicillin and streptomycin.
   - By this method cornea can be stored for 4 days.
   - MK medium has a protective effect on the endothelium compared to moist chamber.
2. Chondroitin-sulphate enriched media.
3. Corneal storage medium (CSM).
4. Dexol medium.
5. Optisol medium.
6. Likoral medium.
7. Pro-cell medium.
8. Honey preservation medium.

C. Long-term Storage:

A. By organ culture method: Cornea can be stored upto 30 days.

B. Cryopreservation: Upto indefinite time. Its advantages are:
   a. Presence of disease can be excluded in the donor.
   b. Tissue matching is possible.
   c. Endothelial count can be checked.

Penetrating Keratoplasty

It is the replacement of **full-thickness of the cornea.**

Types

1. Depending on size: Complete and partial.
2. Depending upon site: Central and eccentric.

Common Indications of PK

1. Keratoconus.
2. Aphakic/Phakic bullous keratopathy **(Most common indication).**
3. Corneal opacity.
4. Corneal dystrophy.

Lamellar Keratoplasty (LK)

It is the replacement of partial thickness of the cornea.

Types

A. Inlay lamellar keratoplasty/Keratophakia: A partial thickness of the recipient cornea is removed by lamellar dissection and replaced by partial thickness of donor cornea.

Common Indications:

1. Large descematocele.
2. Stromal ulcer except fungal.
3. Superficial scar.
4. Pterygium.
5. Corneal tumours.
6. Perforation.

Deep LK: It's a type of LK in which the plane of dissection is just anterior to the descements membrane.

B. Onlay lamellar keratoplasty (Epikeratoplasty/Epikeratophakia): In this procedure, epithelium is debrided and a small peripheral lamellar dissection is done on the recipient cornea and the donor material is secured on the prepared recipient bed.

Common Indications: It is mainly used for refractive purpose.

1. Aphakia.
2. Myopia.
3. Keratoconus.
4. Keratoglobus.

C. Others:

1. **Onlay Limbal Transplantation:** It is done in cases of post chemical burns, Stevens-Johnson syndrome, Chronic contact lens use, Limbal tumours and post irradiation.
2. **Sclerokeratoplasty:** In this method the whole of cornea alongwith partial thickness sclera is transplanted. It is indicated when total corneal pathology extends from limbus to limbus.
3. **Endokeratoplasty:** In this method only the central portion of cornea is substituted, hence a good alternative to conventional PK in cases of endothelial decompensation.

CORNEAL DEGENERATIONS

A. Age-Related Degenerations:

Arcus senilis: It is bilateral lipid deposition circumferentially around the limbus in form of a band. It occurs in old age or patients of hyperlipoproteinemia.

B. Lipid Keratopathy:

It can be of two types:

i. **Primary lipid keratopathy**
   - Rare.
   - It occurs spontaneously in an **avascular** cornea.

ii. **Secondary lipid keratopathy**
   - More common.
   - It is due to previous ocular injury or disease which results in corneal vascularisation **(Commonly due to herpes simplex and herpes zoster disciform keratitis).**
   - White or yellowish corneal stromal deposits consisting of cholesterol, fats and phospholipids associated with vascularisation.
   - It is a progressive condition which causes deterioration of vision.

Treatment:

1. Control of inflammatory disease.
2. Resorption of lipid deposits by Argon laser photocoagulation to the feeder vessels (which are identified by fluorescein angiography).

3. Keratoplasty, if laser therapy is not effective.

C. Band-Shaped Keratopathy:

It is a common disorder characterized by deposition of calcium salts in the sub-epithelial space and anterior portion of Bowman's membrane.

Etiology:

a. Chronic iridocyclitis (particularly in children–JRA).

b. Idiopathic: In elderly.

c. Pthisis bulbi.

d. Increased serum calcium or phosphorus levels.

Clinical Features:

Calcium deposition characteristically showing interpalpebral distribution of the lesions with a clear space separating the sharp margin of the band from the limbus.

Treatment:

1. Chelation
   a. Sodium versenate.
   b. EDTA (1.5%–2.5%).
   c. Sodium acetate.
2. Excimer laser lamellar keratectomy.

D. Spheroidal Degeneration

- **Also called "Corneal Elastosis" or "Climatic Droplet Keratopathy" (CDK).**
- Amber coloured spheroidal granules or droplets composed of protein in superficial corneal stroma in interpalpebral strip, beginning from periphery.
- It varies in severity from localized mistiness to large nodules.
- Severe visual impairment.
- Sequelae: Corneal opacity.

Treatment:

a. Epithelial debridement.

b. Superficial keratectomy.

c. Keratoplasty:
   - Lamellar.
   - Penetrating.

E. Salzmann's Nodular Degeneration

Etiology: It occurs secondary to chronic keratitis especially trachoma and phlyctenulosis.

Clinical Features:

1. Superficial stromal opacities, grey in colour which form nodules and elevate the corneal epithelium.

2. Base of nodule may be surrounded by epithelial iron deposits.

Treatment: Same as spheroidal degeneration.

PERIPHERAL CORNEAL DISORDERS

A. Dellen

It consists of localized area of corneal thinning which occurs as a result of localized tear film instability.

Causes:

1. Raised limbal lesion.
2. Hard contact lens.
3. Idiopathic in elderly.

Treatment:

1. Elimination of cause.
2. Lubricants and patching to enhance corneal rehydration.

B. Marginal Keratitis

- **Also called Catarrhal ulcer.**
- Caused by hypersensitivity reaction to staphylococcus exotoxins (patients of chronic staphylococcal blepharitis).

Treatment:

1. Short course of topical steroids.
2. Treatment of associated blepharitis.

C. Phlyctenulosis or Phlyctenular Keratoconjunctivitis

Corneal phycten may lead to **Fascicular ulcer** which may then form **Ring ulcer.**

D. Mooren's Ulcer

- It is a peripheral ulcerative keratitis caused by ischemic necrosis due to vasculitis of limbal vessels (caused by the enzymes-collagenase and proteoglyconase produced from adjacent conjunctiva).
- It is of two types:
  1. *Limited form:* Usually unilateral and mostly affects elderly.
  2. *Progressive form:* Usually bilateral and mostly affects young individuals.

Sequelae:

1. Vascularised thin opaque cornea.
2. Secondary cataract.
3. Perforation of cornea: Is rare.

Treatment:

1. Topical steroids.
2. Systemic therapy:
   a. Steroids.
   b. Cyclosporin.
   c. Cytotoxic drugs.
3. Conjunctival Excision: Excision is done 3 mm from the limbus and parallel to the ulcer.

MISCELLANEOUS KERATOPATHIES

1. Vortex Keratopathy

Also called **Cornea Verticillata.**

Clinical Features: Symmetrical, bilateral, grayish or golden corneal epithelial deposits which appear in vortex fashion from point below the pupil and swirl outwards sparing the limbus.

Etiology:

a. Fabry's disease (Glycolipidosis).
b. Chloroquine.
c. Amiodarone.
d. Amodiaquine.
e. Meperidine.
f. Indomethacin.
g. Chlorpromazine.
h. Tamoxifen.

2. Neurotrophic Keratopathy

1. In anaesthetic cornea.
2. Loss of neural influences causes edema and exfoliation of epithelial cells by altering their metabolic activity.
3. **Causes:**
   a. HSV.
   b. HZO.
   c. DM.
   d. Leprosy.
   e. Section of 5th nerve.

   Neuroparalytic keratitis occurs due to seventh nerve palsy.

3. Exposure Keratopathy

It is caused by improper wetting of the corneal surface by the pre corneal tear film because of inability of the lids to resurface the cornea with each blink.

Etiology:

1. *Facial nerve palsy:* VII nerve supplies the orbicularis muscle and is responsible for the closure of eyelids. Hence its

paralysis causes lagophthalmos; which leads to exposure keratitis.

2. Severe proptosis.
3. Scarring of the eyelids.

Clinical Features:

1. Inferior punctate epitheliopathy.
2. Severe ulceration which leads to neovascularization.
3. Infection.
4. Perforation.

Treatment:

1. Artificial tears during the day and instillation of ointment and taping of eyelids at night.
2. Lid surgery, if lagophthalmos is permanent.

4. Photophthalmia or Snow Blindness

It is characterized by the occurrence of multiple epithelial erosions due to the effect of ultraviolet rays specially from 311u to 290u. UV rays reflected from the snow can lead to this condition hence the term–snow-blindness. *Photoretinitis is in turn a macular burn which occurs due to infrared rays.*

Pathogenesis: Ultraviolet rays cause desquamation of corneal epithelium.

Presentation is after 4–5 hours.

Clinical Features:

1. Severe burning pain.
2. Lacrimation.
3. Photophobia.
4. Blepharospasm.
5. Swelling of palpebral conjunctiva and retrotarsal folds.
6. Multiple fluorescein positive spots on cornea.

Prophylaxis: Crookers glass should be used by those who are at high risk like welding workers, cinema operators.

Treatment:

1. Cold compresses.
2. Pad and bandage with topical antibiotics.
3. Oral analgesics.
4. Tranquiliser for apprehensive patients.

CORNEAL DYSTROPHY

Group of spontaneous appearing, usually inherited, bilateral, stationary or slowly progressive corneal alterations that develop in absence of inflammation.

Classification

Anterior Dystrophies:

A. Epithelial Corneal Dystrophies:

- Either asymptomatic or present as recurrent corneal erosions.
- It is of 3 types:

1. Microcystic dystrophy

- Most common.
- Also called **Map dot—finger print dystrophy.**

Treatment:

1. Management of recurrent erosions.
2. Keratoplasty.

2. Reis-Bucklers' dystrophy

- Honeycomb cornea due to ring shaped opacities.
- If visual acuity greatly impaired, keratoplasty is needed.

3. Meesman's dystrophy

- Tiny epithelial cysts which extend to limbus and most numerous in interpalpebral area.
- **Treatment:** Keratoplasty.

B. Stromal Dystrophies:

a. **Lattice:** It is associated with systemic amyloidosis. There are interlacing spider like deposits of amyloid in the stroma.

b. **Macular:** It is associated with *mucopolysaccharoidosis*. There are grayish opacities consisting of glycosaminoglycans in the stroma, cornea in between the opacities is cloudy. It is least common, and there is significant impairment of vision. *Unlike other stromal dystrophies, it is* ***autosomal recessive*** *and also involves the peripheral cornea.*

c. **Granular:** There are white, discreet granules in the anterior and axial cornea.

d. **Fleck:**

- It is a stromal dystrophy.
- Also called *Speckled corneal dystrophy*.
- It is a congenital condition, stationary throughout life.
- Patient is asymptomatic and vision is not affected.
- Corneal sensitivity may be normal or reduced.
- Numerous oval or round, pleomorphic grayish white opacities located throughout all layers of the corneal stroma.

C. Posterior Dystrophies or Endothelial Dystrophies:

1. Fuch's endothelial dystrophy.
2. Posterior polymorphous dystrophy.

Endothelial Corneal Dystrophy

- Also called Fuch's Endothelial Dystrophy.
- Slowly progressive bilateral disease of old age common in women.

Clinical Features:

a. Increased number of central endothelial protuberances (**corneal guttatae**) which spread towards the periphery.

b. Edema of central stroma with blurring of vision; due to endothelial decompensation. It may lead to bullous keratopathy. This latter results in corneal opacity with degenerative pannus.

Treatment:

1. Hypertonic agents like sodium chloride 5% drops or ointment.
2. Lowering of IOP.
3. Soft bandage contact lens in bullous keratopathy.
4. Penetrating keratoplasty in advanced stage.

D. Ectatic Dystrophies

a. Keratoconus.

b. Posterior keratoconus.

c. Keratoglobus.

d. Pellucid marginal degeneration.

CORNEAL PIGMENTATIONS

1. Melanin pigments, e.g., Krukenberg's spindle.
2. Chalcosis: Deposition of copper.
3. Siderosis: Deposition of iron.
4. Argyrosis: Deposition of silver.
5. Hematogenous pigmentation commonly due to hyphema.
6. Silicosis: Deposition of silicon.
7. Cystinosis: Deposition of cysteine.

Argyrosis

- It causes deep brown staining of conjunctiva and cornea.
- It occurs due to prolonged application of silver salts in treatment of chronic conjunctivitis especially trachoma.
- It is due to permanent impregnation of the elastic fibres, and particularly descements membrane with metallic silver.

Mustard gas exposure has not been documented as the cause of brown discoloration of cornea.

MICROCORNEA

- Horizontal diameter is less than 10 mm since birth.
- Isolated anomaly—rare.
- Associated with:
  a. Nanophthalmos—normal small eyeball.
  b. Microphthalmos—abnormal small eyeball.

MEGALOCORNEA

- Horizontal diameter at birth > 12.0 mm (instead of 10 mm).
- > 13 mm after 2 years of age.
- It occurs due to defective growth of the optic cup, which leaves large space for development of the cornea.
- **It is associated with Marfan's syndrome.**

CORNEA PLANA

It's a rare congenital anomaly in which cornea is comparatively flat. It may be associated with microcornea. It usually results in marked astigmatic refractive error.

CORNEAL VASCULARISATION

It may be superficial or deep. Superficial vascularisation occurs due to proliferation from limbal vessels and deep vascularisation occurs due to proliferation from anterior ciliary artery.

Causes of Superficial Vascularisation

1. Trachoma.
2. Phlyctenular keratoconjunctivitis.
3. Superficial corneal ulcers.
4. Rosacea keratitis.

Causes of Deep Vascularisation

1. Interstitial keratitis.
2. Disciform keratitis.
3. Deep corneal ulcers.
4. Sclerosing keratitis.
5. Chemical burns.

Pannus: When superficial keratitis is associated with white cuff of cellular infilteration it is termed as pannus.

SLE (SYSTEMIC LUPUS ERYTHEMATOSUS)

Ocular Features

1. Punctate epithelial keratopathy: **Most common.**
2. Keratoconjunctivitis sicca.
3. Scleritis.
4. Retinal vasculitis.
5. Optic neuropathy.

RHEUMATOID ARTHRITIS

It is a seropositive arthritis and does not present as uveitis.

Ocular Features of RA

1. *Sclerosing keratitis:* Thickening and opacification of corneal stroma.
2. Peripheral corneal thinning **(called *"contact lens cornea"*):**
   a. It is an acute and severe melting of cornea.
   b. It may or may not be associated with inflammation.
   c. It results in descematocoele formation.
3. Acute stromal keratitis.
4. Keratoconjunctivitis sicca.
5. Scleritis–Non-inflammatory; necrotizing called: **"Scleromalacia perforans".**

NEET DRILL

1. It forms the anterior 1/6th of the outer fibrous coat of the eyeball.
2. Anterior surface is elliptical with the horizontal diameter of 11.75 mm and vertical diameter of 11 mm.
3. Posterior surface is circular with the average diameter of 11.5 mm.
4. Thickness at the centre is 0.5 mm–0.6 mm and at the limbus 0.67 mm–1 mm.
5. Optic zone of the cornea is central 5 mm of the cornea. The anterior radius of curvature is 7.8 mm and posteriorly it is 6.5 mm.
6. Refractive power of the cornea is 43D–45D. It is 3/4th of the total refractive power of the eye which is 60D.
7. Refractive index of the cornea is 1.37.
8. Corneal epithelium is stratified squamous.
9. The number of endothelial cells at birth is 6000 cell/mm^2. The cell count falls by 26% by first year and another 26% in the next 11 years.
10. In adults the normal number of endothelial cells are 2500–3000 cells/mm^2.
11. Megalocornea is the adult diameter of > 13 mm diameter.
12. Microcornea is the adult diameter of < 10 mm.
13. Corneal decompensation occurs when the total endothelial cells are <500 cells/mm^2 (i.e., when more than 75% of the cells are lost).
14. The water content of the cornea is around 80%. In corneal edema hydration becomes > than 80%, and transparency is lost.
15. Stroma comprises 90% of the corneal thickness.
16. Primary metabolism in the cornea is aerobic metabolism.
17. KF ring on the descements membrane of the cornea is reversible.
18. Snow blindness is caused by UV-B rays (285 nm–315 nm). Hence UV-B is more dangerous than UV-A rays.
19. Satellite nodules are feature of: Fungal keratitis.
20. Corneal tattooing is done by gold for brown colour and platinum for black color, but platinum is preferred.
21. Corneal epithelium is derived from surface ectoderm whereas the stroma and endothelium is derived from neural crest.
22. Most common nerve involved in HZO is frontal nerve.
23. Band-shaped keratopathy is caused by sarcoidosis as there is hypercalcemia.

24. Urrets–Zavalia syndrome is a triad of fixed dilated pupil, iris atrophy and secondary glaucoma. It occurs after keratoplasty in patients of keratoconus.
25. Total number of endothelial cell loss in DLEK, i.e., deep lamellar endothelial keratoplasty is 20%–25%.
26. Most common stromal dystrophy is lattice and most common corneal dystrophy is microcystic.
27. Least common corneal dystrophy is macular.
28. Arcus senilis occurs due to lipid deposition in the stroma of the cornea.
29. Percentage of acyclovir used for treating viral keratitis is 3% acyclovir eye ointment given 5 times/day.
30. Treatment of choice of fungal keratitis is Natamycin.
31. Bacterial keratitis resembling fungal infection is Nocardia.
32. Masson Trichome is used to stain granular dystrophy.
33. Most common infection after keratoplasty is staphylococcus epidermidis.
34. Minimal no. of endothelium cells required in a corneal graft is 1500–2000 cells/mm^2.
35. Congo red is used to stain lattice stromal dystrophy.
36. Colloidal iron and Alcian blue is used to stain Macular corneal dystrophy.
37. In Reis-Buckler dystrophy, the pathology lies in bowman's membrane.
38. Corneal dystrophy which is Autosomal Recessive: Macular.

MULTIPLE CHOICE QUESTIONS

1. Which of the following is the drug of choice for treatment of corneal ulcers caused by filamentous fungi?

A. Itraconazole
B. Natamycin
C. Nystatin
D. Fluconazole

2. Which of the following stromal dystrophy is a recessive condition?

A. Lattice dystrophy
B. Granular dystrophy
C. Macular dystrophy
D. Fleck dystrophy

3. Afferent component of corneal reflex is mediated by:

A. Vagus nerve
B. Facial nerve
C. Trigeminal nerve
D. Glossopharyngeal nerve

4. Enlarged corneal nerves may be seen in all of the following except:

A. Keratoconus
B. Herpes simplex keratitis
C. Leprosy
D. Neurofibromatosis

5. Which of the following statement is true regarding acanthamoeba keratitis?

A. For the isolation of the causative agent, corneal scraping should be cultured on a nutrient agar plate
B. The causative agent, Acanthamoeba is a helminth whose normal habitat is soil
C. Keratitis due to Acanthamoeba is not seen in the immunocompromised host
D. Acanthamoeba does not depend upon a human host for the completion of its life-cycle

6. Contact lens wear is proven to have deleterious effects on the corneal

physiology. Which of the following statements is incorrect in connection with contact lens wear?

A. The level of glucose availability in the corneal epithelium is reduced

B. There is reduction in hemidesmosomes density

C. There is increased production of CO_2 in the epithelium

D. There is reduction in glucose utilization by corneal epithelium

7. **A 12 years old girl with tremors and emotional liability has a golden brown discoloration of descements membrane. The most likely diagnosis is:**

A. Fabry's disease

B. Wilson's disease

C. Glycogen storage disease

D. Acute rheumatic fever

8. **Which of the following will be the most important adjuvant therapy in a case of fungal corneal ulcer?**

A. Atropine sulphate eye ointment

B. Dexamethasone eye drops

C. Pilocarpine eye drops

D. Lignocaine eye drops

9. **Snow blindness is caused by:**

A. Ultraviolet rays

B. Infrared rays

C. X-rays

D. Microwaves

10. **Corneal sensation is lost in:**

A. Herpes simplex

B. Conjunctivitis

C. Fungal infection

D. Trachoma

11. **Steroids are contraindicated in:**

A. Phylctenular conjunctivitis

B. Vernal conjunctivitis

C. Mooren's ulcer

D. Dendritic ulcer

12. **Dendritic ulcer is caused by:**

A. Mycetoma

B. Herpes simplex

C. Staphylococcus

D. Pneumococcus

13. **Satellite nodule on corneal ulcer is seen due to:**

A. Fungal B. Bacterial

C. Viral D. Mycoplasma

14. **Corneal transparency is maintained by all except:**

A. Hydration of corneal epithelium

B. Wide separated collagen fibres

C. Unmyelinated nerve fibres

D. Mitotic figures in the central cornea

15. **Corneal endothelium ion-exchange pumps are inhibited by:**

A. Inhibition of anaerobic glycolysis

B. Activation of anerobic glycolysis

C. Activation of cAMP phosphodiesterase inhibitors

D. Interference with electron chain transport

16. **Band-shaped keratopathy is caused by:**

A. Amyloid

B. Calcium

C. Monopolysaccharides

D. Lipid

17. **In human corneal transplantation, the donor tissue is:**

A. Synthetic polymer

B. Donated human cadaver eyes

C. Donated eyes from live human beings

D. Monkey eyes

18. A 56-year-old man has painful weeping rashes over the upper eyelid and forehead for the last 2 days along with ipsilateral acute punctate keratopathy. About a year back, he had chemotherapy for non-Hodgkin's lymphoma. There is no other abnormality. Which of the following is the most likely diagnosis?

A. Impetigo

B. Systemic lupus erythematosus

C. Herpes zoster

D. Pyoderma gangrenosum

19. A young man aged 30 years, presents with difficulty in vision in the left eye for the last 10 days. He is immunocompetent, a farmer by occupation, comes from a rural community and gives history of trauma to his left eye, with vegetative matter, 10–15 days back. On examination, there is an ulcerative lesion in the cornea, whose base has raised soft creamy infiltrates, ulcer margin is feathery and hyphate. There are a few satellite lesions also. The most probable aetiological agent is:

A. Acanthamoeba

B. Corynebacterium diphtheriae

C. Fusarium

D. Streptococcus pneumoniae

20. A 17 years old girl with keratitis and severe pain in the eye came to the hospital and Acanthamoeba keratitis was suspected. The patient gave the history of following four points. Out of these which is not a risk factor for acanthamoeba keratitis?

A. Extended wear contact lens

B. Exposure to dirty water

C. Corneal trauma

D. Squamous blepharitis

21. Chandresh Kumar, 15 years old boy has history of injury to the eye resulting in vegetative foreign body in the eye. Standard plating media did not yield any growth, but required addition of E col. Microscopic examination showed macrophage like structure. Culture did not yield any bacteria. Most likely cause is:

A. Acanthamoeba B. Virus

C. Chlamydia D. Aspergillus

22. Recurrent corneal erosion is a feature of:

A. Keratoglobus B. Keratoconus

C. Glaucoma D. Corneal dystrophy

23. Causes of corneal vascularisation:

A. Transplant rejection

B. Infection

C. Contact lens use

D. Corneal dystrophy

24. Features of fungal ulcer:

A. Symptoms more than signs

B. Dry ulcer

C. Diffuse corneal oedema

D. Hyphated margins

25. Features of vernal keratitis are:

A. Papillary hypertrophy

B. Follicular hypertrophy

C. Herbert's pits

D. Trantas' spots

E. Ciliary congestion

26. Clinical features of Vitamin A deficiency:

A. Color blindness
B. Bitot's spots
C. Xerophthalmia
D. Corneal opacity
E. Accommodation defects

27. Corneal nerves are visible in:

A. Diabetes
B. Leprosy
C. Corneal ulcer
D. Keratoconus

28. Corneal epithelium consists of:

A. Columnar epithelium
B. Stratified epithelium and keratinized
C. Pseudostratified and non-keratinized
D. Stratified and non-keratinized
E. Transitional epithelium

29. Herpes zoster ophthalmicus is a predictor of:

A. Leukemia B. Lymphoma
C. HIV D. Disseminated T.B.

30. Rx of dendritic ulcer:

A. Acyclovir B. Idoxuridine
C. Steroid D. Tetracycline
E. Trychophyton

31. Ophthalmia neonatorum is commonly caused by:

A. H. influenzae B. Staphylococcus
C. TRIC D. Gonococcus

32. True about keratoconus:

A. Munson sign seen
B. Protrusion of anterior cornea
C. Protrusion of posterior cornea
D. Fleisher's sign positive

33. Which of the following organism can penetrate the normal cornea?

A. Gonococcus
B. Pseudomonas
C. Diphtheria
D. Streptococcus
E. Staphylococcus epidermidis

34. True about keratoconus:

A. Increased curvature of cornea
B. Astigmatism
C. K.F. ring
D. Thick cornea
E. Soft contact lens is used

35. Which of the following is true about dendritic ulcer?

A. Caused by herpes simplex virus
B. Topical corticosteroid given suppresses the symptoms
C. Oral acyclovir is effective in treatment
D. Topical acyclovir is effective in treatment
E. Heals spontaneously

36. Treatment of photophthalmia:

A. Flush with saline
B. Apply pad and bandage
C. Topical antibiotics
D. Steroid eye drops

37. In keratoconus all are seen except:

A. Munson's sign
B. Thinning of cornea in center
C. Distortion of corneal reflex at center
D. Hypermetropic refractive error found

38. Avascular coat in eye is:

A. Sclera B. Cornea
C. Retina D. Choroid

39. Keratometer is used to assess:

A. Thickness of cornea

B. Refractive power

C. Astigmatism

D. Curvature of cornea

40. Brown skin cornea is seen in:

A. Siderosis

B. Mustard gas exposure

C. Chalcosis

D. Argyrosis

41. Ulcus serpens results from infection by:

A. Gonococcus

B. Pseudomonas pyocyanea

C. Pneumococcus

D. Proteus vulgaris

42. All are complications of herpes zoster ophthalmicus except:

A. Keratitis

B. Keratoconjunctivitis sicca

C. Uveitis

D. Necrotising retinitis

43. In bullous keratopathy there is damage to:

A. Epithelium

B. Stromal layer

C. Endothelium

D. Basal lamina

44. Pachymeter is useful to:

A. Study corneal endothelium

B. Study thickness of cornea

C. Measure depth of anterior chamber

D. Measure field of vision

45. Most common viral infection of the cornea is:

A. Herpes simplex

B. Herpes zoster

C. Adenovirus

D. Molluscum contagiosum

46. Most common presenting feature of Acanthamoeba infection is:

A. Eye discharge

B. Redness

C. Painful eye

D. Photophobia

47. Which of the following is not true about fungal keratitis?

A. Satellite lesions

B. Unsterile hypopyon

C. Symptoms more than sign

D. Most common cause is Aspergillus

48. Examination of the surface of cornea is done by:

A. Pachymeter

B. Specular microscopy

C. Gonioscope

D. Corneal topography

49. In infective keratitis, which of the following is not done?

A. Tarsorrhaphy

B. Keratoplasty

C. Paracentesis

D. Chemical cauterization

50. Hypopyon is seen in:

A. Pneumococcal infection

B. Gonococcal infection

C. Fungal infection

D. All of the above

51. Which of the following is not true about herpes keratitis?

A. Recurrent

B. Virus lies dormant in trigeminal ganglion

C. Primary infection usually self limiting

D. Topical steroids accelerate the recovery

52. Specular microscopy is done for:

A. Measuring depth of anterior chamber

B. Measuring angle of anterior chamber

C. Examining corneal endothelium

D. Measuring corneal curvature

53. Corneal guttata is seen in:

A. Endothelial corneal dystrophy

B. Epithelial corneal dystrophy

C. Corneal abrasion

D. Vitamin A deficiency

54. Exposure keratitis is seen in paralysis of cranial nerve:

A. III B. IV

C. V D. VII

55. Herpetic corneal ulcer is diagnosed by:

A. Giemsa stain

B. ELISA

C. Cell culture/PCR

D. Rose Bengal stain

56. Copper deposition in K.F. ring is seen in:

A. Descements membrane

B. Endothelium

C. Stroma

D. Epithelium

57. Maximum vision loss will occur in:

A. Central leucoma

B. Central nebula

C. Adherent leucoma

D. Peripheral leucoma

58. Band shaped keratopathy is caused by:

A. Vitamin D intoxication

B. Neuroparalytic keratitis

C. Facial palsy

D. Diabetes

59. Steroids are contraindicated in dendritic ulcer because of increased chance of:

A. Perforation B. Corneal ulcer

C. Glaucoma D. Cataract

60. To measure anterior chamber depth, Pachymeter uses the following Purkinje-Samson images:

A. I and II B. II and III

C. III and IV D. I and IV

61. Type of contact lenses used in bullous keratopathy:

A. Soft (Bandage Soft)

B. Hard

C. Gas permeable

D. All of the above

62. A patient with corneal opacity shows improved vision with stenopic slit at 45°. The optical iridectomy should be performed at:

A. 45° B. 90°

C. 135° D. 180°

63. Fleischer's ring is seen in:

A. Intraocular copper containing foreign body

B. Intraocular iron containing foreign body

C. Wilson's disease

D. Keratoconus

64. Common cause of exposure keratitis is:

A. Tuberculosis B. Syphilis

C. Leprosy D. AIDS

65. Hypopyon ulcer is treated by all except:

A. Atropine

B. Antibiotic

C. Antifungal

D. Pad and Bandage

66. Thickened corneal nerves are seen in:

A. TB

B. Leprosy

C. Keratoconus

D. Both B and C

67. Which of the following is a corneal epithelial dystrophy?

A. Dot print B. Macular

C. Granular D. Lattice

68. Munson sign is seen in:

A. Keratconus B. Keratoglobus

C. High myopia D. Keratoplasty

69. A soft contact lens wearer developed pain and itching of the eye and shows a reticular pattern on the corneal epithelium. The cause could be:

A. Corneal dystrophy

B. Acanthamoeba

C. Pseudomonas

D. Recurrent

70. Most common causative organism of corneal ulcer:

A. Pneumococci B. Staphylococci

C. Streptococci D. Fungi

71. Dellen is:

A. Localised thinning of peripheral cornea

B. Raised lesions in coneolimbal junction

C. Age related macular degeneration

D. Marginal keratitis

72. Earliest symptom in corneal ulcer:

A. Loss of sensation

B. Photophobia

C. Pain

D. Diminished vision

73. Treatment of choice in leucoma of cornea is:

A. Lamellar keratoplasty

B. Penetrating keratoplasty

C. Tattooing

D. Laser excision

74. For transplantation cornea is preserved in:

A. Modified MK medium

B. Cryopreservation

C. Dexol medium

D. All of the above

75. Interstitial keratitis in an 8 years old girl can occur in all of the following conditions except:

A. Tuberculosis

B. Leprosy

C. Filaria

D. Syphilis

76. Cornea melts without inflammation in:

A. Gout

B. Keratomalacia

C. SLE

D. Rhematoid arthritis

77. 0.1 to 0.2 mm nebular corneal opacity is treated by:

A. Penetrating keratoplasty

B. Lamellar keratoplasty

C. Laser excision

D. Tattooing

78. Corneal layer responsible for detergescence:

A. Bowman's membrane
B. Endothelium
C. Descements membrane
D. Epithelium

79. A 28 years old male complains of glare in both eyes. The cornea shows whorl like opacities of the epithelium. He also gave history of long-term treatment with amiodarone. The most likely diagnosis is:

A. Terrains marginal degeneration
B. Cornea verticillata
C. Band shaped keratopathy
D. Arcus juvenilis

80. The following bacteria can invade intact corneal epithelium except:

A. Neisseria gonorrhoea
B. Haemophilus influenzae
C. Staphylococcus aureus
D. Listeria

81. Penetrating keratoplasty is least effective in:

A. Pterygium
B. Keratoconus
C. Bullous keratopathy
D. Corneal dystrophy

82. Endothelial cell of cornea is derived from:

A. Mesoderm
B. Ectoderm
C. Endoderm
D. Neural crest

83. EDTA is used in treatment of:

A. Band shaped keratopathy
B. Lipid keratopathy
C. Neurotrophic keratopathy
D. All of the above

84. In Fanconi's disease, deposits in cornea is due to:

A. Cystine B. Copper
C. Gold D. Iron

85. Drug not deposited in cornea:

A. Gold
B. Chloroquine
C. Amiodarone
D. Antimony

86. Stocker's line are seen in:

A. Pterygium
B. Pinguecula
C. External hordeolum
D. Congenital ocular melanosis

87. The organism that penetrates the normal cornea is:

A. Pneumococcus
B. Pseudomonas
C. Gonococcus
D. Chlamydia trachomatis

88. In human corneal transplantation, the donor tissue is:

A. Synthetic polymer
B. Donated human cadaver eyes
C. Donated eyes from live human beings
D. Monkey eyes

89. Dendritic ulcers are caused by:

A. Gonococcus
B. Aspergillus
C. Herpes simplex
D. Adenovirus

90. Corneal dystrophies are:

A. Autoimmune in etiology
B. Associated with vascularity

C. Associated with systemic diseases

D. Hereditary

91. Bullous keratopathy can result from:

A. Keratoplasty

B. Chemical injury

C. Corneal dystrophy

D. Cataract surgery

92. Photophthalmia is caused by:

A. Excimer lasor

B. Ultraviolet rays

C. Infra-red rays

D. Pan retinal photocoagulation

93. Treatment of persistent epithelial defect is:

A. Corneal graft

B. Local steroids

C. Soft contact lens

D. Tarsorrhaphy

94. Ulcus serpens is caused by:

A. Pseudomonas pyocynaceous

B. Cornybacterium

C. Pneumococcus

D. Gonorrhoea

95. All of the following occur in herpes zoster ophthalmicus except:

A. Pseudodendritic keratitis

B. Anterior stromal invasion

C. Sclerokeratitis

D. Endothelitis

96. What is percentage of endothelial cell loss during Descement's membrane stripping in automated penetrating keratoplasty?

A. 0–5%

B. 10–15%

C. 30–40%

D. 50–60%

97. Corneal dystrophies are degenerations that are usually:

A. Primary and bilateral

B. Primary and unilateral

C. Primary, bilateral, with systemic involvement

D. Primary, unilateral, without systemic involvement

98. An immunocompetent male presents with difficulty in vision. He gives history of vegetative material fallen in affected eye. On examination corneal ulcer with feathery margin and creamy exudate seen. Few satellite lesions were also noted. Likely diagnosis is:

A. Fusarium

B. Acanthamoeba

C. Pneumococci

D. Corynebacterium

99. A regular contact lens user presents with complains of redness, photophobia and blurring of vision in one eye for more than 2 weeks, which was not responding to normal treatment. On examination cornea shows ring shaped lesion along with some overlying epithelial defect. Probable diagnosis would be:

A. Fungal keratitis

B. Viral keratitis

C. Acanthamoeba keratitis

D. Bacterial ulcer

100. Which of the following topical eyedrops cannot be used in a patient with keratitis?

A. Fluorometholone

B. Olopatadine

C. Methylcellulose

D. Chlorophenicol

101. The combination of a fixed dilated pupil with iris atrophy and secondary glaucoma following penetrating keratoplasty is known as:

A. Kaufmann's syndrome

B. Urrets-Zavalia syndrome

C. Benedict's triad

D. Posmann-Schlosmann syndrome

102. Under hypoxic conditions, which of the following substances is strongly implicated as a cause of corneal edema?

A. Lactate

B. Glycogen

C. Carbon dioxide

D. Pyruvate

103. A diagnosis of fungal corneal ulcer is not made if there is presence of:

A. Marked photophobia and pain compared to signs

B. Sloughing corneal ulcer

C. Fixed hypopyon

D. Presence of hyphae on KOH mounts

104. A patient presents to the OPD and a diagnosis of fungal keratomycosis is made. Which of the following drugs would be effective in him?

A. Doxycycline

B. Silver sulfadiazine

C. Vancomycin

D. Linezolid

105. Not an absolute contraindication for corneal transplantation is:

A. subacute sclerosing panencephalitis

B. Rabies

C. Tubercular meningitis

D. Death due to unknown cause

106. Band-shaped keratopathy shows deposition of which of the following?

A. Melanin B. Iron

C. Amyloid D. Calcium

107. Which organismal infection is highly virulent and may cause corneal ulcer perforation within 48 hours?

A. Herpes simplex

B. Pseudomonas

C. Staphylococci

D. Aspergillus

108. Circumcorneal neovascularization is observed in deficiency of:

A. Vitamin D B. Thiamine

C. Riboflavin D. Biotin

109. A patient gives a history of chuna falling into his eyes. All of the following would be a part of his immediate management except:

A. Irrigation of both eyes with copious amounts of normal saline

B. Frequent sodium citrate drops

C. Thorough slit-lamp examination on presentation

D. Removal of chuna particles by double eversion of upper eyelids

110. In herpes zoster ophthalmicus least involved nerve is:

A. Facial

B. Infraorbital

C. Lacrimal

D. Nasociliary

111. Which organism can penetrate the intact cornea?

A. N. meningitidis

B. Pseudomonas

C. Staphylococcus

D. Klebsiella

112. Neuroparalytic keratitis is due to which cranial nerve?

A. 3rd nerve B. 5th nerve
C. 6th nerve D. 7th nerve

113. Steroids are contraindicated in:

A. Uveitis
B. Herpetic keratitis
C. Bacterial keratitis
D. None

114. Corneal ulcer resembling fungal ulcer is seen in infection with which of the agents?

A. Nocardia asteroids
B. Mycobacterium
C. Klebsiella pneumonia
D. Chlamydia trachomatis

115. A 33 years old male came with pain and watering in the right eye for 36 hours. On examination a 3 × 2 cm corneal ulcer is seen with elevated margins, feathery hyphae, finger like projections and minimal hypopyon in cornea. What is the likely causative organism?

A. HSV-1
B. Aspergillosis
C. Acanthamoeba
D. Pseudomonas

116. A diagnosis of fungal corneal ulcer is not made if there is presence of:

A. Marked photophobia and pain compared to signs
B. Sloughing corneal ulcer
C. Fixed hypopyon
D. Presence of hyphae on KOH mount

117. A patient presents to the OPD and a diagnosis of fungal keratomycosis is made. Which of the following drugs would be effective in him?

A. Doxycycline
B. Silver sulfadiazine
C. Vancomycin
D. Linezolid

118. Not an absolute contraindication for corneal transplantation is:

A. Subacute sclerosing panencephalitis
B. Rabies
C. Tubercular meningitis
D. Death due to unknown cause

119. Universal marker of limbal epithelial stem cells:

A. Elastin
B. Keratin
C. Collagen
D. ABCG2

120. Which stain is used for diagnosis of Granular dystrophy of cornea?

A. Masson trichome
B. Congo red
C. Colloidal iron
D. Pas

121. All of the following drugs cause amorphous whorl like corneal opacities except:

A. Amiodarone
B. Chloroquine
C. Indomethacin
D. Chlorpromazine

ANSWER AND EXPLANATION

1. b Natamycin is most effective against Aspergillus fumigates and other hyphate fungi.

2. c All the corneal dystrophies are autosomal dominant except Macular dystrophy.

3. c Sensory supply to the eye is by trigeminal nerve.
4. a In keratoconus, corneal nerves are prominent due to thinning of the cornea and not due to thickening of the corneal nerves.
5. d Acanthamoeba is a ubiquitous protozoa, cultured in non-nutrient agar with E. coli. Keratitis is rare but can occur in soft contact lens users and immunocompromised patients.
6. a Contact lens use decreases the oxygen supply to the cornea and hence it is the glucose utilization which is hampered and not the glucose supply.
7. b Golden brown discolouration is the Kayser-Fleicher ring in patients of Wilson's disease.
8. a Corneal ulcer whether fungal or due to any other cause, can affect the uvea causing associated uveitis. Hence Atropine is given.
9. a Snow blindness also called Photophthalmia is UV injury to the eye. It causes corneal epithelial erosion.
10. a Pathognomic feature of viral keratitis is decreased corneal sensation.
11. d Steroids are contraindicated in any infective pathology of the cornea.
12. b DU is a feature of herpes simplex. A dendritic ulcer has knobbed ends.
13. a Satellite nodules are small lesions away from the main ulcer. It is a feature of fungal corneal ulcer.
14. a Hydration of any layer of the cornea is the most important factor to decrease the transparency of the cornea.
15. b Activation of the anaerobic glycolysis leads to accumulation of lactic acid which causes metabolic acidosis leading to the inhibition of the endothelium pump.
16. b Band-shaped keratopathy is accumulation of calcium on the cornea.
17. b Donor cornea is taken from the cadaveric eyes.
18. c Herpes zoster is characterized by skin lesions, eye lesions and trigeminal neuralgia.
19. c Fungal corneal ulcer is common in farmers and most commonly occurs due to trauma by a vegetative matter.
20. d Squamous blepharitis is not a risk factor of Acanthamoeba keratitis. It occurs due to dandruffs in the head.
21. d Aspergillus fumigates is the most common fungus infecting cornea in India.
22. d Reccurrent corneal erosion is a feature of epithelial corneal dystrophy.
23. a,b,c Corneal vascularisation is not a feature of corneal dystrophies. Corneal dystrophy is an idiopathic spontaneous change with no inflammatory component.
24. b,d In fungal corneal ulcer signs are more than symptoms.
25. a,d Vernal keratitis is characterized by only papillary reaction, no follicular reaction.
26. b,c Vitamin A deficiency causes epithelial xerosis. Patient complains of night blindness.
27. b,d In leprosy there is thickening of the nerves whereas in keratoconus there is thinning of the cornea.
28. a,d Corneal epithelium is stratified columnar non-keratinized.

29.	a,b,c,d	HZO is more common in immunocompromised patients.
30.	a,b	Other antivirals are: Trifluorothymidine and Adenine Arabinoside.
31.	b,c,d	Ophthalmia neonatorum is any conjunctivitis within one month of age.
32.	a,b,c,d	Keratoconus is conical protrusion of both anterior and posterior cornea.
33.	a,c	Organisms that can penetrate the normal cornea are: chlamydia, gonorrhea, haemophilus and listeria.
34.	a,b	KF ring is a feature of chalcosis whereas Fleischers ring is a feature of keratoconus.
35.	a,d	Steroids are contraindicated in dendritic ulcer. Oral therapy is not needed in simplex infection; it is required in zoster infections.
36.	b,c	Photophthalmia presents as corneal epithelial erosions and is treated by pad and bandage with antibiotic ointment.
37.	d	Protrusion of the cornea will lead to myopia and not hypermetropia.
38.	b	Both cornea and lens are avascular structures of the eye.
39.	c,d	Thickness of the cornea is measured by pachymetry whereas refractive power is seen by retinoscopy.
40.	a,c,d	Brown skin cornea is the brown discoloration of the cornea. It occurs due to deposition of gold, silver and can also be seen in oculodermal melanocytosis.
41.	c	Pneumococcus causes 'Hypopyon Corneal Ulcer'.
42.	b	KCS is dry eye due to aqueous layer deficiency. It is generally associated with connective tissue disorders.
43.	a	Fluid-filled bullae are formed on the epithelial layer of the cornea due to endothelial dysfunction.
44.	b	Corneal endothelium is studied by specular microscopy.
45.	a	Herpes simplex is more common than Herpes zoster.
46.	c	Pain in acanthamoeba keratitis is disproportionately large due to perineural invasion.
47.	c	Signs are more than symptoms in fungal ulcers.
48.	d	Corneal curvature is measured by both corneal topography and keratometry.
49.	a	Eye should never be patched or covered by tarsorrhaphy in infective pathology.
50.	d	Pus cells in the anterior chamber are known as hypopyon whereas blood in the anterior chamber is called hyphema.
51.	d	Steroids are contraindicated in infective pathology. It is given in herpes infection when there is only disciform keratitis, with no stromal or epithelial involvement.
52.	c	Both quantity and morphology of the endothelial cells are assessed by specular microscopy.
53.	a	Corneal guttatae are collagenous protruberances on the central endothelial cells seen in Fuch's endothelial dystrophy.
54.	d	7th nerve palsy leads to lagophthalmos which causes exposure keratitis.
55.	c	PCR is the best method to diagnose the viral infections.

56.	a	KF ring is seen in descements membrane whereas Fleischers ring is iron deposition in the epithelial layer.
57.	b	Nebular corneal opacity diffracts light and hence disturbs the functioning of the clear cornea leading to marked dimunition of vision.
58.	a	BSK occurs in hypercalcemia. Vitamin D aids in the absorption of the calcium.
59.	b	Giving steroids in dendritic ulcer, leads to geographical ulcer which can later lead to perforation.
60.	b	Image II is the image formed on the back surface of the cornea, whereas image III is formed on the anterior surface of the lens.
61.	a	Bandage contact lens is a soft contact lens used for therapeutic purpose.
62.	a	Iridectomy should be done at the angle of improved vision where corneal opacity is not disturbing the vision. It will act as an additional pupil.
63.	d	Fleischers ring is formed at the base of the cone in patients of keratoconus.
64.	c	Leprosy causes lagophthalmos and also decreases the corneal sensation leading to exposure keratopathy.
65.	d	We should never patch the eye in infective pathology. Patching is done in corneal epithelial erosions.
66.	b	Thickening of the corneal nerves is seen in leprosy and NF-1.
67.	a	Epithelial dystrophies are–Microcystic (i.e., dot print), Meesmans and Reis-buckler.
68.	a	Munson sign is V shaped deformity of the lower lid on looking down, due to conical protrusion of the cornea.
69.	b	Points in favour of acanthamoeba are–soft lens user, pain and reticular pattern in the epithelial layer.
70.	b	Most common cause of infection is staphylococcus.
71.	a	Dellen is a localized thinning of the peripheral cornea which occurs due to raised limbal lesions, or due to hard contact lens or can be idiopathic. It occurs due to instability of the tear film.
72.	b	Photophobia occurs due to trigeminal nerve.
73.	b	Leucoma is a full thickness scarring and hence we do penetrating keratoplasty (i.e., full thickness replacement of the cornea). Lamellar keratoplasty is a partial thickness replacement of the cornea.
74.	d	McKaufmann medium and Dexol are used for intermediate term storage, whereas cryopreservation is a method of long term storage.
75.	c	Other causes of IK are sarcoidosis and Cogans syndrome (IK with deafness).
76.	b	Keratomalacia is melting of the cornea due to vitamin A deficiency.
77.	b	Normal thickness of the cornea is 0.5–0.6 mm. Hence a nebular opacity involving upto 0.1–0.2 mm can be managed by lamellar keratoplasty.
78.	b	It is the pump function of the endothelial cells which is responsible for maintaining the cornea in a dehydrated state.
79.	b	Cornea verticillata is also known as Vortex keratopathy. It occurs due to chloroquine, amiodarone, tamoxifen and Fabry's disease.

80. c Haemophilus can also penetrate the intact cornea.

81. a PK is not needed in pterygium. The best prognosis of PK is in keratoconus followed by corneal dystrophies and bullous keratopathy.

82. d Corneal epithelium is derived from surface ectoderm whereas stroma and endothelium from neural crest.

83. a Chelation is the choice of treatment of band-shaped keratopathy. EDTA and sodium versenate are used.

84. a Fanconi's disease is a pathology of renal tubules. Also called infantile nephropathic cystinosis, it is characterized by corneal crystal (cystine) accumulation and pigmentary retinopathy.

85. d Gold deposition in the cornea is known as chrysiasis. Amiodarone and chloroquine causes vortex keratopathy.

86. a Stocker's line is iron deposition at the head of the pterygium.

87. c Other organisms that penetrate the intact cornea are: diphtheria, haemophilus and listeria.

88. b Donor cornea should be taken out from the cadaveric eyes preferably after 6 hours but may be extended till 12 hours.

89. c Dendritic ulcers are ulcers with knobbed ends caused by HSV.

90. d Corneal dystrophies are all autosomal dominant except for macular dystrophy which is autosomal recessive.

91. d Most common cause of bullous keratopathy is postoperative. It is also a feature of endothelial dystrophy, i.e., Fuchs endothelial dystrophy.

92. b Photophthalmia is also known as "Snow-Blindness".

93. c Bandage contact lenses are soft contact lenses used for therapeutic purpose. It shields the epithelium from the lid movements.

94. c Ulcus serpens is the ulcer of pneumococcus, and progresses in a serpentine manner.

95. c All four options given in the question are correct but since sclerokeratitis is least common, we mark it as the answer.

96. c DSAEK is a procedure which involves stripping of the diseased endothelium and descements membrane with the donor graft which comprises endothelium, descements membrane and a small strip of posterior stroma. This donor graft is harvested with a automated keratome. Since no sutures are required, postop refractive error is least and the rehabilitation time is less compared to conventional penetrating keratoplasty (PK). The endothelial loss is more compared to PK and ranges from more than 20% to 25%, hence we mark the answer c.

97. a Mostly corneal dystrophies are primary and bilateral. Since not all dystrophies are associated with systemic disease, hence we mark the answer as a.

98. a The history of trauma by a vegetative matter, feathery margins of the cornea and satellite nodules, all are strongly suggestive of a fungal infection in the cornea. Common etiological agents are Aspergillus fumigatus and fusarium.

99. c Infection in contact lens user not responding to the normal treatment, most probable diagnosis is acanthamoeba keratitis. Also acanthamoeba can present either as a ring lesion or pseudodendrites.

100. a Steroids are contraindicated in keratitis except when it is allergic in origin.

101. b It is a rare complication after keratoplasty in patients with keratoconus. The rise of intraocular pressure postoperatively leads to iris ischemia due to occlusion of iris root vessels; this causes the fixed dilated pupil with iris atrophy. Patients of keratoconus have some iris abnormality, which predisposes them to this complication.

102. a In hypoxic conditions, there is anaerobic glycolysis, which leads to lactic acid accumulation and hence metabolic acidosis. This causes inhibition of endothelial Na/K pump causing corneal edema.

103. a In fungal keratitis signs are more than symptoms.

104. b Topical silver sulphadiazine ointment is the new drug for keratomycosis.

105. c All the other three options are absolute contraindication. Meningitis of unknown cause is also an absolute contraindication.

106. d Calcium deposition in form of a band on the cornea between epithelium and bowman's membrane is band shaped keratopathy.

107. b Pseudomonas.

108. c If there is mild damage of corneal epithelium, it needs more nutrition for repair, but if there is riboflavin deficiency, then respiratory enzymes to epithelium is insufficient leading to neovascularisation. Abnormal blood vessels are seen in the limbus. Diagnosis is confirmed by blood test and marked improvement in symptoms on treatment with riboflavin.

109. c Slit lamp examination should not be the IMMEDIATE management. In alkali injury, when sodium citrate is given, it chelates with calcium and in low calcium environment, polymorphonuclear cells secrete less proteolytic enzymes, hence ulceration is less. Ideally a combination of ascorbate and citrate is given.

110. a Most commonly involved nerve is frontal nerve.

111. a Both N gonorrhoea and N meningitidis can penetrate intact cornea.

112. d Neuroparalytic keratitis occurs due to seventh nerve palsy.

113. c In herpes simplex infection, if patient presents only with disciform keratitis, with no involvement of epithelium or endothelium then we can give steroids under antiviral cover.

114. a In nocardia keratitis, the initial presentation resembles fungal keratitis and needs laboratory investigations.

115. b Feathery hyphae, and finger like projections, are diagnostic of fungal.

116. a Signs are more than symptoms in fungal keratitis.

- It is commonly due to *Aspergillus*, *Fusarium*, or *Candida albicans*.
- The slough in these ulcers is dry in appearance with feathery

borders, surrounded by a yellow line of demarcation which gradually deepens into a gutter, and there may also be a hypopyon.

- The hypopyon, if present is thick and immobile, and is due to direct invasion into the anterior chamber of fungal hyphae enmeshed in thick exudates.

117. b Silver sulfadiazine is a new line of treatment and very effective for fungal keratitis.

118. c It is not an ABSOLUTE contraindication.

119. d It is the universal marker for limbal stem cells.

120. a In granular dystrophy there are hyaline deposits which stain with Masson trichrome.

In macular dystrophy there are depositions of glycosaminoglycans that stain with colloidal iron or alcian blue.

In lattice dystrophy there are amyloid deposits that stain with Congo Red.

121. d All the options are correct but least common is chlorpromazine. So let's mark that. Vortex keratopathy or cornea verticillata is a whorl like deposition of the drug on the cornea. It is an innocuous condition and does not cause diminution of vision.

RECENTLY ADDED QUESTIONS

1. The cause(s) of hypopyon may include: (PGI)

A. Retinitis pigmentosa
B. Fungal keratitis
C. Episcleritis
D. Gonococcal keratitis
E. Multiple sclerosis

2. Stenopic slit is used for all except:

A. Fincham's test
B. Determine the axis of cylinder
C. Corneal tattooing
D. Iridectomy

3. A 33-year-old male came with pain and watering in the right eye for 36 hours. On examination a 3 × 2 cm corneal ulcer is seen with elevated margins, feathery hyphae, finger like projections and minimal hypopyon in cornea. What is the likely causative organism?

A. HSV-1
B. Aspergillosis
C. Acanthamoeba
D. Pseudomonas

4. Decreased corneal sensitivity is seen in: (PGI)

A. Acanthamoeba keratitis
B. Herpes simplex keratitis
C. Viral keratitis
D. Leprotic involvement
E. Post-keratoplasty

5. Which of the following is used as an adjuvant therapy for fungal corneal ulcer?

A. Atropine eye drops
B. Pilocarpine eye drops
C. Dexamethasone
D. Lidocaine

6. Which of the following is the marker for limbal stem cells?

A. ABCG2

B. P63

C. PAX 6

D. Cadherin

7. Which of the following is the most common fungal infection of the eye seen in an HIV positive patient?

a. Aspergillus

b. Candida

c. Toxoplasma

d. Rhinosporidium

8. True regarding fungal corneal ulcer is/are all except: (PGI)

A. Flat and mobile hypopyon

B. Satellite lesions around the ulcer

C. Mucopurulent discharge may be seen

D. Fungi penetrate into the anterior chamber without perforation

E. Wessley ring present

ANSWERS OF RECENTLY ADDED QUESTIONS

1. b,d Hypopyon is the accumulation of neutrophils in the lower angle of anterior chamber. It usually indicates iritis, i.e., anterior uveitis.

   Causes include iris infections caused by:
   - Corneal ulcers/Keratitis (Most common cause): Bacterial as well as fungal.
   - TB.
   - HSV and VZV infections.
   - Lyme disease.
   - Psoriatic arthritis.
   - Behcet's disease.

2. c Corneal tattooing is done to colour the corneal opacity. Which is not hampering the vision and is only a cosmetic problem. It is done by gold and platinum.

3. b Aspergillosis: A corneal ulcer with feathery hyphae and minimal hypopyon, the cause has to be fungus.

4. a,b, c,d, e **Causes of reduced corneal sensitivity:**
   - Herpes simplex keratitis.
   - Viral keratitis.
   - Neuroparalytic keratitis.
   - Leprosy.
   - Cocaine abuse.
   - Surgical trauma.
   - Multiple sclerosis.
   - Riley-Day syndrome.
   - Acanthamoeba keratitis.

   Post endothelial keratoplasty, full corneal sensitivity is not regained.

5. a Atropine is useful for the associated uveitis along with keratitis.

6. a ABCG2 and ABCB5 are known limbal stem cell markers.

7. b Candida: Fungal species known to cause keratitis in HIV/AIDS patients include Candida albicans and Aspergillus. Cryptococcus neoformans is another fungus that can cause eye problems.

   Candida albicans is the most common causative organism and is prevalent among IV drug users.

8. a **Fungal corneal ulcer:**
   - Mostly caused by Aspergillus, followed by Candida and fusarium.
   - Symptoms same as bacterial corneal ulcer but less marked.

- Signs include:
  - Dry-looking, grey-white ulcer with rolled out margins.
  - A sterile immune ring of Wessley.
  - Delicate, feather-like extensions into the stroma, under the intact epithelium.
  - A big hypopyon, which is thick and immobile.
  - Multiple satellite lesions.
  - Fungi can penetrate the anterior chamber without perforation.
  - Corneal vascularization is absent.

IMAGE-BASED QUESTIONS

1. **The diagnosis is:**

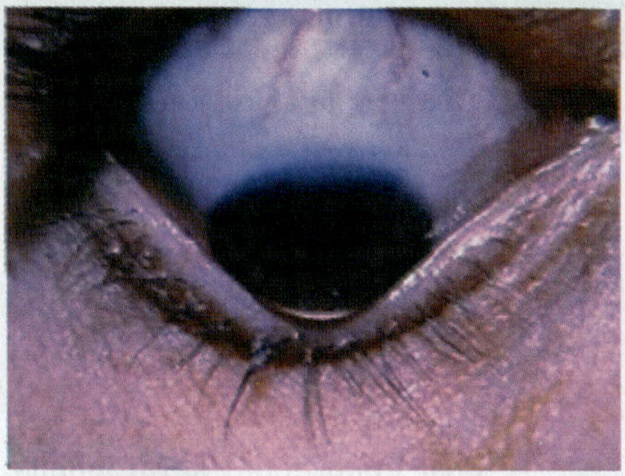

A. Ectropion
B. Keratoconus
C. Keratoglobus
D. Symblepharon

2. **The diagnosis is:**

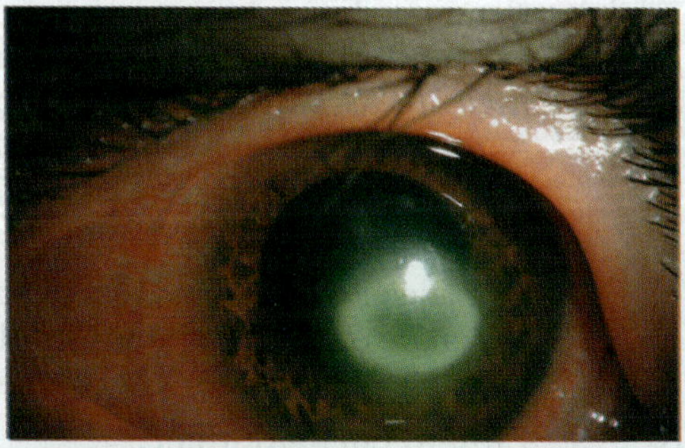

A. Bacterial keratitis
B. Fungal keratitis
C. Acanthamoebal keratitis
D. Viral keratitis

3. **Calcium deposition is:**

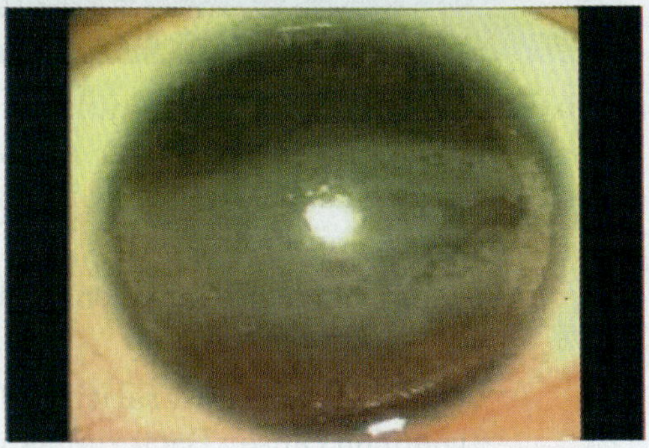

A. Epithelial B. Sub-epithelial
C. Stromal D. Endothelial

4. **The following patient presented with pain, redness, photophobia and dimunition of vision. He gave the history of trauma by a twig. What is the treatment of choice?**

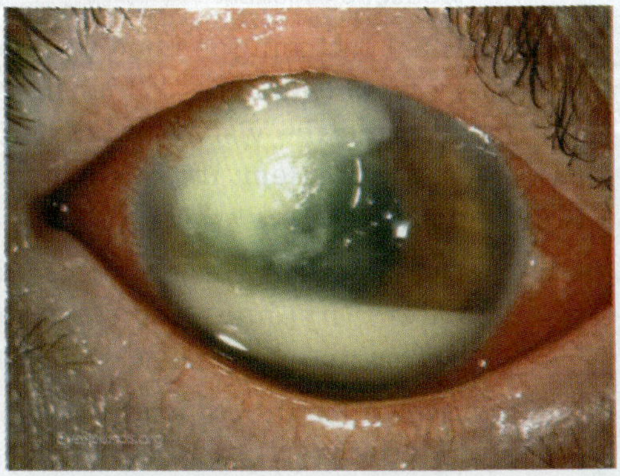

A. Ciplox eye drops B. Natamycin
C. Fluconazole D. Acyclovir

5. **The treatment is:**

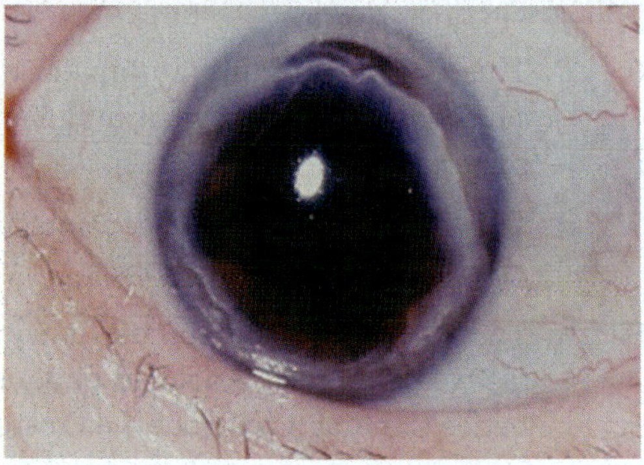

A. Antibiotics B. Steroids
C. Antivirals D. Antifungals

6. **The cause is:**

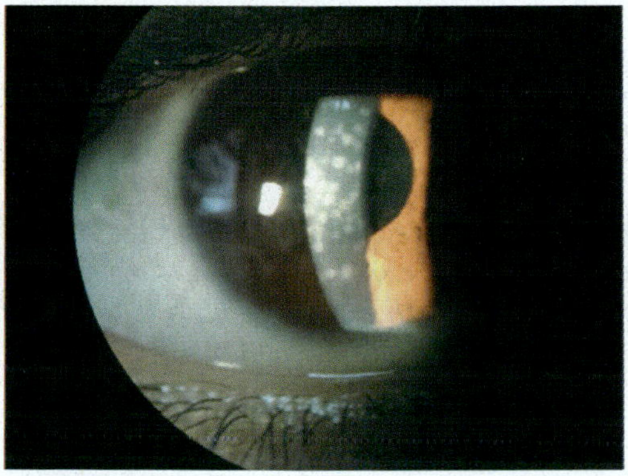

A. Adenovirus B. Herpes zoster
C. Both D. None

7. **The following instrument is used for:**

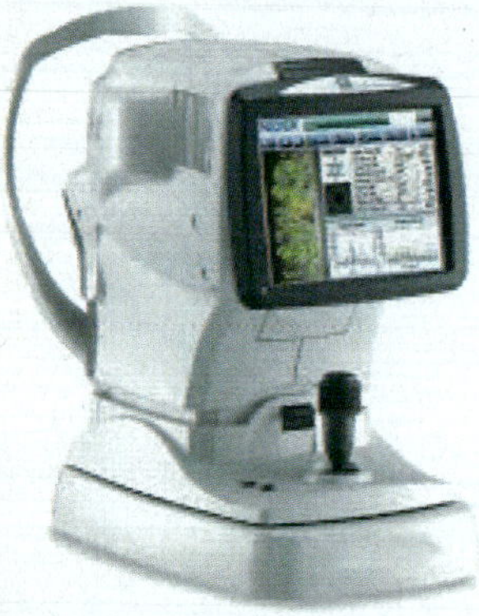

A. Pachymetre
B. Keratometre
C. Corneal topography
D. Specular microscopy

8. **The diagnosis is:**

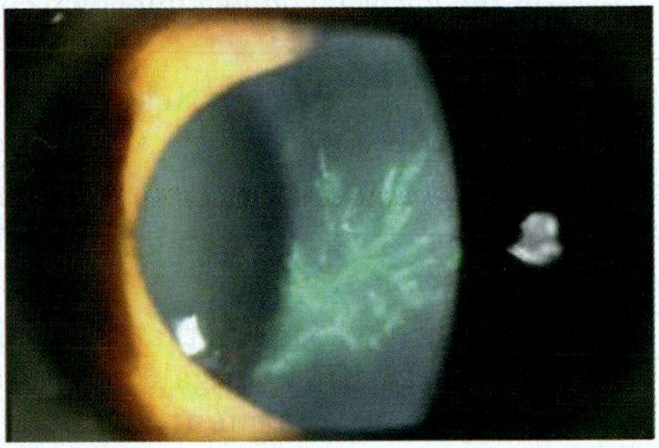

A. Herpes simplex
B. Herpes zoster
C. Adenovirus
D. Coxsackie virus

9. **The instrument is:**

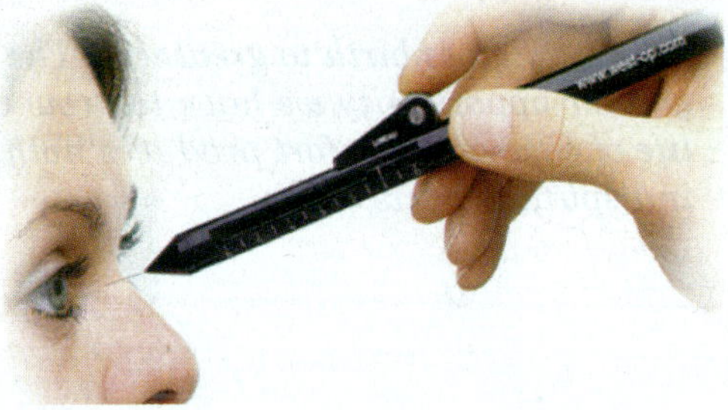

A. Tonopen B. Syringing
C. Aesthesiometer D. Tonography

10. **In the following patient suffering from keratoconus, the diagnosis is:**

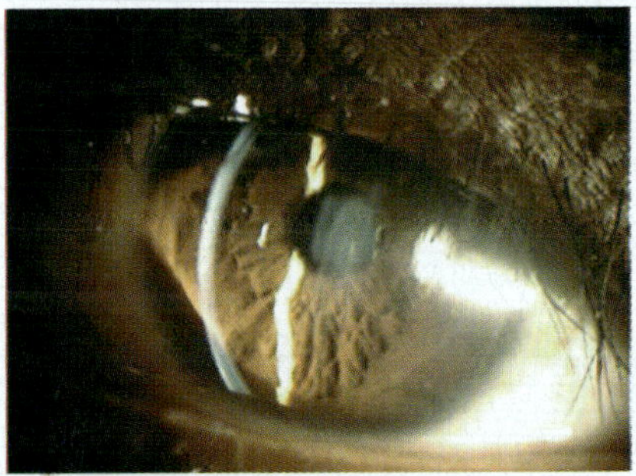

A. Munsons sign B. Scissors reflex
C. Rizutti's sign D. Vogts striae

ANSWERS OF IMAGE-BASED QUESTIONS

1. b The slide depicts "v" shaped deformity of the lower lid on looking down called MUNSONS SIGN.
2. c It's a ring ulcer of acanthamoeba keratitis.
3. b This is band-shaped keratopathy due to calcium deposition and is deposited sub-epithelial.
4. b The history suggests that the patient is suffering from fungal keratitis and hence the treatment of choice is natamycin.
5. b The above clinical slide is Moorens ulcer which has autoimmune etiology and hence the treatment is steroids.
6. c This is a slide of nummular keratitis caused by both adenovirus and herpes zoster.
7. d This is specular microscopy used to examine the endothelial cells.
8. b The above slide shows pseudo dendrites (as we cannot see knobbed ends) and hence the diagnosis is herpes zoster.
9. c The slide shows aesthesiometer that is used to see the corneal sensation.
10. c Rizutti's sign: Light thrown temporally falls in an arrow head pattern on the nasal limbus.

GUIDANCE

Adversity gives birth to greatness. The greater the challenges and difficulties we face, the greater opportunity we have to grow and develop as people. A life without adversity, a life of ease and comfort produces nothing and leaves us with nothing. This is one of the indisputable facts of life.

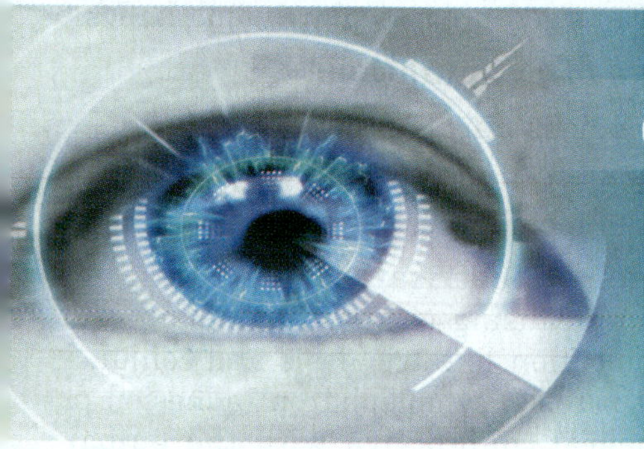

CHAPTER 4

Conjunctiva

Anatomy of Conjunctiva

Histologically, conjunctiva consists of three layers:

1. Epithelium.
2. Adenoid layer.
3. Fibrous layer.

Layers of Conjunctiva

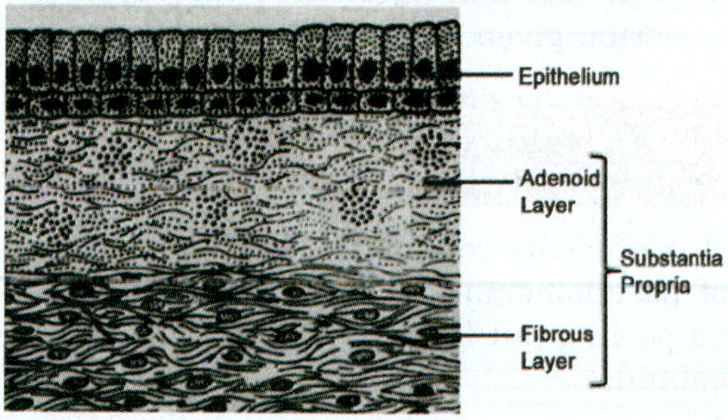

Fig. 4.1

Epithelium

This layer consists of:

a. Layer of epithelial cells.

b. *Goblet cells:* These are present between the epithelial cells in all regions of conjunctiva. These are mucin-secreting glands. **The maximum density of goblet cells is on nasal bulbar conjunctiva and then in inferior fornix.**

c. *Melanocytes.*

d. *Langerhans cells:* They are not phagocytic but function in antigenic presentation, lymphokine and prostaglandin production.

Adenoid layer: It is also called lymphoid layer; and consists of fine connective tissue reticulum in the meshes of which lie lymphocytes.

Fibrous layer: It consists of meshwork of collagenous and elastic fibres. It contains vessels and nerves of conjunctiva. **Adenoid layer and fibrous layer are collectively known as propria.**

Conjunctivitis: Inflammation of the conjunctiva, i.e., conjunctivitis is defined as conjunctival hyperaemia associated with discharge which may be watery, mucoid, mucopurulent or purulent.

Clinical Features:

- Conjunctival congestion.
- FB sensation.
- Mild photophobia.
- Irritation and discomfort in eye.
- Discharge.
- Blurring of vision and halos (if mucopurulent discharge).
- Chemosis.

- Petechial haemorrhages (pneumococcal etiology).
- Subconjunctival haemorrhages (Enterovirus-70, Adenovirus, Coxsackie virus A-24).

Etiology:

It may be bacterial, viral, chlamydial, or allergic in origin.

Bacterial conjunctivitis: Staphylococcus aureus is the most common cause of bacterial conjunctivitis. It is also the most common organism associated with hordeolum and with phlyctenular conjunctivitis. Other organisms are: staphylococcus epidermidis, streptococcus pneumoniae (pneumococcus which causes subconjunctival haemorrhages), streptococcus haemolyticus which causes pseudomembrane formation, cornybacterium diptheriae which causes membranous conjunctivitis.

ACUTE MEMBRANOUS CONJUNCTIVITIS

It is conjunctivitis with true membrane formation usually on palpebral conjunctiva. When the membrane is peeled it bleeds.

Etiology:

1. Corynebacterium diphtheriae.
2. Occasionally by virulent type of streptococcus haemolyticus.

Clinical Features:

It usually affects children between 2 and 8 years, who are not immunized against diphtheriae. It is divided into three stages:

1. Stage of Infiltration:

A. Lids are swollen and hard with scanty conjunctival discharge.

B. Conjunctiva is covered by grey-yellow membrane which bleeds and leaves a raw area on peeling.

C. Enlarged preauricular lymph nodes.

2. Stage of Suppuration:

A. Copious purulent discharge.

B. Pain is less and there is sloughing of the membrane.

3. Stage of Cicatrisation: It is a stage of healing causing cicatrisation leading to complication like trichiasis and conjunctival xerosis, symblepharon (adhesion of palpebral conjunctiva with the bulbar conjunctiva) and entropion.

Treatment:

1. Penicillin eye drops given half hourly.
2. Antidiphtheric serum given hourly.
3. Atropine eye ointment and broad spectrum antibiotic ointment at night.
4. Intramuscular injection of penicillin for ten days.
5. Intramuscular injection of anti-diphtheric serum given stat.

PSEUDOMEMBRANOUS CONJUNCTIVITIS

It is an acute conjunctivitis with formation of pseudomembrane which does not bleed on peeling but leaves an intact conjunctiva behind.

Etiology:

1. C. diphtheriae of low virulence.
2. Streptococcus haemolyticus.
3. H. influenzae.
4. Herpes simplex.
5. Severe adenoviral infections.
6. Gonococcal infection.
7. Autoimmune conjunctivitis.

Treatment:

1. Topical antibiotics and ointment.

2. Irrigation of conjunctiva.
3. No steroids and bandage.
4. Anti-inflammatory and analgesic drugs.

VIRAL CONJUNCTIVITIS

Typical viral lesion is a keratoconjunctivitis.

Etiology:

a. Adenovirus.
b. HSV.
c. Herpes zoster.
d. Pox virus.
e. Myxo virus.
f. Paramyxo virus.

ADENOVIRAL KERATOCONJUNCTIVITIS

Usually affects children with URI.

Causes:

- Pharyngoconjunctival fever (PCF).
- Epidemic keratoconjunctivitis (EKC).

Clinical Features:

1. *Conjunctivitis*
   - Watering, discomfort, photophobia.
   - Follicular response.
   - Preauricular adenopathy.
   - Severe cases:
     - Subconjunctival haemorrhage.
     - Chemosis.
     - Pseudomembranes.
2. *Keratitis.*

ANGULAR CONJUNCTIVITIS

Also called "Diplobacillary conjunctivitis".

Etiology:

Causative organism is **Moraxella Axenfeld**. It is rarely caused by Staphylococcus aureus.

Moraxella are diplobacilla and have been found in nasal tract of healthy persons.

Clinical Features:

Congestion of conjunctiva at intermarginal strip especially at inner and outer canthi with excoriation of skin at these angles.

Complications:

a. Blepharitis.
b. Clear, shallow corneal ulcers associated (rarely) with hypopyon.

Treatment:

1. Oxytetracycline eye ointment.
2. Zinc lotion – It acts by inhibiting the proteolytic ferment.
3. Zinc oxide ointment at night.

TRACHOMA

- It is also called **"Egyptian Ophthalmia"**.
- It is caused by Chlamydia trachomatis–**serotypes, A, B, Ba, C.**
- **Serotypes D-K:** They cause **Adult Inclusion Conjunctivitis**, also called **"Swimming-pool Conjunctivitis".**
- It is a leading cause of preventable blindness in the world.
- **SAFE-Strategy**–It stands for Surgery, Antibiotics, Facial cleanliness, Environment. It is the strategy used to control the disease in the community. Chemotherapy can be given in two ways:

A. *Mass treatment or Blanket treatment:* It is given when the prevalence then of moderate to severe trachoma is greater than 5% in children under 10 years. The drug given is Azithromycin.

B. *Selective treatment:* The whole population at risk is screened and treatment is applied only to persons with active trachoma.

Clinical Features:

1. It is a disease of children and presents as intense itching and watering.
2. Conjunctival reaction is both follicular and papillary.

O/E:

1. Sago-grain-like follicles on the upper palpebral conjunctiva.
2. Herberts follicles on the superior limbus. In the scarring stage it cicratizes into herberts pits.
3. In later stage, there is a linear scarring at sulcus subtarsalis called Arlt's line.

Pathology of Trachoma

Chlamydia trachomatis is epitheliotrophic and seen typically in conjunctival scrapings in colony form in the epithelial cells as **Halberstaedter-Prowazek inclusion bodies.** The inclusion is first composed of numerous *Initial bodies.* These divide until eventually the cell becomes filled with innumerable *Elementary bodies* embedded in carbohydrate matrix to form the *Inclusion body.* There is lymphocytic infiltration involving the whole of adenoid layer of the parts of conjunctiva affected. Special aggregations of lymphocytes form follicles. These follicles tend to show necrosis and contain large multinucleated cells (*Lebers' cells).* In long standing cases, fibrous tissues form around follicles giving rise to cicatricial bands.

Sequelae of Trachoma

1. *Lids*

- Trichiasis.
- Entropion.
- Tylosis.
- Ptosis.
- Madarosis.
- Ankyloblepharon.

2. *Conjunctiva*

- Concretions.
- Pseudocyst.
- Xerosis.
- Symblepharon.

3. *Cornea*

- Corneal opacity.
- Corneal ectasia.
- Corneal xerosis.
- Total corneal pannus.

4. *Other Sequelae*

- Chronic dacryocystitis.
- Chronic dacryoadenitis.
- Rarely secondary glaucoma due to scarring of episcleral drainage channel.

Complication: The only complication of trachoma is corneal ulcer which may occur due to rubbing by concretions or trichiasis with superimposed bacterial infection.

WHO CLASSIFICATION OF TRACHOMA

- *TF:* Trachomatous follicular inflammation of **more than five follicles**, larger than 0.5 mm on the upper tarsus.
- *TI:* Trachomatous intense inflammation with thickening, obscuring over 50% of large, deep, tarsal vessels.
- *TS:* Trachomatous (conjunctival) cicatrization with white lines, bands or sheets of fibrosis in the tarsal conjunctiva

characteristically, they are glistening and fibrous in appearance with straight, angular or feathered edges.

- *TT:* Trachomatous trichiasis of at least one in turning eye lash or evidence of recent removal.
- *CO:* Corneal opacity obscuring at least part of the pupil margin and causing a visual acuity of less than 6/18.

This classification may be remembered as:

MNEMONIC

FISTO

Treatment:

The choice of treatment in trachoma is tetracycline. There are two types of regimes mentioned:

1. *Topical Regime:* It consists of tetracycline 1% or erythromycin 1% ointment given QID or 20% sulphacetamide given QID alongwith ointment given at night.
2. *Systemic Regime:* Oral tetracycline or oral erythromycin given QID or oral doxycycline is given BD or single dose of Azithromycin can be given.

ADULT INCLUSION CONJUNCTIVITIS

- It is a type of acute follicular conjunctivitis associated with mucopurulent discharge. It usually affects the sexually active young adults.
- Inclusion conjunctivitis is caused by serotypes D to K of chlamydia trachomatis.
- The primary source of infection is urethritis in males and cervicitis in females.
- The transmission of infection may occur to eyes either through contaminated fingers or more commonly through contaminated water of swimming pool. (Hence called **"swimming pool conjunctivitis"**).

Ophthalmia Neonatorum

Neonatal conjunctivitis (Ophthalmia neonatorum) is defined as a conjunctival inflammation that occurs during the *first month of life:*

Etiology:

A. Chlamydial.

B. Gonococcal.

C. Miscellaneous.

Chlamydial conjunctivitis: Presentation is between 5–14 days after birth with an **acute mucopurulent conjunctivitis:**

Ocular complication: Superior corneal pannus, conjunctival scarring, corneal opacity.

Systemic complication: Otitis, rhinitis, pneumonitis.

Treatment:

Systemic erythromycin, topical tetracycline.

GONOCOCCAL CONJUNCTIVITIS

It is transmitted from mother during delivery.

Presentation is after 1–3 days with **hyper-acute purulent conjunctivitis** associated with chemosis and sometimes membrane or pseudomembrane formation.

Treatment is topical and systemic penicillin.

MISCELLANEOUS CONJUNCTIVITIS

1. *Chemical conjunctivitis:* It occurs due to instillation of 1% silver nitrate, given to prevent infective conjunctivitis (called

"credes method") or by antibiotic used as prophylaxis against gonococcal infection.

Clinical feature: Presents with mild conjunctival hyperaemia which lasts no longer than 24 hours.

2. *Simple bacterial conjunctivitis:* Most frequently by staphylococcus aureus.
3. *Herpes simplex:* By type-2 HSV (due to maternal infection). It presents as: Blepharoconjunctivitis and keratitis.

Sticky eye: It is not a separate clinical entity and refers to the condition where eye becomes sticky due to discharge.

ACUTE HAEMORRHAGIC CONJUNCTIVITIS

- By Enterovirus–70, Member of picorna–virus group.
- **Disease is:**
  1. Highly contagious.
  2. Self-limiting and resolves in 7 days.

Clinical Features:

1. Bilateral profuse watery discharge.
2. Palpebral follicles.
3. Subconjunctival haemorrhage.

Treatment:

No Effective Treatment.

- **Other etiological agents are:**
  1. Severe adenovirus infection.
  2. Echo virus—34.
  3. Coxsackie virus—24.

Causes of Subconjunctival Haemorrhage

1. Trauma.
2. Foreign body.
3. Hypertension.
4. Bleeding diasthesis.
5. Pertussis, i.e., whooping cough.
6. Pneumococcal infection.
7. Viral infections.

ALLERGIC CONJUNCTIVITIS

A. Spring Catarrh Or Vernal Keratoconjunctivitis (VKC)

- It's a recurrent, bilateral external ocular inflammation, affecting children and young adults.
- More common in males.
- It's an allergic disorder in which IgE mediated mechanisms play an important role. **There is only papillary reaction with no follicular reaction.**
- VKC is usually after the age of 5 years and the condition eventually resolves around puberty, rarely persisting beyond 25 years of age.
- **C/F**–Symptoms are worse during summer.
  a. Intense ocular itching.
  b. Lacrimation, photophobia, foreign body sensation and blurring.
  c. **Thick mucus discharge:** *ROPY*.
  d. Rarely ptosis.
- **O/E**—It is of three main clinical types:
  i. **Palpebral VKC:** Papillary hypertrophy most marked in superior palpebral conjunctiva. In severe case: **'Cobblestone appearance'** is seen (which are flat topped polygonal papillae).
  ii. **Limbal VKC:** Limbal papillary hypertrophy. These papillae have white superficial spots called **"Horner Trantas Spots"**. It is

composed predominantly of eosinophils.

iii. **Mixed form:** Both limbal and palpebral conjunctiva are involved.

- **Corneal Changes in VKC:**
  a. *Punctate epitheliopathy:* It constitutes microerosions.
  b. *Macroerosions.*
  c. *Plaque:* It is the desiccated mucus over the epithelial macroerosions.
  d. *Subepithelial scarring:* It is generally in form of a ring.
  e. *Pseudogerontoxon:* It resembles Arcus senilis, which is also called gerontoxon, hence the name. It is also called **"Cupids bow".**
  f. Keratoconus may be associated.

Treatment:

1. *Topical steroids:* Preferably Fluoromethalone.
2. *Sodium cromoglycate:* 2% drops.
3. *Lodoxamide 0.1% drops:* It is superior to sodium cromoglycate.
4. *Acetylcysteine 5% drops:* In treatment of plaques, because it has mucolytic property.
5. *Lamellar keratectomy:* It removes the plaques and speeds the process of re-epithelisation.

B. Phlyctenular Keratoconjunctivitis

- Also called **Phlyctenulosis.**
- Predominantly affects children.
- **Etiology:** Allergy due to non-specific delayed hypersensitivity reaction to staphylococci, tuberculosis or other endogenous bacterial antigens.
- **Clinical feature:** Small pinkish-white nodule near the limbus, surrounded by hyperaemia called phlycten. **Corneal phlycten** leads to **Fascicular ulcer** which can later transform into **Ring ulcer.**

D/D: *Scleritis and Episcleritis:* The clinical picture is same but pain is a feature of scleritis and episcleritis. Also the congestion is deep congestion in scleritis and episcleritis whereas in phlyctenular conjunctivitis it is superficial conjunctival congestion.

Treatment:

1. Short course of topical steroids.
2. Any associated staphylococcal blepharitis must be treated.

Xerophthalmia

It is the most common cause of blindness in children.

Ocular manifestations of vitamin A deficiency include not only the structural changes affecting the conjunctiva, cornea and retina but also biophysical disorders of retinal rods and cone function. **Vitamin A deficiency, i.e., xerophthalmia causes epithelial xerosis and not parenchymatous xerosis.**

Etiology:

Dietary deficiency of vitamin A or its defective absorption.

New WHO Classification of Xerophthalmia

XN	Night blindness.
X1A	Conjunctival xerosis.
X1B	Bitots' spots.
X2	Corneal xerosis.
X3A	Keratomalacia affecting less than one-third of corneal surface.
X3B	Keratomalacia affecting more than one-third of corneal surface.
XS	Corneal scar due to xerophthalmia.

XF Xerophthalmic fundus.

Treatment:

1. Local ocular therapy

a. Topical artificial tears.

b. If keratomalacia present, full-fledged treatment on the lines of bacterial corneal ulcer.

2. Vitamin A therapy

>1 year age

1 lakh IU of Vitamin A I/M injection given on 0, 1, 14th day.

or

2 lakh IU given orally on same schedule.

< 1 year age

Half the dose.

3. Treatment of underlying conditions

- *Treatment of PEM:* Protein Energy Malnutrition.
- Other nutritional disorders like diarrhoea, dehydration and electrolyte imbalance.

WHO Recommendation for Prophylaxis of Xerophthalmia

< 6 months infant (not being breast fed)	50,000 IU orally
6–12 months (< 8 kg)	1 lakh IU orally
> 1 year < 6 years	2 lakh IU orally every 6 months

Revised Schedule Under CSSM (Child Survival and Safe Motherhood)

- First dose (1 lakh IU)—at 9 months along with measles.
- Second dose (2 lakh IU)—at 18 months, along with booster of DPT.
- Third dose (2 lakh IU) at 2 years of age.

Causes of Night Blindness

1. Vitamin A deficiency (Xerophthalmia).
2. High myopia.
3. Retinitis pigmentosa.
4. Late stage of primary open angle glaucoma.
5. Congenital stationary night blindness.
6. Oguchi's disease.
7. Fundus albipunctatus.
8. Favre-Goldmann syndrome.
9. Choroideremia.
10. Gyrate atrophy of choroid.
11. Generalized choroidal atrophy.

Causes of Parenchymatous Xerosis (involving the interstitial layer of conjunctiva)

Cicatrizing disorders	Overexposure to atmosphere
1. Cicatrical pemphigoid	1. Marked proptosis
2. Stevens-Johnson syndrome	2. Facial palsy
3. Trachoma	3. Ectropion
4. Diphtheric membranous conjunctivitis	4. Lack of blinking (coma)
5. Thermal, chemical burns	5. Lagophthalmos due to symblepharon
6. Radiotherapy	

Pre-corneal tear film has three layers:

1. Lipid layer (From Meibomian glands and gland of Zeis).
2. Aqueous layer (From main lacrimal glands (95%) and accessory lacrimal glands of Krause and Wolfring).
3. Mucin layer (From goblet cells and glands of Henle and Manz present in conjunctiva).

Keratoconjunctivitis Sicca (KCS)

It is dry eye primarily resulting from **aqueous layer deficiency** of the tear film.

Types of KCS:

A. **Pure KCS:** Only lacrimal glands are involved.

B. **Sjögren's syndrome:** KCS with Xerostomia, hypergammaglobulinemia, RA and increased ANA. Also termed as **Primary Sjögren's syndrome or Sicca syndrome.**

C. When associated with connective tissue disorders, it is termed as **Secondary Sjögren's syndrome.**

Etiology:

a. Destruction of lacrimal gland due to tumour, inflammation.

b. Meibomian gland dysfunction.

c. Congenital/Surgical absence of lacrimal glands.

d. Blockage of excretory ducts.

e. Destruction of goblet cells in conjunctival scarring conditions.

f. *Neurological lesions*—Familial dysautonomia (Riley-Day Syndrome).

Clinical Features:

1. Irritation, FB sensation, burning, stingy mucus discharge.
2. Severe pain due to filamentary keratitis.

On Examination:

1. **Tear film:**
   - Marginal tear meniscus is concave, small and less than 1 mm.
   - Increase of mucus strands and debris in tear film.
2. **Corneal abnormalities:**
   - Punctate epitheliopathy.
   - Filamentary keratitis.
   - Mucous plaques.

Investigations:

1. **Tear film break-up time:** Normal: 34 secs. Abnormal: <10 secs.
2. **Rose Bengal Staining:** It has affinity for dead cells and mucus.

   In KCS, typical picture is—**Two triangles with base towards limbus.**
3. **Schirmers test:**

   Normal > 15 mm.

   Borderline Between 5 mm and 10 mm.

   Abnormal <5 mm.
4. **Lactoferrin levels in tears:** It decreases in patients of dry eye. The normal levels are 327 mg/dL. Anything less than 90 mg/dL is pathological.
5. **Tear osmolality measurements:** It is the most sensitive indicator of dry eye disease. It increases in patients of dry eye. Normal value is 302 mosm/lt. 310–311 mosm/lt is indicative of early dry eye whereas 312 mosm/lt is indicative of keratoconjunctivitis sicca.

Treatment:

1. **Tear substitutes:**

   Types of Artificial Tears/Tear Substitutes:
   - Polyvinyl alcohol and povidone.
   - Sodium hyaluronate (Healon) – prepared in 1:10 dilution with sterile balanced salt solution.
   - Hydroxypropyl methyl cellulose.
   - Gel tears—composed of high molecular weight cross linked polymers of acrylic acid.
   - Patients own serum, diluted with preservative free normal saline.
2. **Mucolytic agents:** 5% Acetylcysteine drops.

3. **Topical cyclosporine: It is an immunomodulator and is helpful to treat dry eye due to autoimmune etiology. It enhances the secretion of tears from the lacrimal gland.**
4. **Reduction of tear drainage:** Punctal occlusion.
   - *Temporary:* It is done by cauterizing it with heat cautery.
   - *Permanent:* It is done with silicone plugs.

Ocular Lesions of Measles

1. Catarrhal conjunctivitis.
2. *Koplik's spots* on conjunctiva.
3. Corneal ulceration due to Xerophthalmia.
4. Optic neuritis.
5. Retinitis.

Ocular Features of Mumps

1. Acute Dacryocystoadenitis.
2. Uveitis.
3. Keratitis.
4. Conjunctivitis.

Ocular Manifestations of Chickenpox

Though both Varicella (Chickenpox) and Zoster are different manifestations of the same virus, there is no evidence that Zoster, i.e., HZO Herpes Zoster Ophthalmicus can be caused by contact with patients of Chickenpox.

Chickenpox in expectant mothers can produce the following ocular abnormalities:

- Horners syndrome.
- Optic nerve hypoplasia.
- Chorioretinitis.
- Cataract.

CONJUNCTIVAL DEGENERATIONS

A. Pinguecula

- Yellow white deposits on the bulbar conjunctiva adjacent to the limbus.
- **Histology:** Degeneration of collagen fibres of conjunctival stroma with thinning of epithelium and calcification.

B. Pterygium

- It is a triangular sheet of fibrovascular tissue which invades the cornea. It occurs due to exposure to dust and ultraviolet rays.
- Deposition of iron in corneal epithelium anterior to advancing head of pterygium is called **"Stocker's line"**.

Treatment:

a. Surgical excision with autograft. Autograft is the most reliable method of preventing the recurrences in cases of pterygium.

b. Postoperative use of beta-Radiation, topical Thiotepa or Mitomycin-C may also be effective in prevention of recurrence. Mitomycin-C may also be used preoperatively.

C. Concretions

Small yellow white deposits present in palpebral conjunctiva.

D. Retention Cyst

- Asymptomatic thin walled lesion containing clear fluid. It is due to obstruction of Krauses gland.
- **Other conjunctival cysts are:**

  a. *Lymphangiectasis:* Dilatation of lymph spaces.

  b. *Implantation cyst:* Occur following squint surgery.

  c. *Hydatid cyst* or cysticercosis cyst.

  d. *Lymphangioma:* It is a solitary multilocular cyst.

NEET DRILL

1. Percentage of tetracycline used in trachoma is 1%.
2. In Credes method the percentage of silver nitrate used is 1%.
3. Pterygium is more common nasally.
4. Bitot's spot is more common temporally.
5. Conjunctival cysts are typically seen in cysticercosis.
6. SAFE strategy is indicated when the prevalence of trachoma follicles in a community is >10%. If it is between 5–10%, only FE is followed, i.e., facial hygiene and environmental cleanliness whereas < 5%, nothing is done.
7. Percentage of erythromycin ointment given in trachoma is 1%.
8. 20% sulphacetamide can also be given for the treatment of trachoma.
9. In Schirmer's test if wetting of the tear strip is < 5 mm, it is severe dry eye.
10. BUT test is considered positive if it is <10 secs.
11. Gonococcal infection in ophthalmia neonatorum presents after 1–3 days of birth whereas chlamydial infection presents between 5 and 14 days.
12. Density of goblet cells is maximum on inferonasal conjunctiva.
13. Dose of vitamin A in xerophthalmia is: > 1 year: 1 lakh IU injection on 0,1,14th day whereas in <1 year, we half the dose.
14. Trachoma is caused by strain A, B, Ba and C of Chlamydia trachomatis whereas the strain D-K causes adult inclusion conjunctivitis which is also called **swimming pool conjunctivitis**.
15. Most common conjunctival tumour is squamous cell carcinoma and in children it is naevus.
16. Dose of azithromycin in blanket therapy is 1 gm for adults and 20 mg/kg for children.
17. Phenol Red Thread Test is used to check the tear volume just like schirmers test.
18. Earliest feature of vitamin A deficiency is nyctalopia.
19. Causes of swimming pool conjunctivitis are chlamydia and adenovirus.
20. Phlyctenular keratoconjunctivitis is type IV hypersensitivity reaction.
21. Vernal keratoconjunctivitis is type I hypersensitivity reaction.
22. PERFECT SURGERY is done for pterygium, with NO recurrence. It stands for Pterygium Extended Resection Followed By Extended Conjunctival Transplantation.
23. Complication of trachoma is only one, i.e., corneal ulcer.
24. Pinguecula is more common nasally.

MULTIPLE CHOICE QUESTIONS

1. **A child of 8 kg has Bitot's spots in both eyes. Which of the following is the most appropriate schedule to prescribe vitamin A to this child?**
   A. 2 lakh units IM on day 0, 14
   B. 1 lakh units IM on day 0, 14
   C. 2 lakh units IM on day 0,1 and 14
   D. 1 lakh units IM on day 0, 1 and 14
2. **Maximum density of goblet cells is seen in:**
   A. Superior conjunctiva
   B. Inferior conjunctiva

C. Temporal conjunctiva

D. Nasal conjunctiva

3. Arlt's line is seen in:

A. Vernal keratoconjunctivitis

B. Pterygium

C. Ocular pemphigoid

D. Trachoma

4. A recurrent bilateral conjunctivitis occurring with the onset of hot weather in young boys with symptoms of burning, itching and lacrimation with polygonal raised areas in palpebral conjunctiva is:

A. Trachoma

B. Phlyctenular conjunctivitis

C. Mucopurulent conjunctivitis

D. Vernal keratoconjunctivitis

5. The vitamin A supplement administered in "Prevention of Nutritional Blindness in Children Programme" contain:

A. 25,000 IU/ml B. 1 lakh IU/ml

C. 3 lakh IU/ml D. 5 lakh IU/ml

6. Unilateral watery discharge from the eye of a newborn with no edema or chemosis is due to:

A. Chlamydia

B. Gonococcus

C. Sticky eye

D. Chemical conjunctivitis

7. Horner Trantas spots are seen in:

A. Vernal conjunctivitis

B. Phlyctenular conjunctivitis

C. Angular conjunctivitis

D. Follicular conjunctivitis

8. Which microorganism does not cause haemorrhagic conjunctivitis?

A. Adenovirus B. Coxsackie–24

C. Enterovirus–70 D. Papilloma virus

9. Herbert's pits are seen in:

A. Trachoma

B. Spring catarrh

C. Phlyctenular conjunctivitis

D. Sarcoidosis

10. Pterygium is:

A. An inflammatory response

B. A connective tissue disorder

C. An infection

D. Associated with vitamin A deficiency

11. True about chalazion:

A. Chronic non-specific inflammation

B. Lipogranulomatous inflammation

C. Acute inflammation

D. Suppurative inflammation

12. In the grading of trachoma, trachomatous inflammations follicular is defined as the presence of:

A. Five or more follicles in the lower tarsal conjunctiva

B. Three or more follicles in the lower tarsal conjunctiva

C. Five or more follicles in the upper tarsal conjunctiva

D. Three or more follicles in the upper tarsal conjunctiva

13. Chlamydia trachomatis serovars D-K cause:

A. Arteriosclerosis

B. Trachoma

C. Lymphogranuloma venereum

D. Urethritis

14. "Cobblestone appearance" is seen in:

A. Spring catarrh

B. Viral conjunctivitis

C. Phlyctenular conjunctivitis
D. Bacterial conjunctivitis

15. All are features of trachoma, except:
A. Circumcorneal congestion
B. Follicle
C. Cicatrization
D. Keratitis

16. Tear film is absent in:
A. Herpes keratitis
B. Keratoconjunctivitis sicca
C. Dacryoadenitis
D. Acute conjunctivitis

17. Features of vernal keratitis are:
A. Papillary hypertrophy
B. Follicular hypertrophy
C. Herberts pits
D. Trantas spots
E. Ciliary congestion

18. Epithelial lining of conjunctiva:
A. Sq keratinized
B. Sq non-keratinized
C. Pseudostratified
D. Columnar
E. Transitional

19. Ophthalmia neonatorum is caused by:
A. Gonorrhoea B. H. Influenzae
C. Chlamydia D. Pseudomonas
E. Staph aureus

20. Parenchymatous xerosis of conjunctiva is caused by:
A. Trachoma
B. Vitamin A deficiency
C. Vernal catarrh
D. Phlyctenular keratoconjunctivitis
E. Alkali burns

21. Staphylococcal conjunctivitis is associated with all except:
A. Corneal margin infiltration
B. Phlyctenular conjunctivitis
C. Vernal conjunctivitis
D. Hordeolum
E. Follicular conjunctivitis

22. Keratomalacia is associated with:
A. Measles B. Mumps
C. Rubella D. Diarrhoea
E. Chickenpox

23. Seen in Vernal Catarrh are:
A. Papillary hypertrophy
B. Follicles
C. Pannus formation
D. Fascicular ulcer
E. Ropy discharge

24. Keratomalacia:
A. Occurs due to vitamin A deficiency
B. Relatively benign condition
C. First feature of vitamin A deficiency
D. Also seen in retinitis pigmentosa

25. Seen in trachoma are/is:
A. Papillary hypertrophy
B. Follicles
C. Pannus formation
D. Herberts pits
E. Ropy discharge

26. Angular conjunctivitis is caused by:
A. Moraxella B. Virus
C. Bacteroides D. Fungus

27. Phlycten is due to:

A. Exogenous allergy

B. Endogenous allergy

C. Viral keratitis

D. Fungal keratitis

28. Acute haemorrhagic conjunctivitis is seen with:

A. Adenovirus B. Pneumococcus

C. Haemophilus D. Staphylococcal

29. Pseudomembranous conjunctivitis is caused by:

A. Gonococcus

B. Staphylococcus

C. Streptococcus

D. Keratoconjunctivitis sicca

30. Which of the following is not a feature of vernal conjunctivitis?

A. Maxwell Lyon sign

B. Trantas spots

C. Follicles

D. Perilimbal papillary hypertrophy

31. Acute conjunctivitis is caused by all except:

A. Adenovirus B. CMV

C. Enterovirus-70D. Coxsackie-24

32. Nodule at limbus, hyperaemia of conjunctiva and photophobia. Diagnosis is:

A. Scleritis

B. Koeppe's nodule

C. Conjunctivitis (Phlyctenular)

D. Bussaca's nodule

33. All of the following viruses involve eye except:

A. Herpes zoster B. Herpes simplex

C. Echo D Adenovirus–8

34. WHO grading (X 3a) for Xerophthalmia indicates:

A. Corneal xerosis

B. Keratomalacia

C. Corneal ulcer

D Conjunctival xerosis and Bitot's spot

35. Complication of trachoma:

A. Trichiasis

B. Corneal opacity

C. Cataract

D. Vitreous haemorrhage

36. Following are embryological remnants except:

A. Bergmeister's papilla

B. Epicapsular stars

C. Mittendorf's dot

D. Posterior embryotoxon

37. Artificial tears is produced by:

A. Methyl cellulose

B. Polyvinyl alcohol

C. Hyaluronate

D. All of the above

38. Night blindness is due to:

A. Vitamin A deficiency

B. Myopia

C. Retinitis pigmentosa

D. All of the above

39. The following is not a feature of conjunctivitis:

A. Irritation B. Discharge

C. Redness D. Pain

40. Steroids are used in all except:

A. Vernal conjunctivitis

B. Phlyctenular conjunctivitis

C. Acute dacryocystitis

D. Acute iridocyclitis

41. Trachoma causes:

A. Mechanical ptosis

B. Trichiasis

C. Entropion

D. All of the above

42. Blindness in a child is most commonly due to:

A. Keratomalacia

B. Congenital cataract

C. Glaucoma

D. Injuries

43. Percentage of silver nitrate used in Credes method:

A. 0.5% B. 1%

C. 1.5% D. 2%

44. H.P. inclusion bodies in trachoma are seen is:

A. Extracellular B. Intracytoplasmic

C. Intranuclear D. None of the above

45. Type IV hypersensitivity to Mycobacterium tuberculosis antigen may manifest as:

A. Iridocyclitis

B. Polyarteritis nodosa

C. Phyctenular

D. Giant cell arteritis

46. Subconjunctival haemorrhage occurs in all conditions except:

A. Passive venous congestion

B. Pertussis

C. Trauma

D. High intraocular tension

47. The normal pH of tear is:

A. 5.7 B. 7.5

C. 6.5 D. 7.9

48. All are seen in stage III trachoma except:

A. Tarsal epitheliofibrosis

B. Herberts pits

C. Disappearance of Bowman's membrane

D. Trichiasis

49. A malnourished child from poor socio-economic status, residing in overcrowded and dirty areas presents with a nodule around limbus with hyperemia of conjunctiva. Other significant findings were axillary and cervical lymph adenopathy:

A. Phylectenular conjunctivitis

B. Foreign body granuloma

C. Scleritis

D. Episcleritis

50. Which of the following is false regarding acute conjunctivitis?

A. Vision is not affected

B. Cornea is infiltrated

C. Pupil is not affected

D. Topical antibiotics is the treatment of choice

51. Conjunctiva in Vitamin A deficiency shows:

A. Hyperplasia of squamous epithelium

B. Actinic degeneration

C. Macrophage infiltration

D. Hyperplasia of goblet cells

52. Which of the following is true about pterygium?

A. Associated with infrared radiation exposure

B. Probe can be passed underneath the pterygium at the limbus

C. There is elastotic degeneration with Descemet's membrane distortion

D. Bare sclera technique of treatment has 30–80% recurrence

53. Treatment of phlyctenular conjunctivitis is:

A. Systemic steroids

B. Topical steroids

C. Antibiotics

D. Miotics

54. All of the following are cause of night blindness except:

A. Oguchi

B. Vitamin A deficiency

C. High myopia

D. Devics disease

55. Vitamin A supplementation in a 10-month-old child with xeropthalmia is:

A. One dose of 1 lakh units

B. Two doses of 1 lakh units

C. Three doses of 1 lakh units

D. Two doses of 2 lakh units

56. Circumcorneal congestion is not seen in:

A. Acute bacterial conjunctivitis

B. Acute iritis

C. Acute glaucoma

D. Scleritis

57. Alkali injury to eye cause:

A. Globe perforation

B. Retinal detachment

C. Optic neuritis

D. Symblepharon

58. All are true about membranous conjunctivitis except:

A. Easy to peel

B. Caused by corynebacterium

C. May lead to cicatrisation

D. May cause corneal ulceration

ANSWER AND EXPLANATION

1.	d	If patient is more than one year of age, we give 1 lakh IU of injection Vitamin A on 0,1,14 days. If age is <1 year then we half the dose.
2.	d	Goblet cells form the mucin layer of the tear film. They are maximum nasally and least superiorly.
3.	d	Arlt's line is a linear scarring on the upper palpebral conjunctiva in patients of trachoma.
4.	d	VKC is an allergic conjunctivitis due to exogenous antigen, common in male children.
5.	b	1 lakh IU is given on 0, 1 and 14th day.
6.	d	Chemical conjunctivitis occurs due to silver nitrate eye drops given in children to prevent gonorrhea infection (CREDES METHOD).

7.	a	Horner Trantas spots are eosinophils. It is seen on the hypertrophied papilla in the upper limbus.
8.	d	Other causes of haemorrhagic conjunctivitis are Echo virus –34. Bacterial causes are–Haemophilus and pneumococcus.
9.	a	Herbert's pits are cicatrized follicles on the upper limbus.
10.	b	Pterygium is subconjunctival fibrovascular growth encroaching on the cornea.
11.	b	Chalazion is a lipogranulomatous inflammation of the meibomian gland.
12.	c	The pneumonic is FIST-O.
13.	c	Lymphogranuloma venereum can later cause adult inclusion conjunctivitis. Most common mode of infection is through swimming pool; hence it is also called swimming pool conjunctivitis.
14.	a	Cobblestone appearance is severe papillary hyperplasia in upper palpebral conjunctiva.
15.	a	Trachoma is characterized by conjunctival congestion. Ciliary congestion is not a feature of conjunctivitis.
16.	b	KCS is deficiency of the aqueous layer of tear film.
17.	a,d	See Q.7.
18.	b	Conjunctival epithelium is squamous non-keratinized.
19.	a,c, e	Other causes of ophthalmia neonatorum are herpes simplex and chemical conjunctivitis.
20.	a,e	Xerosis due to vitamin A deficiency is epithelial xerosis whereas parenchymatous xerosis occurs due to cicatrizing (scarring) conditions of the conjunctiva.
21.	c,e	Vernal conjunctivitis is allergic and not infective.
22.	a,d	Both measles and diarrhea manifest as vitamin A deficiency leading to xerophthalmia.
23.	a,e	Pannus is corneal neovascularisation. Fascicular ulcer is a feature of phyctenular conjunctivitis.
24.	a	Night blindness is the first feature of vitamin A deficiency and is also a feature of RP.
25.	a,b, c,d	In trachoma there is both follicular and papillary reaction.
26.	a	Both Moraxella and staph aureus cause angular conjunctivitis.
27.	b	Endogenous allergens in phyctenular conjunctivitis are staph aureus and TB.
28.	a,b, c	Haemorrhagic conjunctivitis is conjunctivitis with subconjunctival haemorrhages.
29.	a,b, c	In Pseudomembranous conjunctivitis, the inflammatory membrane does not bleed on peeling.
30.	c	Maxwell Lyon sign is presence of eosinophils in the ropy discharge.
31.	b	Ocular manifestation of CMV is posterior uveitis.
32.	c	Nodule at the limbus is called phlycten.
33.	c	All the options are correct but since the least common is Echo virus, we will mark it as the answer.
34.	b	X3a is keratomalacia involving less than 1/3rd of the cornea.
35.	b	There is only one complication of trachoma, i.e., corneal ulcer leading to corneal opacity.
36.	d	Posterior gerontoxon is a prominent schwalbe's line whereas anterior

embryotoxon is the other name of arcus senilis.

37. d All are the different kinds of artificial tears.

38. d Another cause is late stage of POAG.

39. d Pain is not a common feature but will occur only in severe conjunctivitis.

40. c Acute dacryocystitis is an infective condition and is treated by antibiotics.

41. d All are sequelae of trachoma due to scarring.

42. a Most common cause of childhood blindness is vitamin A deficiency.

43. b Credes method is used to prevent gonococcal infection in a newborn.

44. b Halbersteidter Prowasek bodies are intracytoplasmic inclusion bodies.

45. c Most common allergic ocular manifestation of TB is phlyctenular keratoconjunctivitis.

46. d Other causes are–Hypertension and bleeding diasthesis.

47. b pH of tear is–7.4.

48. d Stage III is the scarring stage.

49. a The history suggests that the child has TB and due to endogenous allergy, he is suffering from phlyctenular conjunctivitis. The nodule around the limbus is called the phlycten.

50. a Among all the four options, option A seems the most appropriate as any corneal infilteration will lead to decreased vision, though in conjunctivitis it is commonly reversible.

We cannot agree totally with option D as the question does not mention the cause of conjunctivitis.

51. a In vitamin A deficiency, there is metaplasia of squamous epithelium and goblet cell atrophy.

52. d It is associated with exposure to ultraviolet rays. There is elastotic degeneration with Bowman's membrane distortion not descements membrane.

Probe cannot be passed underneath, and this feature helps to differentiate between pterygium and pseudopterygium.

Pseudopterygium may mimic the appearance of pterygia, since it is a fibrovascular scar arising in the bulbar conjunctiva that extends onto the cornea.

53. b It's an endogenous allergy treated by anti-allergic and mild topical steroids.

54. d Devics disease is optic neuritis with myelitis. It is also called neuromyelitis optica.

55. c The three doses are given on 0, 1 and 14th day. In less than 1 year age—oral dose is 1 lakh IU whereas injectable is 50,000 IU.

56. a In conjunctivitis we get conjunctival congestion.

57. d Symblepharon is adhesion of bulbar conjunctiva with palpebral conjunctiva.

58. a A true membrane bleeds on peeling.

RECENTLY ADDED QUESTIONS

1. Identify the image shown:

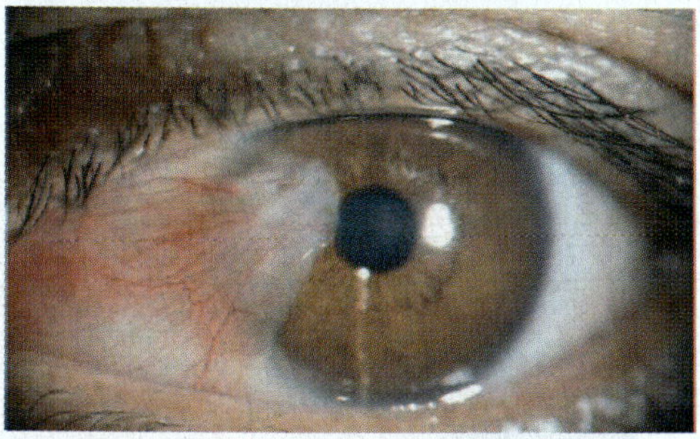

A. Pinguecula

B. Pterygium

C. Bitots' spot

D. Conjunctivitis

2. Which conjunctivitis results in blindness in neonates?

A. Chemical conjunctivitis

B. Chlamydia

C. Neisseria

D. Adenovirus

3. Which of the following enterovirus causes hemorrhagic conjunctivitis?

A. E70 B. E72

C. E69 D. E71

4. True regarding adenovirus-induced conjunctivitis is/are: (PGI)

A. Single stranded DNA virus

B. Incubation period is 6-10 days

C. Supportive treatment indicated

D. Ganciclovir is the drug of choice

E. True membrane lining the lower fornix and palpebral conjunctive usually present

ANSWERS OF RECENTLY ADDED QUESTIONS

1.	b	Pterygium is a subconjunctival fibrovascular tissue encroaching the cornea. It is most commonly seen on nasal side.
2.	c	Gonorrhoeal conjunctivitis can complicate as corneal perforation.
3.	a	Other causes of haemorrhagic conjunctivitis are coxsackie 24, adenovirus and echo virus 34.
4.	b, c	Adenoviral conjunctivitis is caused by dsDNA virus. Adenovirus of strains types 7, 8 and 19. Incubation period is about 6-10 days. The conjunctivitis so produced begins in one eye and spreads to the other. Pseudomembrane formed in lower fornix in severe cases. Treatment is mainly supportive. Cidofovir may be helpful in severe cases.

IMAGE-BASED QUESTIONS

1. **The diagnosis is:**

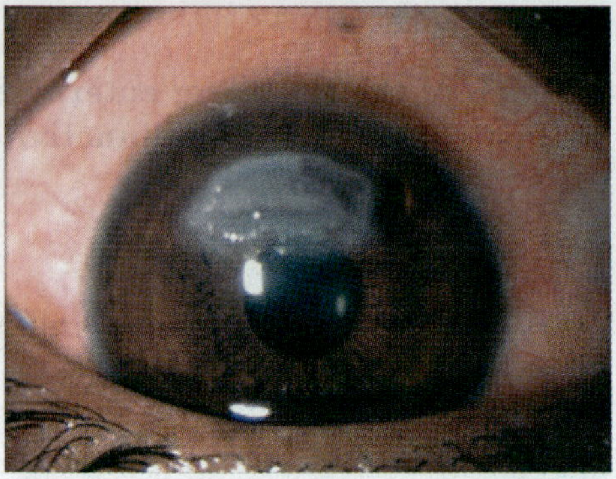

A. Bacterial ulcer B. Mooren's ulcer
C. Shield ulcer D. Fungal ulcer

2. **The diagnosis is:**

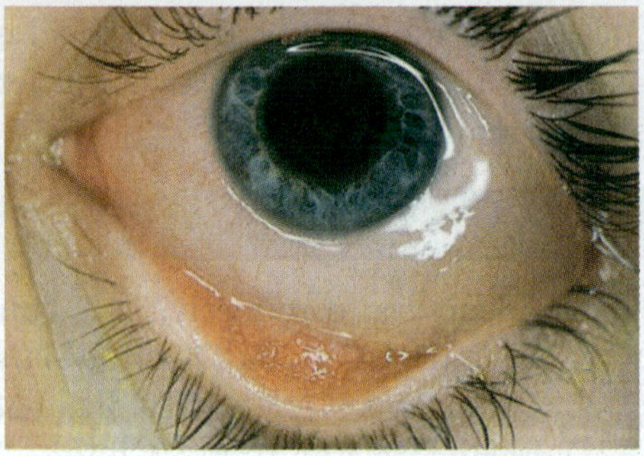

A. Concretions B. Congestion
C. Chemosis D. Cyst

3. **The diagnosis is:**

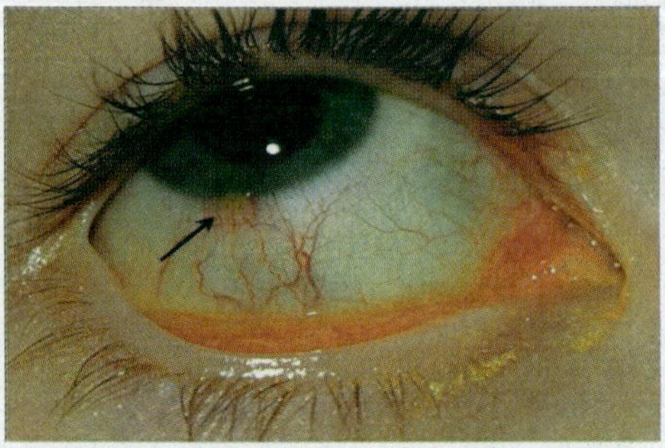

A. Phlyctenular keratoconjunctivitis
B. Vernal keratoconjunctivits
C. Conjunctival cyst
D. Bitot's spot

4. **The diagnosis is:**

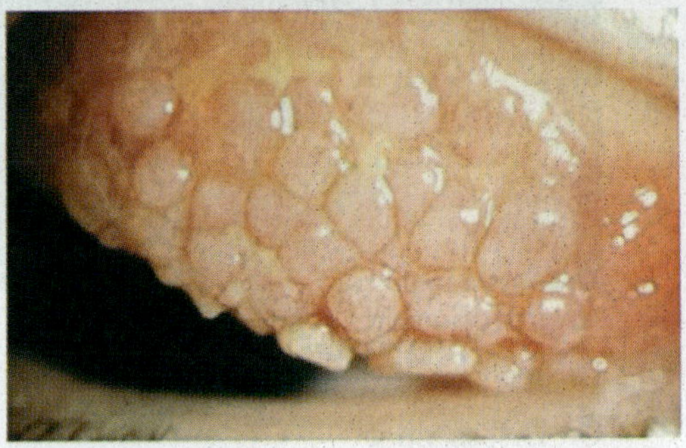

A. Trachoma
B. Vernal KC
C. Contact lens overwear
D. Chemosis

5. **The diagnosis is:**

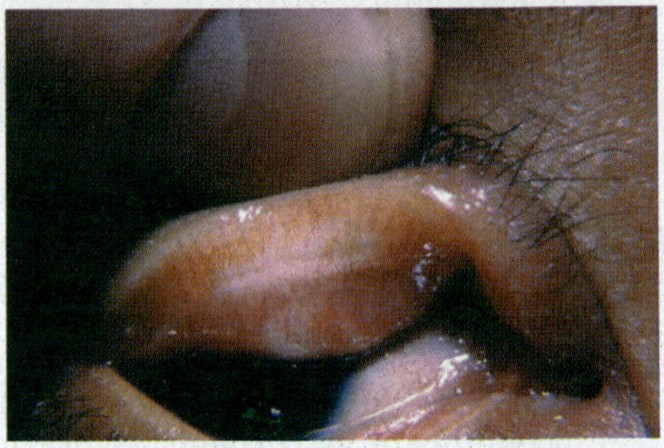

A. Trachoma B. Vernal KC
C. Phyctenular KC D. Chemical burn

6. **The treatment of choice is:**

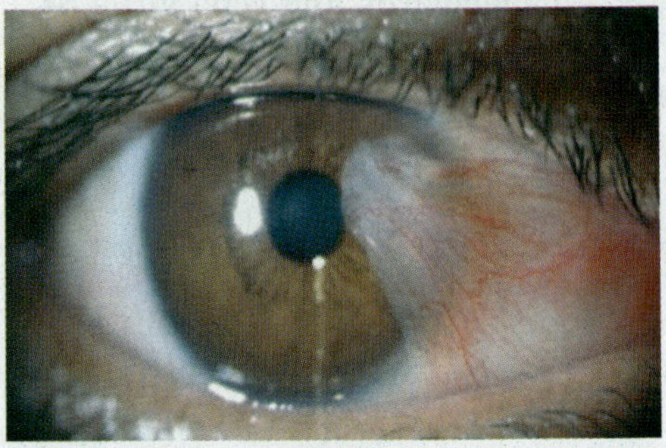

A. Bare – sclera technique
B. Excision with mitomycin-C
C. Excision with autografting
D. PERFECT surgery

7. The most common organism is:

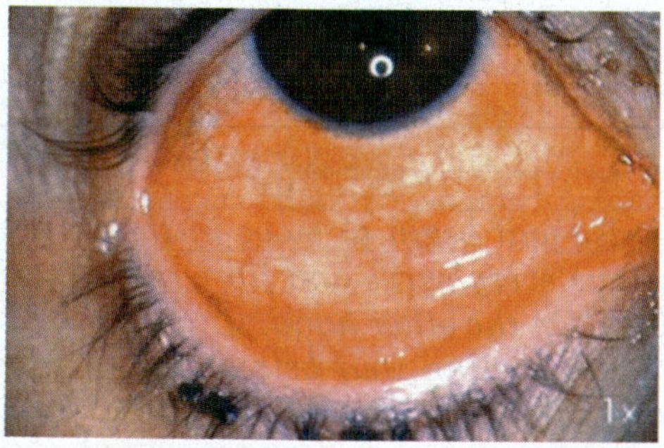

A. Enterovirus-70 B. Coxsackie-24
C. Echo virus-34 D. Adenovirus

8. The etiological agent is:

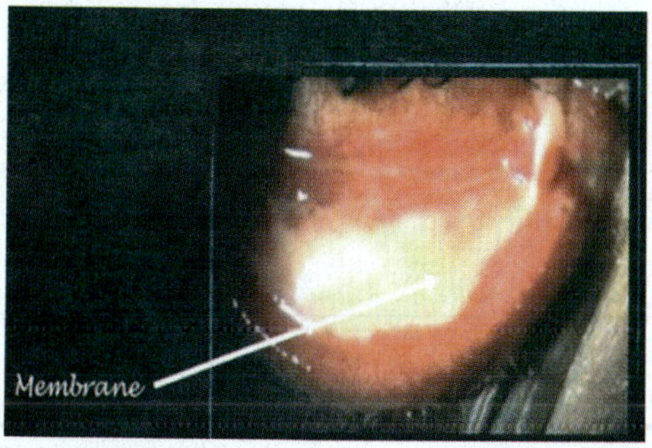

A. Adenovirus
B. Staphylococcus
C. Streptococcus
D. Corynebacterium diphtheria

9. The cause is:

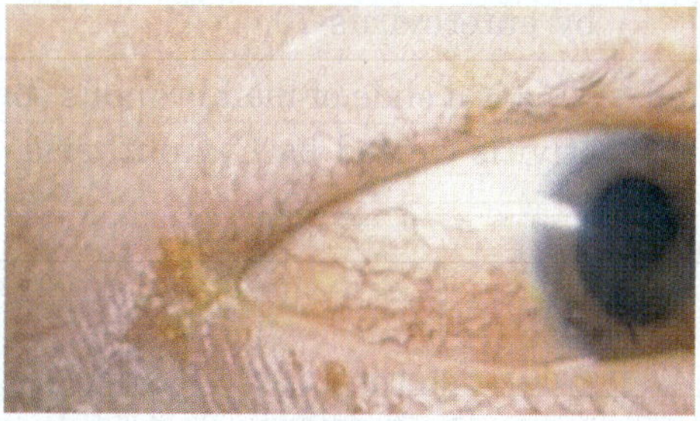

A. Moraxella axenfeld
B. Moraxella lacunata
C. Moraxella catarrhalis
D. All of the above

10. All are secondary signs except:

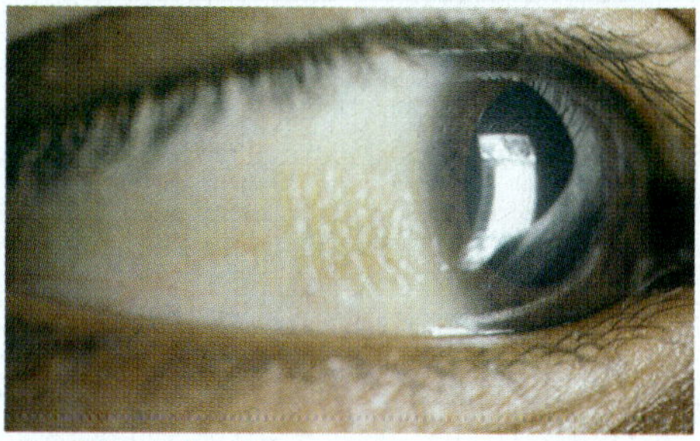

A. Nyctalopia
B. Corneal scarring
C. Xerophthalmic fundus
D. Conjunctival xerosis

ANSWERS OF IMAGE-BASED QUESTIONS

1. c This is shield ulcer seen in vernal keratoconjunctivitis.
   Shield ulcer: Plaque containing mucus and fibrin covers the epithelial defect—this leads to impairment of epithelial healing leading to formation of shield ulcer.
2. c Chemosis is edema of the conjunctiva.
3. a This is a phlycten caused by endogenous allergy by either staphylococcus or tuberculosis.
4. b This is "cobblestone appearance" which is due to severe epithelial hyperplasia seen in vernal keratoconjunctivitis.
5. a The slide shows Arlts line – which is linear scarring due to trachoma.
6. d PERFECT stands for pterygium extended resection followed by extended conjunctival transplantation. The recurrence in this surgery is zero.

7. a This is a slide of haemorrhagic conjunctivitis caused by all the following organisms. Most commonly by enterovirus-70.

8. d This is a slide of membranous conjunctivitis caused by C diphtheria.

9. d This is angular conjunctivitis caused by Moraxella and staphylococcus.

10. d The slide shows Bitots' spot, which is extreme conjunctival xerosis.

Secondary signs are the signs which may be seen in some other conditions other than xerophthalmia.

GUIDANCE

When your determination changes, everything else will begin to move in the direction you desire. The moment you resolve to be victorious every nerve and fibre in your being will immediately orient itself towards your success. On the other hand, if you think "This is never going to work out", then at that instant every cell in your being will be deflated and give up the fight, and then everything really will move in the direction of failure.

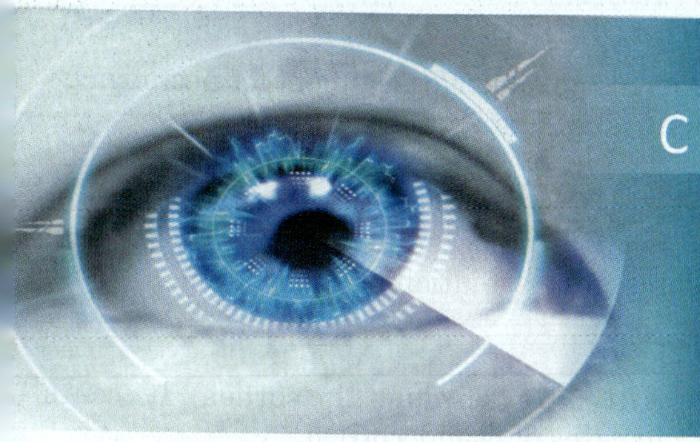

CHAPTER 5

Sclera and Episclera

EPISCLERITIS

- It is a common benign self-limiting recurrent disorder frequently affecting young adults.
- It never progresses to true scleritis.
- It is of two types:
  a. Simple.
  b. Nodular.

Clinical Features:

1. Unilateral mild discomfort.
2. Watering.
3. Tenderness to touch.

On Examination:

1. Simple—Sectoral or diffuse redness.
2. Nodular—Nodule with surrounding injection.

Treatment:

1. Mild case—No treatment.
2. Topical steroids and/or topical NSAIDS.
3. In recurrent case:
   a. Oral Flurbiprofen (100 mg tds).
   b. Oral Indomethacin (50 mg BD).

SCLERITIS

It is a granulomatous inflammation of the scleral coat of the eye.

Thinnest at the size of muscle insertions, more posteriorly than anteriorly.

Layers of sclera

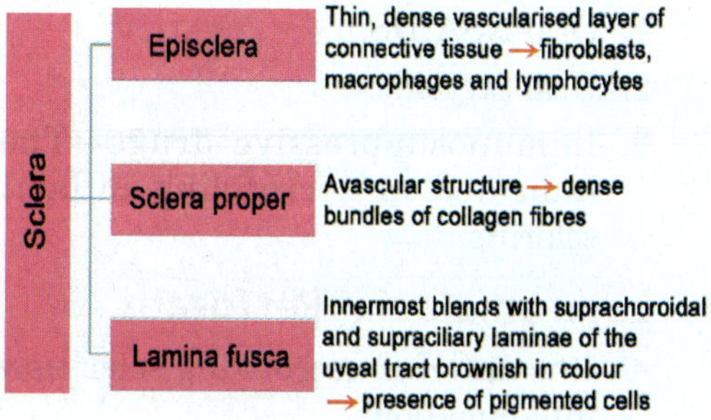

Fig. 5.1

Classification of Scleritis

Anterior Scleritis:

1. *Non-Necrotizing*
   - Diffuse.
   - Nodular.
2. *Necrotizing*
   - With inflammation.
   - Without inflammation.

Posterior Scleritis:

1. *Non-Necrotizing*
   - Diffuse.
   - Nodular.
2. *Necrotizing with inflammation.*
3. *Surgically induced scleritis.*

Associated Systemic Diseases in Scleritis

Patients of particularly necrotizing scleritis may have one of the following systemic diseases:

A. Rheumatoid arthritis.

B. Connective tissue vascular disorders like Polyarteritis nodosa, Systemic lupus erythematosus, Wegener's granulomatosis.

C. *Miscellaneous:*
   1. Relapsing Polychondritis.
   2. Herpes Zoster.

Treatment:

1. Oral NSAIDS.
2. Oral Steroids.
3. Immunosuppressive drugs—These are indicated in necrotizing inflammatory scleritis.

Scleromalacia Perforans

- It is anterior necrotising scleritis without inflammation.
- Common in women with long-standing seropositive rheumatoid arthritis.

Clinical Features:

1. Asymptomatic and starts with yellow necrotic scleral patch.
2. Large areas of exposed uvea due to scleral thinning.
3. Spontaneous perforation is rare, unless intraocular pressure is elevated.

Treatment:

There is no effective treatment for necrotizing–non-inflammatory scleritis.

Staphyloma

It is an ectatic condition of the eyeball alongwith herniation of uveal tissue.

Types:

1. **Anterior** (Through the cornea): It occurs in cases of pseudocornea.
2. **Intercalary staphyloma** (Through the limbus): It occurs in peripheral corneal ulcer.
3. **Ciliary** (Through the area of ciliary body, 2–3 mm from the limbus): It occurs in scleritis, perforating injury and absolute glaucoma.
4. **Equatorial** (Through the choroidal region): It occurs in scleritis and pathological myopia.
5. **Posterior staphyloma** (It is behind the equator): It is a feature of pathological myopia. It also occurs in posterior scleritis and perforating injuries.

   Blue sclera: It is a generalized blue discoloration of sclera due to thinning.

Causes:

1. Osteogenesis imperfecta.
2. Ehlers-Danlos syndrome.
3. Pseudoxanthoma elasticum.
4. Buphthalmos.
5. Healed scleritis.

NEET DRILL

1. Sclera is thinnest posterior to the muscle insertion.
2. The most common type of staphyloma is: posterior staphyloma.

MULTIPLE CHOICE QUESTIONS

1. **The following ocular structure is not derived from surface ectoderm:**

   A. Crystalline lens

   B. Sclera

C. Corneal epithelium

D. Epithelium of lacrimal glands

2. **The most common systemic association of scleritis:**

A. Ehlers-Danlos syndrome

B. Disseminated systemic sclerosis

C. Rheumatoid arthritis

D. Giant cell arteritis

3. **Scleromalacia perforans is a complication of:**

A. Rheumatoid arthritis

B. Sarcoidosis

C. Tuberculosis

D. Herpes zoster

4. **Most common cause of posterior staphyloma is:**

A. Glaucoma

B. Retinal detachment

C. Iridocyclitis

D. High myopia

5. **Blue sclera is seen in:**

A. Alkaptonuria

B. Ehlers-Danlos syndrome

C. Osteogenesis imperfecta

D. Kawasaki syndrome

6. **Sclera is thinnest at:**

A. Limbus B. Insertion of recti

C. Posterior pole D. Equator

7. **Weakest area of sclera:**

A. Behind insertion of rectus muscle

B. Equator

C. Limbus

D. Infront insertion of rectus

8. **Blue sclera is seen in all of the following conditions *except*:**

A. Keratoconus

B. Marfan's syndrome

C. Osteogenesis imperfecta

D. Rheumatoid arthritis

ANSWER AND EXPLANATION

1.	b	Sclera is derived from neural crest and mesoderm.
2.	c	45% of patients with scleritis have associated systemic disease like connective tissue disorders (Polyarteritis nodosa, Wegener's granulomatosis and SLE), Rheumatoid Arthritis, Herpes Zoster etc. It is most frequently associated with Rheumatoid Arthritis.
3.	a	Scleromalacia perforans, i.e., necrotizing anterior uveitis without inflammation, seen in patients of rheumatoid arthritis.
4.	d	Staphyloma is an ectatic condition of the eyeball with herniation of uveal tissue. Posterior staphyloma is a feature of axial myopia, where the eyeball is excessively long.
5.	b,c	Blue sclera is thin sclera so that the uveal tissue is visible. It is seen in patients of connective tissue disorders.
6.	b	The thinnest part of sclera is posterior to the insertion of muscles.
7.	a	Thickness of sclera anterior to the muscle insertion is 0.6 mm whereas posterior to the muscle insertion it is 0.3 mm.
8.	a	All other options are associated with blue sclera.

RECENTLY ADDED QUESTION

1. **A 21-year-old patient with glaucoma presents with bulging cornea. What is the diagnosis?**
   A. Staphyloma
   B. Granular dystrophy
   C. Keratoconus
   D. Keratomalacia

ANSWER OF RECENTLY ADDED QUESTION

1. a It is an ectatic condition of eyeball with herniation of uveal tissue.
   Staphyloma occurs in response to the inflammatory or degenerative changes in the eye which result in weakening of the eyeball. The presence of increased IOP contributes to the formation of staphyloma.

IMAGE-BASED QUESTIONS

1. **The diagnosis is:**

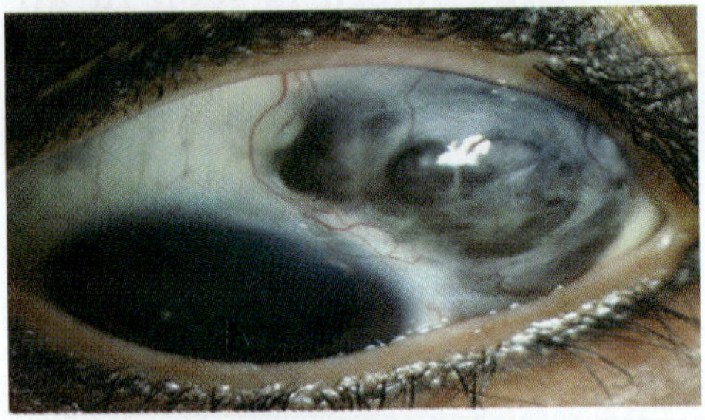

   A. Osteogenesis imperfecta
   B. Pseudoxanthoma elasticum
   C. Ehlers-Danlos syndrome
   D. Scleromalacia perforans

2. **The diagnosis is:**

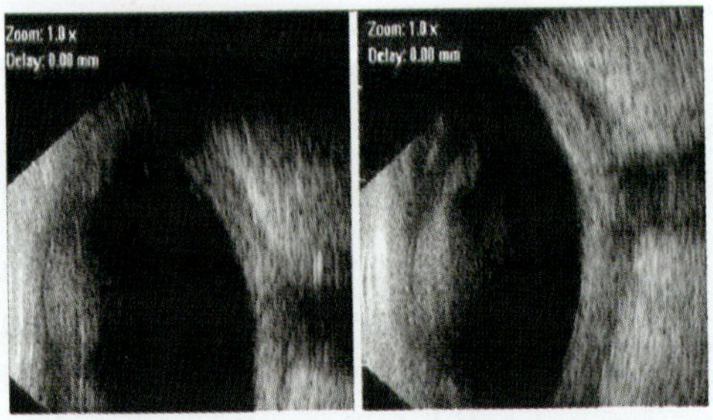

   A. Normal B scan
   B. Posterior scleritis
   C. Retinal detachment
   D. Floaters

3. **The diagnosis is:**

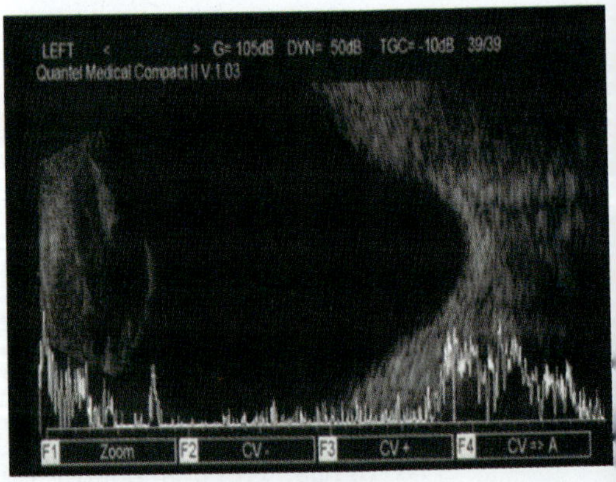

   A. Vitreous haemorrhage
   B. Posterior staphyloma
   C. Equatorial staphyloma
   D. Floaters

ANSWERS OF IMAGE-BASED QUESTIONS

1. d The above is a slide of scleromalacia perforans which is necrotizing anterior scleritis without inflammation.
2. b The above slide shows 'T' sign of posterior scleritis due to accumulation of fluid in the subtenons space.
3. b The above slide shows posterior staphyloma which is the most common type of staphyloma.

GUIDANCE

Position and Appearances are irrelevant. The important thing is to carry out our personal duty, our commitment, no matter what anyone else may say. This is a life of true victory, a life of unsurpassed nobility and fulfillment.

CHAPTER 6

Uveitis

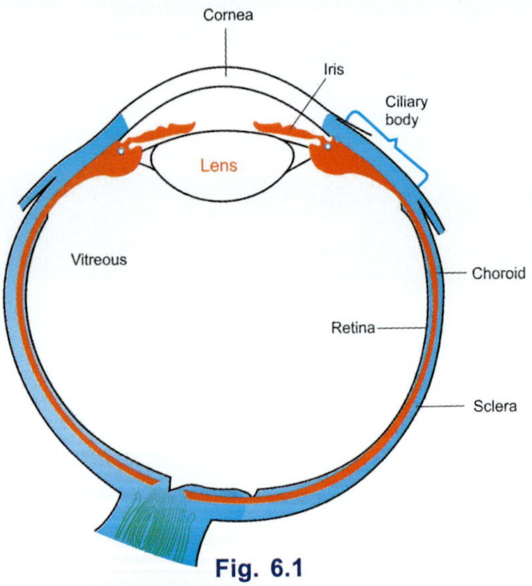

Fig. 6.1

IRIS

1. It is a circular disc, 12 mm in diameter with an aperture of 3–4 mm called pupil.
2. **Iris is thinnest at its root.**
3. *Anterior Surface:* It is divided into ciliary zone and pupillary zone by a zig-zag line called **Collarette** (represents attachment of pupillary membrane).

Microscopic Structure of Iris

Four layers from anterior to posterior are:

1. Anterior limiting membrane.
2. Iris stroma (It contains vessels, nerves, sphincter pupillae and dilator pupillae).
3. Anterior epithelial layer.
4. Posterior pigmented epithelial layer.

Ciliary Body: It is also called dangerous area of the eye as its trauma leads to severe immune reaction against uveal antigen leading to sympathetic ophthalmitis.

1. It's a forward continuation of choroid at ora serrata and is triangular in cut section.
2. It is divided into two parts:
   a. *Pars plicata.*
   b. Pars plana.

Microscopic Structure of Ciliary Body

1. Supraciliary lamina (outermost condensed stroma, consists of pigmented collagen fibres).
2. Stroma (consists of longitudinal or meridional, circular and radial fibres and vascular stroma having major arterial circle).
3. Layer of pigmented epithelium.
4. Layer of non-pigmented epithelium.
5. Internal limiting membrane.

Choroid: From without inwards it is divided into three layers:

1. **Suprachoroidal lamina:** It is a thin membrane of condensed collagen. The space between this membrane and the sclera is called suprachoroidal space which contains long and short posterior ciliary arteries.
2. **Stroma:** It constitutes of loose collagenous tissue. Its main bulk is formed of vessels which are arranged in three layers namely:
   A. Layer of large vessels, i.e., Haller's layer.
   B. Layer of medium vessels, i.e., Sattler's layer.
   C. Layer of choriocapillaris which nourishes the outer layer of retina.
3. **Basal lamina, i.e., Bruch's membrane:** It lies adjacent to RPE layer of the retina.

Blood Supply of Uveal Tract

Arterial Supply:

Uveal tract is supplied by three sets of arteries:

1. **Short posterior ciliary arteries:** It arises from ophthalmic artery as 2 trunks. Each trunk divides into 10–20 branches. These pierce the sclera around optic nerve and supply the choroids in segmental manner.
2. **Long posterior ciliary arteries:** They are two in no. Nasal and Temporal, pierce the sclera medial and lateral to optic nerve, travel in suprachoroidal space, reach ciliary muscle. At anterior end of ciliary muscle, these anastomose with each other and with anterior ciliary arteries to form **"Major Arterial Circle" (Circulus Ateriosus Major).**
3. **Anterior ciliary arteries:** They arise from muscular branches of ophthalmic artery (7 in no.), travel anteriorly in episclera, giving branches to sclera, limbus and conjunctiva, pierce sclera at limbus, enter the ciliary muscle and anastomose with two long posterior ciliary arteries to form **"circulus arteriosus major"** near root of the iris. Many branches from this circle run readily towards pupillary margin where they anastomose to form **"Circulus arteriosus minor".**

Venous Drainage

1. Anterior ciliary veins carry blood only from ciliary muscles.
2. Smaller veins from sclera carry blood from sclera.
3. **Venae verticosae** (vortex veins or posterior ciliary veins): They are four in no., at 5 O'clock, 7 O'clock, 11 O'clock and 1 O'clock. 2 superior vortex veins open in superior ophthalmic vein and 2 inferior veins in inferior ophthalmic vein.

   It drains:

   a. Whole of choroid.
   b. Receive small veins from optic nerve head.
   c. Sometimes small veins from retina.
   d. Anterior tributaries come from iris, ciliary processes, ciliary muscles and anterior part of choroid.

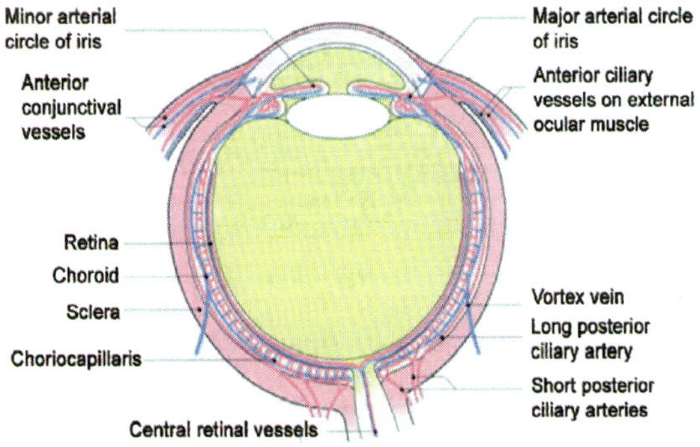

Fig. 6.2

UVEITIS

It is defined as the inflammation of the uveal tract.

Classification of Uveitis

a. Anatomical:

- *Anterior uveitis:* It is the inflammation of iris and pars plicata part of the ciliary body.
- *Intermediate uveitis:* It is the inflammation of the pars plana part of the ciliary body.
- *Posterior uveitis:* It is the inflammation of the choroid.
- *Panuveitis:* It is the inflammation of all parts of the uveal tissue.

b. Clinical:

- Acute uveitis.
- Chronic uveitis.

c. Pathological:

- Granulomatous.
- Non-granulomatous.

Masquerade syndrome: It denotes any condition which mimicks uveitis.

Causes are:

1. Intraocular lymphoma.
2. Retinoblastoma.
3. Choroidal melanoma.
4. Leukemia.
5. Amyloidosis.

Anterior Uveitis

It is the inflammation of the iris (iritis) and anterior part of ciliary body, i.e., pars plicata (iridocyclitis).

Clinical Features:

1. Photophobia, pain, redness, decreased vision, lacrimation (It never presents as a mucopurulent discharge).
2. Circumcorneal (ciliary) congestion.
3. **Keratic precipitates (KP):** They are proteinaceous deposits on the back of the cornea. They are fine and grey in non-granulomatous inflammation and mutton fat in granulomatous inflammation.

Types:

a. Mutton-Fat KPs:

- In granulomatous uveitis.
- Consist of macrophages, lymphocytes, plasma cells. These group into epithelioid cells.
- They have greasy quality hence called Mutton-Fat KPs.

b. Medium White and Small KPs:

- Sharply defined, white to beige-white in colour.
- In non-granulomatous uveitis.
- Mainly composed of lymphocytes.

c. Pigmented KPs:

- When the KPs phagocytose pigment; they become pigmented.
- These indicate an old chronic inflammatory process.

d. Stringy Keratic Precipitates:

- Consist of fine, thin lines on the endothelial surface appearing as intermeshing network.
- These are precipitated fibrin and not cellular deposits.

e. Red Keratic Precipitates:

- Consist of RBCs.
- In frank hyphema.

- Hyphema occurs more frequently in viral (especially herpetic) uveitis.

4. **Iris nodules** (feature of granulomatous inflammation):
   a. *Koeppe nodules:* It is at the pupillary border.
   b. *Busacca nodule:* It is at the base of the iris.
5. **Aqueous cells:** They are the inflammatory cells in the aqueous humour. It is the sign of active inflammation.
6. **Aqueous flare:** It is due to leakage of proteins in the anterior chamber from the iris capillaries.
7. **Constricted pupil: Miotic pupil is a pathognomic feature of uveitis:** In anterior uveitis, the pupil becomes small and reacts sluggishly due to iris edema, cellular infiltration of the stroma and effect of toxins on the nerve endings. Due to compact nature of sphincter muscle, it is more powerful than the dilator muscle which is diffuse and not very specific in action. As a result when iris becomes boggy from edema or cells, the sphincter muscle exerts a correspondingly greater effect than dilator muscle and therefore pupil constricts. When permanent synechiae form, they cause an irregular distortion of the pupil. This irregular appearance becomes most marked when pupil is dilated, and termed as **"festooned shaped pupil"**.

   In contrast to the uveitis, pupil in acute angle closure glaucoma is vertically oval dilated.
8. **Posterior Synechiae:** It presents as irregular, festooned-shaped pupil. It may lead to **Secclusio pupillae,** which is the posterior synechiae extending 360°, also called **Ring synechiae**. It will complicate to iris bombe and (PAS) peripheral anterior synechiae causing angle closure glaucoma. Later it may turn into **occlusio pupillae (the whole pupillary space is covered with fibrous tissue).**
9. Inflammatory cells in the anterior vitreous, also called retrolental flare.

Treatment of Anterior Uveitis

1. *Topical mydriatics:* **The primary role of mydriatics is to give rest to the ciliary muscles.** It also prevents the formation of posterior synechiae.
2. Topical steroids.
3. **In case if uveitis is associated with increased intraocular pressure, latanoprost and pilocarpine are contraindicated as anti-glaucoma therapy as they aggravate inflammation.**
4. *Cytotoxic drugs:* It may be indicated in severe cases when the patient does not respond with steroids.

   Indications are:
   a. Behcet's disease.
   b. Sympathetic uveitis: Relative indication.
   c. Intermediate uveitis: Rare indication.
   d. Serpiginous choroiditis.
5. *Immunomodulators:* Cyclosporin.

Intermediate Uveitis or Pars Planitis or Chronic Cyclitis

Idiopathic, insidious, chronic, intraocular inflammation typically affecting young adults.

Clinical Features:

1. Blurred vision.
2. Floaters which increase gradually.

3. Diminished visual acuity, if associated with CME (cystoid macular edema).

O/E:

a. *Anterior chamber:* It may be quiet or few cells and KPs may be present.

b. *Vitritis:* It is characterized by:
   - Inflammatory cells.
   - **Snow balls** or cotton balls: They are inflammatory exudates in the vitreous.
   - Posterior vitreous detachment (PVD).

c. *Mild peripheral periphlebitis:* Sheathing of terminal venules.

d. *Snow-Banking:* **It is the hallmark of pars planitis**. It consists of grey-white inflammatory plaque involving the inferior pars plana; which can only be seen by indirect ophthalmoscopy with scleral indentation.

Complications:

1. CME.
2. Secondary cataract.
3. Tractional RD.
4. Cyclitic membranes.

Differential Diagnosis of Snow-Banking

1. Sarcoidosis.
2. Candidiasis.
3. Multiple sclerosis.
4. Ocular toxocariasis.

Treatment:

It is in a four step approach:

Step 1: Periocular steroid injections, given in form of subtenon injections of triamicilone acetate.

Step 2: Systemic steroid and cytotoxic drugs.

Step 3: Cryotherapy of vitreous base: It damages the blood supply of the inflammatory membrane, i.e., snow banking.

Step 4: Vitrectomy: It aims at decreasing the bulk of inflammation and also the hazy media is removed leading to improvement of vision.

Posterior uveitis: It involves the inflammation of choroid alongwith other associated structures, i.e., vitreous, optic disc, macula, peripheral retina and retinal veins.

Clinical Features:

1. Choroiditis: It presents as yellowish round lesions.
2. Vitritis.
3. Cystoid macular edema.
4. Papillitis.
5. Retinal edema and sometimes associated with papilloedema.
6. Necrotic retinitis as in case of CMV infection.
7. Periphlebitis.

Treatment of Posterior Uveitis

1. Periocular subtenon injections of steroids (Triamcilone acetate).
2. Systemic steroids.
3. Rarely, cytotoxic drugs as mentioned above.

Complications of Uveitis

a. In the Cornea:

- Sclerosing keratouveitis.
- Corneal edema.
- Bullous keratopathy.
- Disciform keratitis.

- Descematocoele.
- Pannus.
- Band-shaped keratopathy.

b. Iris:

- Synechiae.
- Atrophy.
- Rubeosis.

c. Lens:

- Secondary cataract.

d. In the Globe:

- Glaucoma.
- Cyclitic membrane.
- *Pthisis bulbi:* It is the shrinkage of eyeball. In this all the three layers of the eyeball can be distinguished compared with **Atrophic bulbi**. In atrophic bulbi there is shrinkage of eyeball and the layers of the eyeball cannot be distinguished.

e. Posterior Segment:

- *CME (Cystoid macular edema):* It occurs due to release of prostaglandins in the inflammatory process.
- *Retinal detachment:* It does not occur as a complication of anterior uveitis but can occur in other form of uveitis.
- Optic nerve head edema.
- Macular hole.
- Cyclitic membrane formation which leads to cilio-choroidal detachment and finally hypotony.
- Choroidal neovascular membrane.

Causes of Anterior Uveitis

1. Idiopathic anterior uveitis.
2. Sero-negative arthropathies
   - Reiter's syndrome.
   - Ankylosing spondylitis.
   - Psoriatic arthritis.
   - JRA.
3. Inflammatory bowel disease.
4. Fuch's heterochromic cyclitis.
5. Viral (HSV, HZO) keratouveitis.
6. Posner-Schlossman syndrome.

Causes of Panuveitis

1. Sympathetic ophthalmitis.
2. Sarcoidosis.
3. Syphilis.
4. Vogt Koyanagi-Harada syndrome.
5. Tuberculosis.
6. Toxoplasmosis.

Causes of Posterior Uveitis

1. Idiopathic.
2. CMV retinitis.
3. Toxocariasis.
4. Presumed ocular histoplasmosis syndrome.
5. Acute retinal necrosis.
6. White dot syndromes.
7. Eales disease.

Causes of Intermediate Uveitis

1. Idiopathic.
2. Sarcoidosis.
3. Multiple sclerosis.
4. Toxocariasis.
5. Lyme disease.

Causes of Granulomatous Uveitis

1. Sarcoidosis.
2. Sympathetic ophthalmia.

3. Lens-induced uveitis.
4. VKH syndrome.
5. Syphilis.
6. TB.
7. Leprosy.

INVESTIGATIONS

A. Haematological Tests/Serological Tests:

1. *TLC, DLC, ESR:* To see for infections and tumours.

   DLC: Increased neutrophils indicate bacterial infections or immune complexes.
   Eosinophils: Parasitic infections.
   Lymphocytes: Viral, fungal or hypersensitivity reactions.

   Macrophages: Sympathetic ophthalmitis, Phacoanaphylactic reactions.

   Tumour cells: Masquerade syndrome.

2. *Urine analysis:* To see for pus cells; and

   Calcium: To exclude Reiter's syndrome and syphilis.

3. VDRL and FTA-ABS.
4. *ACE titres* (Angiotensin-converting enzyme): The serum levels are raised in patients of sarcoidosis.
5. ELISA and Western Blot to exclude AIDS.
6. *Immunofluorescent tests, ELISA, Indirect Haemagglutination tests and PCR:* To exclude Toxoplasmosis, Toxocariasis and Lyme disease.
7. *ANA:* To check for JRA and connective tissue disorders.

B. Skin Tests: All tests are based on type IV hypersensitivity reactions.

1. TB.
2. Sarcoidosis.
3. Lepromin test.
4. Histoplasmosis skin test.
5. Behcet's disease.

C. Imaging Techniques:

1. *X-ray chest:* TB, Sarcoidosis, old calcified lesions in lungs and spleen is seen in POHS.
2. *X-ray sacroiliac joint:* Ankylosing joint.
3. *X-ray affected joints:* For signs of arthritis.
4. *Skull X-ray:* Calcification in congenital toxoplasmosis.
5. Gallium-67 scan for sarcoidosis.

D. USG: It is needed in hazy media (specially in cases of toxocariasis to exclude other causes of leukocoria).

1. RD.
2. Intraocular tumours.
3. Diffuse retinochoroidal thickening in VKH and Sympathetic ophthalmitis.
4. Parasitic cysts as in cysticercosis.
5. Coats' disease.

E. HLA Typing:

HLA association in uveitis is a very important factor which helps in diagnosis.

a. HLA-B27—Sero-negative arthritis.
b. HLA-B5—Behcet's disease.
c. HLA-DR2—Intermediate uveitis.
d. HLA-DR4—VKH syndrome.

F. Aqueous Tap or Vitreous Biopsy:

Cytology, Histology and antibody estimation to exclude endophthalmitis and toxoplasmosis.

G. Biopsies:

1. *Conjunctival:* Sarcoidosis, Tuberculosis, Leprosy and syphilis.
2. *Lacrimal gland:* Sarcoidosis.
3. *Mucosal (buccal):* Behcet's disease.
4. *Vitreous:* Endophthalmitis and Acute Retinal Necrosis.
5. Syphilitic chancre.

H. Flourescein Angiography or Indocyanine Green Angiography:

1. Any case of anterior or intermediate uveitis with unexplained loss of vision to rule out CME.
2. Posterior uveitis.
3. White dot syndromes.
4. VKH.
5. SO.

I. Special Tests:

1. Audiometry in VKH.
2. Lumbar puncture in intraocular lymphomas and VKH.
3. Gallium scan.

SYSTEMIC ASSOCIATIONS OF UVEITIS

1. Uveitis Associated With Arthritis:

a. *Ankylosing Spondylitis:*

Inflammatory arthritis involving axial skeleton leading to fixed flexion deformity.

- **HLA-B27 associated.**
- Acute, recurrent non-granulomatous iritis.
- Negative RA factor.

b. *Reiter's Syndrome:*

- Constitutes triad of:
  a. Urethritis.
  b. Conjunctivitis.
  c. Sero-negative arthritis.
- **HLA-B27 associated.**
- **Ocular Features:**
  a. Bilateral mucopurulent conjunctivitis.
  b. Acute iritis.
  c. Keratitis.

c. *Psoriatic Arthritis:*

- Psoriasis is idiopathic, erythematous–scaly plaques all over the body.
- Sero-negative arthritis.
- **HLA-B27 associated.**
- **Ocular Features:**
  a. Conjunctivitis.
  b. Acute iritis.
  c. Keratitis.
  d. Secondary Sjögren's syndrome.

d. *Juvenile Chronic Arthritis (JCA):*

It is an idiopathic inflammatory arthritis of at least 3 months, developing in children below age of 16 years.

It is divided into 3 types:

1. Systemic onset.
2. Polyarticular (>5 joints involvement).
3. Pauciarticular (<5 joints involvement).
   - It's a sero-negative arthritis, i.e., **rheumatoid factor is negative.**
   - **It's the pauciarticular arthritis which is associated with uveitis.**

Ocular Features:

Anterior uveitis: It is chronic, non-granulomatous and bilateral (in 70% cases).

Clinical Features:

Asymptomatic and uveitis is detected on routine slit lamp examination.

On Examination:

- White eye with no congestion even in presence of severe uveitis. Hence also called **"White Uveitis"**.
- KPs – Small to medium.
- Hypopyon – Rare.
- Posterior synechiae – Common in long-standing cases.

Complications:

1. Complicated cataract.
2. Band keratopathy.
3. Extensive posterior synechiae.
4. Secondary glaucoma.

Treatment:

Topical steroids, periocular injection of steroids, systemic steroids.

2. Sarcoidosis:

It is an idiopathic, multisystem disorder characterised by presence of non-caseating granulomata in lungs and other organs.

Ocular Features:

It causes granulomatous panuveitis.

1. Sarcoid plaques, sarcoid granulomata on the eyelids.
2. Anterior segment lesion: Involvement of conjunctiva, episclera, sclera.
3. KCS: Due to involvement of lacrimal gland.
4. Anterior uveitis: Chronic granulomatous iridocyclitis.
5. Diffuse vitritis.
6. Snow ball opacities in vitreous.
7. *Fundus Changes:*

   a. Periphlebitis—Advanced stage of vascular sheathing leads to **Candle-wax drippings.**

   b. Retinal granulomata.

   c. Pre-retinal nodules – **Lander's sign.**

   d. Retinal haemorrhages – In acute sarcoid retinopathy.

   e. Choroidal granulomata.

   f. **Optic nerve lesions:**

      1. Disc granuloma.
      2. Neovascularization.
      3. Papilloedema.
      4. Optic atrophy.

3. Behcet's Disease:

1. It is an idiopathic multi-system disorder, affecting young men leading to obliterative vasculitis due to circulating immune complexes.
2. **Clinical Features:**

   a. Oral ulceration.

   b. Recurrent genital ulceration.

   c. Skin lesions.

   d. Eye involvement.

   e. Positive pathergy test.
3. **HLA-B5 associated.**

Ocular Features: Recurrent, bilateral, non-granulomatous, intraocular inflammation affecting either anterior or posterior segment.

Anterior Segment: Acute recurrent iridocyclitis, may be associated with **transient hypopyon.**

Posterior Segment:

a. Diffuse vascular leakage, leading to diffuse retinal edema, CME, disc edema.

b. Periphlebitis.

c. Retinitis: White, necrotic, infiltrates of inner retina, with intraretinal haemorrhage leading to retinal atrophy.

d. Vitritis.

4. Vogt-Koyanagi-Harada Syndrome:

1. Idiopathic multisystem disorder which **typically affects pigmented individuals.**
2. HLA-DR4 associated.
3. **Skin and Hair Changes:**
   a. Alopecia.
   b. Poliosis.
   c. Vitiligo **(suguiras sign).**
4. **Neurological Features:**
   a. Irritation.
   b. Encephalopathy.
   c. Auditory symptoms: Tinnitus, Vertigo, Deafness.
   d. CSF: Lymphocytosis.
5. **Ocular Features:**
   a. Chronic granulomatous iridocyclitis.
   b. *Posterior segment*:
      - Multifocal choroiditis.
      - Multifocal detachment of sensory retina.

5. AIDS: Ocular complications develop in 75% of AIDS patients.

a. **Retinal Microangiopathy: It is the most common ocular manifestation of AIDS.**

Clinical Features:

- Commonly non-infectious.
- It is characterized by cottonwool spots, haemorrhages, microaneurysms. Cottonwool spots resolve spontaneously.

Pathogenesis:

1. Due to immune complex deposition.
2. Due to HIV infection of retinal vascular endothelium.

b. **Opportunist Infections:**

1. **CMV Retinitis: Most common secondary infection in AIDS.**

   a. *Central Retinitis:*

   Dense, white, well-demarcated geographical area of retinal necrosis, along the vascular arcades, with retinal haemorrhages in the area of necrosis or along its leading edge. This whole picture is described as **"Sauce and Cheese Retinopathy".**

   b. *Peripheral Retinitis:*
   - It has the same picture but is less demarcated.
   - The infection spreads slowly along vascular arcades in a **brushfire-like fashion** and leads to retinal atrophy, optic atrophy and retinal detachment.

   Treatment:
   1. I/V Gangcyclovir.
   2. I/V Foscarnet.
   3. Intravitreal Gangcyclovir implants.

2. **Pneumocystis Carinii Choroiditis:**

   a. Pneumocystis carinii, is an opportunistic protozoan parasite and is the major cause of morbidity and mortality in AIDS.

   b. **C/F:** Choroiditis: Flat, yellow, round lesions located behind the equator.

   Treatment:

   a. I/V Trimethoprim + Sulphamethoxazole.

b. Parental Pentamidine.

3. **Toxoplasma Retinochoroiditis.**
4. **Fungal Infections:**

Cryptococcus neoformans choroiditis: It is the most common fungal infection in AIDS.

a. Asymptomatic creamy choroidal lesions, not associated with vitritis.

b. Optic nerve involvement leads to disc swelling or retrobulbar neuritis. It is usually associated with meningitis.

Histoplasma Capsulatum:

1. It is a rare fungal infection in AIDS patient.
2. It causes POHS–Presumed Ocular Histoplasmosis Syndrome.

Clinical Features—Triad of:

1. Multiple atrophic choroidal spots (histospots).
2. Peripapillary atrophy.
3. Haemorrhagic, disciform maculopathy.

Other fungal infection that involves the posterior segment is: Candidiasis.

5. **Varicella-Zoster Retinitis:** It causes ARN, i.e., acute retinal necrosis. CMV and HSV cause acute retinal necrosis in young and HZO in adults.
6. **Large Cell Intraocular Lymphoma.**

6. Toxoplasmosis: It's an obligate intracellular protozoan, cat is a definitive host and humans, mice are intermediate host.

Mode of Infection: Most commonly is in foetal life and later it reoccurs in old healed chorioretinal scar due to rupture of cyst.

Ocular Features:

a. **Iridocyclitis:**

Granulomatous or non-granulomatous.

b. **Posterior Uveitis:**

1. Focal superficial necrotising retinochoroiditis – **"Headlight in Fog Appearance"**.
2. Deep retinitis (involving outer retinal layer).
3. Granuloma.
4. Papillitis.

Old choroid lesions of toxoplasmosis are seen as punched out lesions with pigmented borders.

Treatment:

1. *Systemic steroids:* In immunocompromised patients, subtenon injections are given.
2. *Clindamycin:* 300 mg four times daily.
3. Sulphonamide therapy.
4. Pyrimethamine.
5. Co-trimoxazole.

Adjunctive Therapy:

1. *Laser photocoagulation:* To limit cell to cell spread of infection by encircling the active lesion.
2. *Cryotherapy:* Used for peripheral lesions where laser is not possible.
3. *Vitrectomy:* If severe opacities.

7. Syphilis

Ocular Features:

a. *Anterior Segment:*

1. Madarosis, primary chancre of conjunctiva, scleritis, interstitial keratitis (affecting stroma of cornea).

Madarosis: Loss of eyelashes and eyebrows, both conditions are termed as madarosis.

2. Acute granulomatous or non-granulomatous uveitis.

b. *Posterior Segment:*

1. **Multifocal chorioretinitis:**

"Salt and pepper fundus" also called "Pseudo-Retinitis Pigmentosa".

Salt and Pepper Fundus: Due to dispersion of pigments in the retina, the picture on ophthalmoscopy appears as salt and pepper and hence the name.

D/D of Salt and Pepper Fundus

1. Rubella.
2. Syphilis.
3. Retinitis pigmentosa sine pigmento.
4. Carriers of albinism.
5. Refsum's disease (Phytanic acid storage disorder).
6. Leber's congenital amaurosis.

2. **Unifocal choroiditis:** Less common.

a. *Juxtapapillary:* Near disc.

b. *Central:* At macula (Macular patch).

Other causes of macular patch:

1. Central choroiditis due to toxoplasmosis.
2. Atrophic choroidal spots due to histoplasmosis (Histiospots).
3. Pathological myopia.
4. Trauma.
5. Macular coloboma.

3. **Neuroretinitis:** Retinal and disc edema with peripapillary (around the disc) cottonwool spots and flame-shaped haemorrhages.

c. *Neuro-Ophthalmic Features:*

1. *Argyll-Robertson pupil:* Light reaction absent and near-reflex present.

2. *Optic-nerve lesions:*

a. Retrobulbar neuritis.

b. *If raised ICT:* Papilloedema.

c. *Perioptic neuritis:* Inflammation of meningeal sheaths of optic nerve, seen in association with syphilitic meningitis.

3. *Ocular motor palsy:* 3rd and 6th.

4. *Visual field defects:* Due to gummatous involvement of brain.

Treatment:

1. 12–24 MU of aqueous penicillin I/V for 10 days followed by 2.4 MU I/M for 3 weeks.
2. Oral tetracycline and oral erythromycin.

8. **Tuberculosis:** It causes chronic granulomatous infection.

Ocular Features:

a. **External Lesions:** It may involve any ocular and periocular structure, i.e., eyelids, conjunctiva, cornea, sclera and orbit.

b. **Uveitis:** There is no specific finding in TB uveitis and the clinical picture is pleomorphic.

1. *Chronic iridocyclitis:*
   - Most frequent feature.
   - Usually Granulomatous.
2. *Choroiditis:* Focal or multifocal.
3. *Retinal vasculitis:*
   - Moderate vitritis.
   - Severe ischemic periphlebitis.
   - Peripheral capillary closure which can lead to neovascularisation.

Treatment:

ATT drugs.

9. Leprosy:

a. Loss of eyebrows and eyelashes (*Madarosis*).

b. Trichiasis.

c. Episcleritis and scleritis.

d. Facial palsy leading to lagophthalmos.

e. Granuloma over cornea.

f. Leperoma over cornea.

g. Interstitial keratitis.

h. Granulomatous uveitis.

i. Posterior uveitis.

j. Optic neuritis.

k. Complicated cataract.

l. If chronic uveitis: Iris pearls, iris atrophy.

10. Fuch's Uveitis Syndrome or Fuch's Heterochromic Cyclitis (FUS)

It's an insidious, *non-granulomatous*, *anterior uveitis* affecting *one eye* of a *middle aged patient*.

Clinical Features:

a. Uniocular blurring of vision secondary to cataract formation.

b. Keratic precipitates are pathognomic as they are small, *stellate and grey-coloured*, scattered throughout the cornea. These KPs never become confluent or pigmented. *Feathery fibrin filaments* may be seen in between the KPs.

c. Aqueous humour:

- Faint flare.
- Few cells.

d. Absence of posterior synechiae.

e. Iris stromal atrophy: It may be associated with patchy atrophy of posterior pigment layer of iris.

f. Heterochromia iridis.

g. Koeppes nodules are occasionally seen.

h. Rubeosis iridis.

i. Enlarged pupil, due to atrophy of iris sphincter.

j. Vitritis.

Complications:

1. Cataract.
2. Glaucoma is usually of open-angle type caused by trabecular sclerosis.

Treatment:

- **No role of topical steroids and mydriatics (as no synechiae is formed).**
- 6 months follow-up to detect glaucoma.

11. Sympathetic Ophthalmitis:

- Very rare, bilateral, *granulomatous, non-suppurative, panuveitis*.
- Occurs after accidental penetrating trauma.
- It involves both eyes. The traumatized eye is referred as the *exciting eye* and the fellow eye is the *sympathizing eye*.
- **65% of cases occur between 2 weeks and 3 months after injury.**
- 90% of cases occur within first year.
- Prodromal symptoms in sympathizing eye are:

  a. Blurring of vision due to loss of accommodation **(The first symptom of sympathetic ophthalmitis).**

  b. Photophobia.

Clinical Features:

1. Anterior Segment:

- Red and irritable eye.
- **Earliest sign:** Retrolental flare, as inflammation starts in ciliary body.

- Koeppe nodules.
- Mutton-fat KPs.
- Posterior synechiae.

2. **Posterior Segment:**
   - **Dalen-Fuch's Nodules:** Small, deep, yellow-white spots scattered throughout the fundus. Dalen-Fuch's nodules consist of **epithelioid cells between retinal pigment epithelium and Bruch's membrane**.
   - Optic nerve head oedema.
   - Sub-retinal oedema.

Complications:

1. Complicated cataract.
2. Secondary glaucoma.
3. Pthisis bulbi.

Treatment:

1. Vigorous steroid therapy by all possible routes of administration.
2. Immunosuppressive therapy with Chlorambucil, Cyclophosphamide or Cyclosporin *in severe steroid-resistant cases*.
3. **Enucleation (not evisceration):** Within 2 weeks of injury will prevent sympathetic uveitis. **Evisceration is contraindicated in this condition, because if any uveal tissue is left behind after evisceration then it will incite the immune reaction and sympathetic ophthalmitis will not be prevented.**

12. River Blindness (Onchocerciasis)

- It is caused by infection by **Onchocerca volvulus, a nematode.**
- It is endemic in Africa and Central and South America.
- Its vector is Blackfly.
- Microfilariae are reproduced in nodules and are spread throughout the body where they incite local inflammation.

Ocular Features:

Route of entry into eye is not clear.

1. *Anterior uveitis:* It causes non-granulomatous anterior uveitis as the earliest sign. Small, white wriggling worm in the anterior chamber may be seen.
2. *Sclerosing keratitis:* It is the major cause of blindness.
3. *Chorioretinitis:* It causes chronic, non-granulomatous chorioretinitis leading to extensive retinal atrophy and scarring. Macula is spared.
4. *Visual field defects* and *Night blindness* are out of proportion to the fundus changes.

Treatment:

Ivermectin: It is given, only to those at high risk of blindness because treatment can lead to severe, acute, systemic, inflammation (*MAZZOTI'S REACTION*) that can cause death. Control of onchocerciasis is included **in Vision 2020 programme.**

Ophthalmia Nodosum

It is a very severe, granulomatous iridocyclitis, **due to caterpillar hair** in the eye. A very large nodule is formed on the iris, and hence the name.

Posner-Schlossman Syndrome

- It is also called **Glaucomatocyclitic crisis/Hypertensive uveitis.**
- It constitutes recurrent attacks of mild anterior uveitis with secondary open-angle glaucoma. Intraocular pressure is usually severely elevated: 40 mm Hg to 60 mm Hg, and the signs of uveitis, i.e.,

KPs are few. This may lead to misdiagnosis as acute angle closure glaucoma.

Treatment:

The aim of treatment is to control uveitis which may lead to decrease in intraocular pressure.

1. Atropine therapy alongwith medical reduction of intraocular pressure.
2. Role of topical steroids is doubtful, as it itself leads to increase in the IOP. Mild steroids may be needed to control uveitis.

Hence the drug of choice in a patient of uveitis with raised intraocular pressure is atropine.

Heterochromia Iridis: (D/D)

1. *Congenital:*
   a. Waardenburg's syndrome.
   b. Horner's syndrome.
   c. Naevus of ota.
   d. Congenital ocular melanocytosis.
2. *Acquired:*
   a. Chronic iritis.
   b. Fuch's heterochromic cyclitis.
   c. Iris naevus or melanoma.
   d. Siderosis.
   e. Rubeosis.
   f. Topical latanoprost.

Ocular Features of Ulcerative Colitis

a. The most common manifestation documented is **Recurrent anterior uveitis (commonly iritis)**. It may be unilateral or bilateral.

b. Patient may have associated Ankylosing spondylitis.

Ocular Features of Crohn's Disease

1. Anterior uveitis.
2. Episcleritis
   (1) Scleritis.
   (2) Optic neuritis.
   (3) Extraocular muscle paresis.
   (4) Lid edema.
   (5) Rarely
   - Retinal vasculitis.
   - Peripheral corneal infiltrates.

Treatment of Uveitis in Inflammatory Bowel Disease

1. Systemic steroids.
2. Oral NSAIDs.
3. Immunomodulator therapy
   - Azathioprine.
   - Cyclosporin.

Whipple's Disease

Ocular Features:

1. Anterior uveitis.
2. Vitritis.
3. Extraocular muscle paresis.
4. Supranuclear ophthalmoplegia.

Treatment:

Antibiotic therapy.

WHITE DOT SYNDROMES

- It is a broad term comprising various uveitic entities characterized by multiple white dots; in retinal pigment epithelium and/or choroids.
- These white dots are microgranuloma composed of lymphocytes and macrophages. **Lymphocytes are mainly T-lymphocytes.**

Causes of White Dot Syndromes

A. Inflammatory:

1. POHS–Presumed Ocular Histoplasmosis Syndrome.
2. MEWDS–Multiple Evanescent White Dot Syndrome.
3. Multifocal Choroiditis.
4. Sympathetic Ophthalmitis.
5. VKH Syndrome.
6. HIV Retinopathy.
7. Serpiginous Choroidopathy.

B. Degenerative:

1. Stargardt's disease.
2. Retinitis punctata albescens.
3. Drusen.

C. Neoplastic:

1. Leukemic retinopathy.
2. Metastatic tumour.
3. Large cell lymphoma (Non-Hodgkin's Lymphoma).

D. Traumatic: Purtscher's Retinopathy.

E. MSC:

1. Drugs like Chloroquine, Tamoxifen.
2. Photocoagulation spots.

NEET DRILL

1. Eales' disease also called periphlebitis retinae presents as recurrent vitreous haemorrhage and is typically a disease of young males.
2. Most common cause of recurrent anterior uveitis in young males: sero-negative arthritis which is associated with HLA B-27.
3. Sarcoidosis causes granulomatous panuveitis, and in the cornea it can cause interstitial keratitis and band-shaped keratopathy.
4. Sign of active inflammation in anterior uveitis is aqueous cells.
5. Choice of treatment of anterior uveitis is topical steroids.
6. Pathognomic feature of pars planitis is snow-banking.
7. JRA associated with uveitis is Pauciarticular, Sero-negative Early Onset JRA.
8. Ciliary muscles are derived from neural crest.
9. Eales' disease is type 4 hypersensitivity reaction.
10. Most common side effect of HAART therapy is Immune Recovery Uveitis.
11. LUMINATE program: Study to find a non-steroidal treatment of uveitis. Drug that is studied is Voclosporin.
12. "Sauce and Cheese Retinopathy" is a feature of CMV retinitis.
13. "Headlight-In-Fog" appearance is a feature of Toxoplasmosis.
14. Candle-wax drippings is a feature of sarcoidosis.
15. Dangerous area of eye is "ciliary body".
16. Juxtapapillary choroiditis is a feature of syphilis.
17. Most common ocular manifestation of TB in uveitis.
18. Most common allergic manifestation of TB is phlyctenular keratoconjunctivitis.

MULTIPLE CHOICE QUESTIONS

1. **Which of the following statements is incorrect about pthisis bulbi?**
   A. The intraocular pressure is increased
   B. Calcification of the lens is common
   C. Sclera is thickened
   D. Size of the globe is reduced
2. **An 18-year-old boy comes to the eye casualty with history of injury with a tennis ball. On examination there is no perforation but there is hyphema. The most likely source of the blood is:**
   A. Iris vessels
   B. Circulus iridis major
   C. Circulus iridis minor
   D. Short posterior ciliary arteries
3. **In a patient with AIDS, chorioretinitis is typically caused by:**
   A. Cytomegalovirus
   B. Toxoplasma gondii
   C. Cryptococcus neoformans
   D. Histoplasma capsulatum
4. **A 26 years old male has miotic pupil, intraocular pressure is 25 mm Hg, normal anterior chamber, hazy cornea with shallow anterior chamber of fellow eye. The likely diagnosis is:**
   A. Acute anterior uveitis
   B. Acute angle closure glaucoma
   C. Senile cataract
   D. Acute open angle glaucoma
5. **All the following diseases are associated with HLA-B27 and uveitis except:**
   A. Behcet's syndrome
   B. Psoriasis
   C. Ankylosing spondylitis
   D. Reiter's syndrome
6. **Sauce and cheese retinopathy is seen in:**
   A. CMV
   B. Rubella
   C. Toxoplasmosis
   D. Congenital syphilis
7. **For acute anterior uveitis, the treatment of choice is:**
   A. Local steroids
   B. Systemic steroids
   C. Local NSAIDS
   D. Systemic NSAIDS
8. **First sign of sympathetic ophthalmia is:**
   A. Retrolental flare
   B. Aqueous flare
   C. Dilated pupil
   D. Constricted pupil
9. **All drugs are used in acute anterior uveitis except:**
   A. Pilocarpine B. Atropine
   C. Timolol D. Propanolol
10. **Dangerous area of eye is:**
    A. Retina B. Sclera
    C. Ciliary body D. Optic nerve
11. **The laser procedure most often used for treating iris neo-vascularisation is:**
    A. Goniophotocoagulation
    B. Laser trabeculoplasty
    C. Panretinal photocoagulation
    D. Laser iridoplasty

12. A 25-year-old male gives a history of redness, pain and mild diminution of vision in one eye for past 3 days. There is also a history of low backache for the past one year. On examination there is circumcorneal congestion, cornea is clear apart from a few fine keratic precipitates on the corneal endothelium, there are 2 + cells in the anterior chamber and the intraocular pressure is within normal limits. The patient is most likely suffering from:

A. Acute attack of angle closure glaucoma
B. HLA B-27 related anterior uveitis
C. JRA associated uveitis
D. Herpetic keratitis

13. Which of these does not feature eye manifestations in association with a sero-negative arthropathy?

A. Psoriasis
B. Rheumatoid arthritis
C. Reiter's syndrome
D. Ankylosing spondylitis

14. What is the most common eye manifestation of allergy to tubercular bacilli?

A. Koeppes nodules
B. Posterior scleritis
C. Phlyctenular conjunctivitis
D. Optic neuritis

15. A 25-year-old lady presents with severe congestion, photophobia and deep anterior chamber in the right eye. The left eye is normal. X-ray pelvis shows sacroilitis. The diagnosis is:

A. Anterior uveitis
B. Posterior uveitis
C. Intermediate uveitis
D. Scleritis

16. Which of the following is the most common infection which causes blindness in adult man?

A. Toxocara
B. Toxoplasma gondii
C. Taenia solium
D. Plasmodium falciparum

17. A boy presents two weeks after an injury of his left eye. He complains of bilateral pain and redness and watering from right eye. What is the probable diagnosis?

A. Endophthalmitis
B. Optic neuritis
C. Sympathetic irritation
D. Sympathetic ophthalmitis

18. In hypertensive patient having acute uveitis to decrease the IOP which drug is used?

A. Pilocarpine B. Latanoprost
C. Iodine D. Timolol

19. Atropine is used in uveitis to:

A. Give rest to ciliary body and iris
B. Increase vascularity that provides antibodies
C. Prevent posterior synechiae formation
D. None

20. All of the following features are seen in pauciarticular JRA except:

A. Cataract B. Keratopathy
C. Scleritis D. Uveitis

21. All are complications of acute anterior uveitis, except:

A. Glaucoma
B. Cataract

C. Macular oedema

D. Retinal detachment

22. Skin depigmentation, bilateral uveitis and tinitus are features of:

A. Vogt-Koyanagi-Harada syndrome

B. Waardenburg syndrome

C. Apert syndrome

D. Werner's syndrome

23. Iridocyclitis is a feature of:

A. Juvenile rheumatoid arthritis with systemic involvement

B. Seropositive, pauciarticular, juvenile rheumatoid arthritis

C. Seronegative, pauciarticular, juvenile rheumatoid arthritis

D. Seropositive, polyarticular, juvenile rheumatoid arthritis

24. All are features of acute anterior uveitis, except:

A. Aqueous flare

B. Shallow anterior chamber

C. Circumcorneal congestion

D. Miosis

25. Dalen Fuch's nodule is seen in:

A. Bacterial endophthalmitis

B. Mycotic endophthalmitis

C. Sympathetic ophthalmia

D. Phacotoxic endopthalmitis

26. River blindness is caused by:

A. Oncocerca volvulus

B. Lymphogranuloma venereum

C. Chlamydia trachomatis

D. Acanthamoeba

27. First symptom of sympathetic ophthalmitis is:

A. Retrolental flare

B. Circumciliary congestion

C. Difficulty in accommodation

D. Photophobia

28. In acute anterior uveitis pupil is:

A. Large and fixed

B. Semidilated

C. Irregular and constricted

D. Oval and fixed

29. Sympathetic ophthalmia is:

A. Bilateral suppurative uveitis

B. Bilateral non-suppurative uveitis

C. Unilateral non-suppurative uveitis

D. Unilateral suppurative uveitis

30. Signs of uveitis:

A. Generalised conjunctival congestion

B. Circumciliary congestion

C. Cells and flare in aqueous

D. Keratic precipitates

31. Common features between sympathetic ophthalmitis and VKH syndrome:

A. Autoimmune etiology

B. Injury

C. Uveitis

D. Vitiligo

32. Uveitis is caused by:

A. TB

B. Staphylococcus

C. Streptococcus

D. E coli

E. Klebsiella

33. The investigations of anterior uveitis for a 25 years old boy are:

A. HLA B27

B. X-ray sacroiliac joint

C. TORCH agent

D. USG abdomen

34. All are seen in acute iridocyclitis except:

A. Pain

B. Ciliary congestion

C. Mucopurulent discharge

D. Small pupil

35. Snow banking is typically seen in:

A. Pars planitis

B. Endophthalmitis

C. Coats' disease

D. Eales' disease

36. Macula involvement is common in:

A. Toxoplasma B. Malaria

C. CMV D. Syphilis

37. In sympathetic ophthalmitis injury is to the:

A. Iris B. Retina

C. Ciliary body D. Sclera

38. Anterior uveitis is seen in:

A. Rheumatoid arthritis

B. HLAB27

C. Ankylosing spondylitis

D. Juvenile rheumatoid arthritis

E. All of the above

39. Most common ocular manifestation of AIDS is:

A. Cottonwool spots

B. Cytomegalovirus retinitis

C. Kaposi sarcoma of conjunctiva

D. Toxoplasmic uveitis

40. Acute retinal necrosis can be caused by:

A. Staphylococcus aureus

B. Cytomegalovirus

C. Streptococcus pyogenes

D. Adenovirus

41. "Headlight—In Fog Appearance" of retina is seen in:

A. Toxoplasmosis

B. Toxocara

C. Herpes

D. Tractional retinal detachment

42. Which of the following is not a feature of granulomatous uveitis?

A. Mutton fat keratic precipitates

B. Koeppe's nodules

C. Involves usually anterior uvea

D. Marked impairment of vision

43. All of the following cause panuveitis except:

A. Ankylosing spondylitis

B. Toxoplasmosis

C. Sarcoidosis

D. Sympathetic ophthalmitis

44. Salt and pepper fundus occurs in:

A. Toxoplasma B. Toxocara

C. Rubella D. Scurvy

45. Nodule in iris not found in:

A. Sarcoidosis

B. Neurofibromatosis

C. Tuberous sclerosis

D. SLE

46. Iris is thinned at:

A. Root of iris

B. Pupillary border

C. Collarette

D. Ciliary body junction

47. Cysts are associated with repeated use of:

A. Pilocarpine B. Eserine

C. Adrenaline D. Timolol

48. All of the following are true regarding sympathetic ophthalmia except:

A. Approximately 65% of cases occur after perforating injury

B. Most of the cases occur within 2 weeks of injury

C. Uveal antigen has been implicated as the responsible exciting agent

D. First symptom is loss of accommodation

49. Ocular complication of ulcerative colitis:

A. Uveitis B. Conjunctivitis

C. Keratitis D. All of the above

50. Sympathetic ophthalmitis affects:

A. Injured eye

B. Sound eye

C. Both the eyes

D. Eye with past history of injury

51. Iris nodules are noted in all except:

A. Hansen's disease

B. Neurofibromatosis

C. Fuch's heterochromic iridocyclitis

D. Tuberculosis

52. Ocular lesion in toxocariasis may be:

A. Posterior pole granuloma

B. Retinal detachment

C. Low grade iridocyclitis

D. All of the above

53. Smooth muscle of iris is developed from:

A. Surface ectoderm

B. Mesoderm

C. Neural crest

D. Neural ectoderm

54. Same between sympathetic ophthalmitis and VKH syndrome is:

A. Both are bilateral granulomatous panuveitis

B. Either of them can be unilateral

C. Both have autoimmune etiology

D. Both A and C

55. Mutton-Fat keratic precipitates are seen in:

A. Granulomatous iridocyclitis

B. Non-granulomatous iridocyclitis

C. Granulomatous choroiditis

D. Non-granulomatous choroiditis

56. Iris bombe is due to:

A. Anterior synechiae

B. Posterior synechiae

C. Peripheral synechiae

D. Ring synechiae

57. All of the following are true regarding acute anterior uveitis in ankylosing spondylitis except:

A. More common in females

B. Recurrent attacks occur

C. Fibrous reaction in anterior chambers

D. Narrowing of joint spaces and sclerosis of the sacroiliac joints

58. All are causes of chronic granulomatous uveitis except:

A. Sarcoidosis

B. Tuberculosis

C. Brucellosis

D. Fuch's heterochromic cyclitis

59. One of the most common complication of iridocyclitis is:

A. Scleritis

B. Secondary glaucoma

C. Band shaped keratopathy

D. Corneal ulcer

60. The correct statement regarding the duration after which sympathetic ophthalmitis develops is:

A. 3 weeks–12 weeks after trauma

B. Within 1 week

C. After 2 months

D. Typically at 10 days

61. In which of the following condition, iridectomy is indicated?

A. Prolapsed iris

B. Closed angle glaucoma

C. As part of cataract extraction

D. Threatening ring synechiae

E. All of the above

62. Total posterior synechia causes:

A. Deep anteriror chamber

B. Shallow anterior chamber

C. Funnel-shaped anterior chamber

D. Festooned pupil

63. Bilateral blindness can result from:

A. Corneal ulcer

B. Open globe injuries

C. Stevens-Johnson syndrome

D. Optic neuritis

64. Ciliary staphyloma can occur in:

A. Corneal ulcer

B. Myopia

C. Scleritis

D. Interstitial keratitis

65. Treatment of uveitis with raised intraocular tension:

A. Timolol B. Pilocarpine

C. Atropine D. Glucocorticoids

66. Which of the following drug is currently used for the prophylaxis of non-infectious uveitis in LUMINATE programme?

A. Cyclosporine B. Vaclosporine

C. Methotrexate D. Infliximib

67. The most common posterior segment pathology responsible for diminished vision in anterior uveitis is:

A. Vitreous floaters

B. Exudative retinal detachment

C. Inflammatory edema

D. Cystoid macular edema

68. A female presented with breathlessness, arthralgia and blurring of vision with granulomatous anterior uveitis. Which is the most likely etiology?

A. Tubercular uveitis

B. HLA-B27 related uveitis

C. Intraocular lymphoma

D. Ocular sarcoidosis

69. A 32-year-old male presents with unilateral diminished vision in the right eye. On examination, there is mild iritis, vitritis and focal necrotic lesion is seen at macula. The most likely diagnosis is:

A. Multiple evanescent white dot syndrome

B. Ocular toxoplasmosis

C. Multifocal choroiditis

D. Ocular sarcoidosis

70. A 35-year-old male on slit lamp shows keratic precipitates and

aqueous flare in his right eye. No synechiae but a complicated cataract is seen. Probable diagnosis would be:

A. Intermediate uveitis

B. Heerfordt's syndrome

C. Subacute iridocyclitis

D. Heterochromic iridocyclitis of Fuch's

71. Drug of choice for anterior uveitis is:

A. Oral steroids

B. Topical steroids

C. Topical antibiotics

D. Atropine

72. After a leisure trip, a patient comes with gritty pain in eye and joint pain. What is the most probable diagnosis?

A. Reiter's syndrome

B. Behcet's syndrome

C. Sarcoidosis

D. SLE

73. Dalen-Fuch's nodule is pathognomic of:

A. Sympathetic ophthalmitis

B. Sarcoidosis

C. Tuberculosis

D. Retinitis pigmentosa

74. Iris pearl are seen in:

A. Sarcoidosis

B. Hansen's

C. Tuberculosis

D. Sympathetic ophthalmitis

75. Anti-cholinergic used in all except:

A. Uveitis

B. Fundus examination

C. OPC poisoning

D. Glaucoma

76. Eales' disease is:

A. Recurrent anterior uveitis

B. Recurrent vitreous hemorrhage

C. Recurrent macular hemorrhage

D. Recurrent subconjunctival hemorrhage

77. Uveoparotitis is seen in:

A. Sarcoidosis B. SLE

C. Scleroderma D. Mumps

ANSWER AND EXPLANATION

1.	a	Pthisis bulbi is a non-seeing eye where there is shrinkage of the eyeball. Intraocular pressure is nil.
2.	b	Iris is weakest at its root, hence any blunt trauma will affect the major arterial circle.
3.	a	The most common opportunistic infection in AIDS is CMV retinitis.
4.	a	Miotic pupil is a feature of uveitis whereas in acute congestive glaucoma the pupil is vertically oval and mid-dilated.
5.	a	Behcet's disease is HLA-B5 and HLA-B51 associated.
6.	a	The necrosis and haemorrhage in the retina seen in CMV infections is described as "sauce and cheese retinopathy".
7.	a	Acute anterior uveitis is treated by topical steroids and topical cycloplegics.
8.	a	Sympathetic ophthalmia is a granulomatous panuveitis due to perforating injury in the other eye.

9. a Pilocarpine increases inflammation and hence is contraindicated in uveitis. Also it constricts the pupil which leads to increased chance of posterior synechiae.

10. c Any trauma to the ciliary body can cause sympathetic ophthalmitis; hence it is considered the dangerous area of the eye.

11. c Iris neovascularisation, i.e., Rubeosis iridis occurs due to hypoxia which starts from the retina. Hence, the choice of treatment is panretinal photo-coagulation.

12. b A red eye, with KPs, cells in the aqueous humour, normal IOP and backache, the most probable diagnosis is uveitis associated arthritis (which is HLA-B27 associated).

13. b Rheumatoid arthritis is seropositive arthritis. Its ocular features are corneal melting, sclerosing keratitis and scleritis.

14. c Phlyctenular conjunctivitis is allergy to endogenous antigen, most commonly staphylococcus aureus and tuberculosis. TB in eye also causes granulomatous panuveitis but it is not the most common manifestation.

15. a It is a case of arthritis associated with uveitis which is a non-granulomatous anterior uveitis.

16. b Most common protozoal infection in adults is toxoplasmosis and in children it is toxocariasis.

17. d Inflammation in the eye due to injury in the other eye is sympathetic ophthalmitis.

18. d Both pilocarpine and latanoprost aggravate inflammation and hence are contraindicated in patients of uveitis.

19. a All the three options are correct. The most important role is rest to the ciliary muscles.

20. c It presents as atypical anterior uveitis as the child does not have pain, redness and photophobia. The child presents with complications which are complicated cataract, secondary glaucoma and band-shaped keratopathy.

21. d Retinal detachment can occur as a complication in intermediate and posterior uveitis but not in anterior uveitis.

22. a VKH syndrome is granulomatous panuveitis with encephalitis, alopecia, tinnitus, vitiligo and poliosis.

23. c JRA is a sero-negative arthritis. It is of three types namely: pauci-articular, polyarticular and systemic onset. Only the pauciarticular arthritis presents with uveitis.

24. b Shallow anterior chamber is a feature of angle-closure glaucoma. In uveitis AC is deep if there is posterior synechiae.

25. c Sympathetic ophthalmitis is a granulomatous inflammation with nodules between Bruchs and retina called Dalen-Fuch's nodules.

26. a Onchocerciasis is also called River Blindness and is caused by a nematode named Onchocerca volvulus.

27. c The first sign is retrolental flare and the first symptom is difficulty

in near vision or accommodation, as the problem initiates from the ciliary body area.

28. c Pupil is constricted in uveitis due to release of toxins from the inflamed uveal tissue and is irregular due to formation of posterior synechiae.

29. b SO is a bilateral uveitis (both exciting and sympathizing eye is involved, non-suppurative, granulomatous panuveitis.

30. b,c,d Congestion in uveitis is ciliary congestion and not conjunctival congestion.

31. a,c Both the uveitis occurs due to autoimmune reaction.

32. a,b,c E coli and Klebsiella is not known to cause uveitis.

33. a,b,c A young male with a history of anterior uveitis should be investigated on the line of arthritis associated uveitis. TORCHS should be done in all patients to exclude infective pathology.

34. c Mucopurulent discharge is a feature of infective conjunctivitis.

35. a,b Snow-banking is an inflammatory membrane on the pars plana and ora serrata.

36. a,d Both toxoplasmosis and Syphilis can involve the central retina.

37. a,c SO is injury to the uveal tissue which incites an autoimmune response against it.

38. b,c,d Rheumatoid arthritis does not present as uveitis.

39. a Most commonly AIDS presents as microangiopathy characterized by cottonwool spots, haemorrhages and microaneurysms.

40. b CMV causes retinal necrosis best described as sauce and cheese retinopathy. Herpes Zoster also causes ARN, i.e., acute retinal necrosis.

41. a There is intense vitritis in patients of toxoplasmosis and the retinochoroiditis seen through it is described as "Headlight-in-fog" appearance.

42. c Granulomatous uveitis is intense inflammation leading to nodule formation and can involve any part of the uveal tissue.

43. a Uveitis due to arthritis is always an anterior uveitis, non-granulomatous.

44. c Salt and pepper fundus is diffuse chorioretinitis characterized by pigmentary disturbance in form of salt and pepper.

45. d Sarcoidosis is a granulomatous inflammation with sarcoid nodules in the conjunctiva, sclera and iris. Lisch nodules are seen in NF-1. In tuberous sclerosis there are hypopigmented spots on the iris. SLE most commonly presents as corneal epitheliopathy.

46. a Iris is weakest at its root.

47. a Prolonged use of pilocarpine can lead to iris cysts. It can also cause myopic shift due to accommodation spasm and in rare cases can also cause retinal detachment.

48. b SO never occurs before two weeks of the injury.

49. a Ulcerative colitis presents as iritis.

50. c SO causes uveitis in both injured eye (i.e., exciting eye) and uninjured eye (sympathizing eye).

51. c Fuch's heterochromic cyclitis is a non-granulomatous inflammation

and hence does not present as nodules.

52. d Toxocariasis causes choroiditis in the central retina and hence is a D/D of leukocoria.

53. d Smooth muscles of the iris are: iris sphincter and dilator pupillae and they develop from neuroectoderm.

54. d Both SO and VKH are granulomatous panuveitis.

55. a Mutton-fat KPs are large in size with greasy look, seen in granulomatous inflammations.

56. d Iris bombe is bowing forward of the iris due to collection of aqueous in the posterior chamber, which occurs due to pupillary block caused by the ring synechiae.

57. a AS leads to non-granulomatous anterior uveitis. It can lead to fixed flexion deformities due to sclerosis of the sacroiliac joint.

58. d Fuch's heterochromic cyclitis is a non-granulomatous uveitis involving the anterior uvea. It presents as atypical anterior uveitis with no redness or pain. The KPs are stellate, i.e., star-shaped.

59. b Uveitis most commonly complicates as secondary glaucoma which can be either angle closure (due to posterior synechiae or peripheral anterior synechiae) or open angle (inflammatory cells block the trabecular meshwork).

60. a Sympathetic ophthalmitis never occurs before 2 weeks of injury.

61. e Prolapsed iris should never be reimposed as there is a risk of infection in the eye. Iridectomy in cataract surgery was a routine in ICCE. It is not done on a regular basis with other procedures, i.e., ECCE and Phacoemulsification.

62. c A total posterior synechiae means when the whole margin of the pupil gets adhered to the lens.

63. d Corneal ulcers and globe injuries are generally unilateral. Stevens-Johnson syndrome causes conjunctival fibrosis, lacrimal dysfunction and keratopathy. It will rarely cause blindness.

64. c Corneal ulcer will lead to anterior staphyloma, whereas in myopia we get posterior staphyloma.

65. c Treatment of uveitis is steroids and cycloplegic. We do not answer steroids as the IOP is raised.

66. b Luminate program is a study conducted by Lux Biosciences, for corticosteroid sparing agent for the treatment of non-infective uveitis. The name of the drug is Luveniq (Voclosporin) which is calcineurin inhibitor and an immunomodulator.

67. d Anterior uveitis if severe may lead to involvement of vitreous leading to vitritis and retina leading most commonly to cystoid macular edema. Since in this question, it is mentioned dimunition of vision, we will mark the answer as CME. This edema is due to inflammation but in option C it has not mentioned inflammatory edema of which part. So the best possible answer is CME. Also option A is vitreous floaters and not vitritis, vitreous floaters is a very broad term as floaters are of numerous types.

68. d The history of the patient with dyspnoea and arthralgia alongwith

granulomatous inflammation, most probable diagnosis is sarcoidosis. Uveitis is not a common occurrence in patients of TB.

69. b The most common protozoal infection in adults is toxoplasmosis.

The most common means of toxoplasmosis infection in the eye is through reactivation of trophozoites, primary infection occurs in the fetal life. The history strongly suggests toxoplasmosis as there is NECROTIC lesion in the retina with vitritis.

70. d Fuch's heterochromic cyclitis is a non-granulomatous anterior uveitis. It's a low-grade chronic cyclitis and hence there is no synechiae formation. The typical feature of this condition is heterochromia iridis. The condition is associated with some disturbance of the sympathetic nerve supply, these nerves control the chromatophores accounting for the depigmentation. Cataract frequently develops with very good operative prognosis.

71. b Treatment of anterior uveitis includes topical steroids and topical cycloplegics.

72. a Joint pain is a feature of Reiter's syndrome. It's a triad of urethritis, arthritis and conjunctivitis.

73. a These nodules are present between Bruch's membrane and RPE.

74. b Iris pearls is characteristic of anterior uveitis in leprosy. It consists of bacilli and monocytes.

75. d Dilatation of pupil can precipitate glaucoma.

76. b Eales' disease is a disease of young males presenting with recurrent vitreous haemorrhage.

77. a Uveitis with parotitis in sarcoidosis is called Heerfordt's syndrome.

RECENTLY ADDED QUESTIONS

1. **The use of highly active anti-retroviral therapy (HAART) is associated with the development of:**
   A. Keratitis
   B. Uveitis
   C. Retinitis
   D. Optic neuritis

2. **Sclera is thinnest at:**
   A. Limbus
   B. Insertion of rectus muscle
   C. Equator
   D. Posterior pole

3. **Crohn's disease is associated with:**
   A. Anterior uveitis
   B. Episcleritis
   C. Conjunctivitis
   D. Scleritis

ANSWERS OF RECENTLY ADDED QUESTIONS

1. b HAART is given in AIDS patients, and has proved to be very effective in decreasing the viraemia and improving the CD count. Incidence

of CMV retinitis is markedly decreased in such patients. But due to the improvement in the immunity, the patient starts developing uveitis.

2. b Sclera is thinnest posterior to the muscle insertions.

3. b Most common ocular feature is episcleritis. Anterior uveitis is another important feature.

IMAGE-BASED QUESTIONS

1. The diagnosis is:

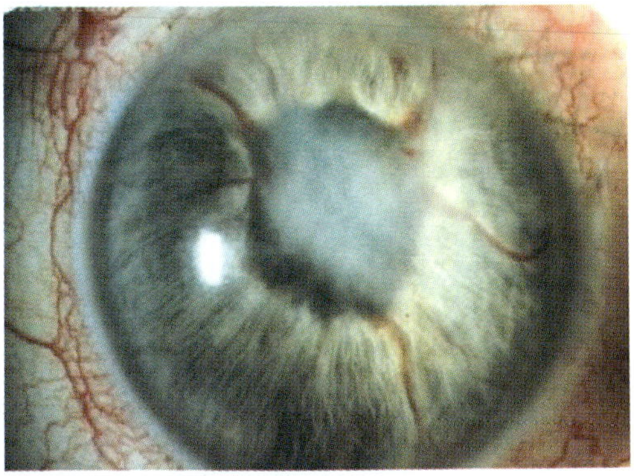

A. Anterior uveitis
B. Endophthalmitis
C. Leukocoria
D. Intermediate uveitis

2. The diagnosis is:

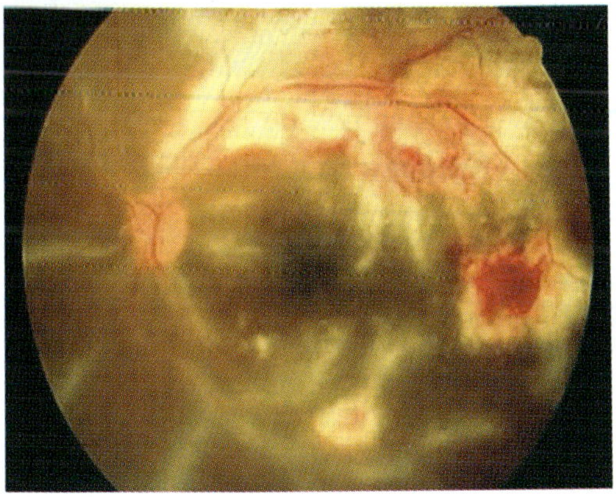

A. Splashed-sauce appearance
B. Snow-banking
C. Sauce and cheese retinopathy
D. Flower petal paten

3. The diagnosis is:

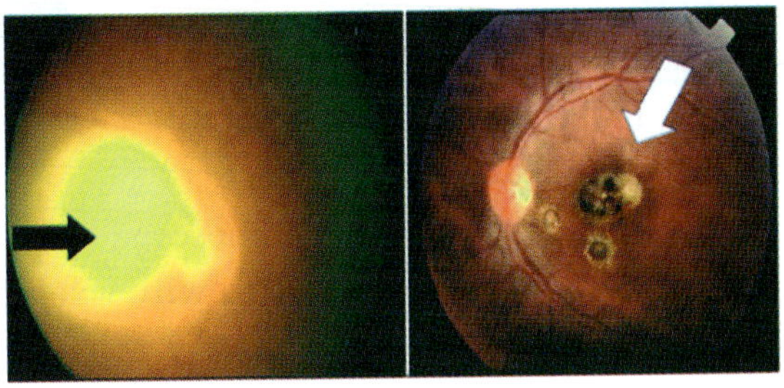

A. Sarcoidosis
B. HIV
C. Toxoplasmosis
D. VKH syndrome

4. The diagnosis is:

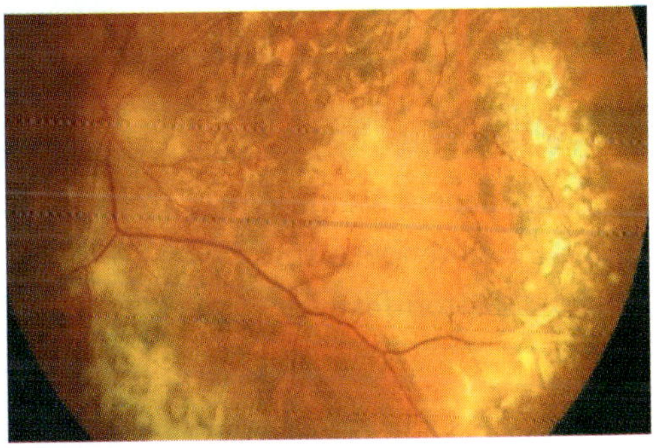

A. Sarcoidosis
B. Eales' disease
C. HIV
D. CMV

5. Which instrument is used for diagnosis in this patient of intermediate uveitis?

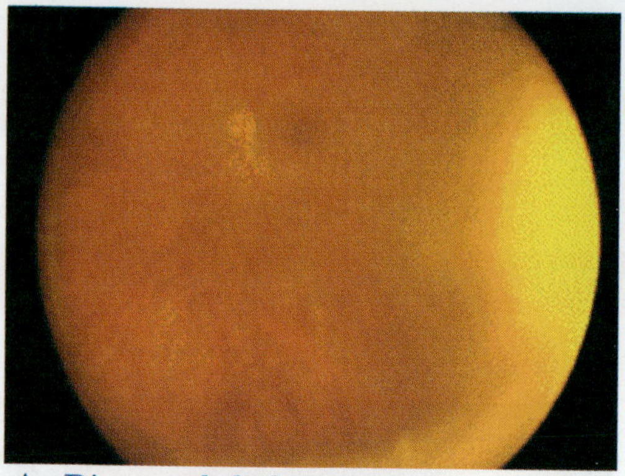

A. Direct ophthalmoscope
B. Indirect ophthalmoscope
C. Distant-direct ophthalmoscope
D. Indirect ophthalmoscope with scleral indentation

6. **The diagnosis is:**

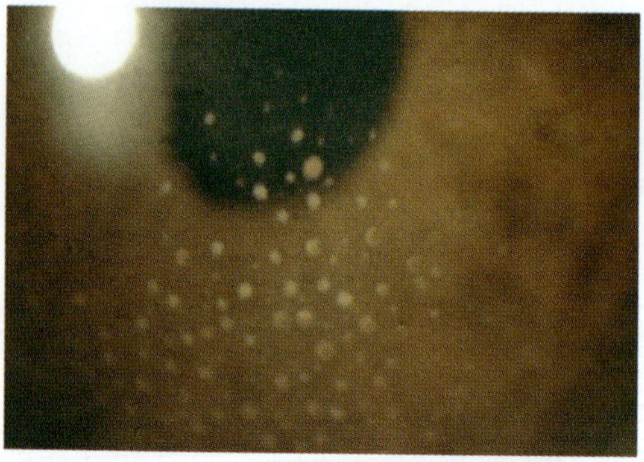

A. Corneal staining
B. Krukenberg spindles
C. Mutton-fat KPs
D. Corneal dystrophy

7. **The slide shows:**

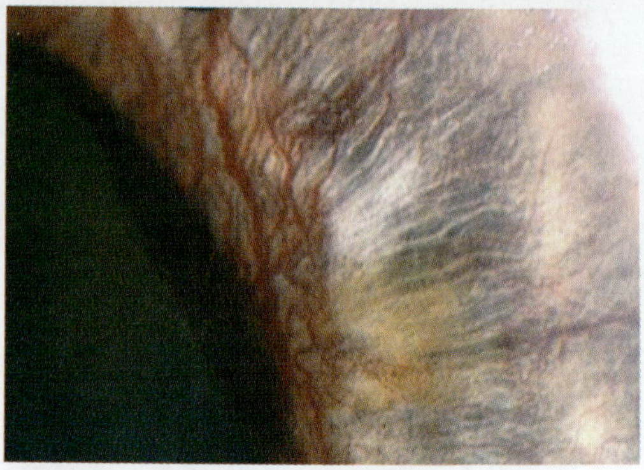

A. Iris schaffing
B. Iris atrophy
C. Iris neovascularisation
D. Heterochromia iridis

8. **The diagnosis is:**

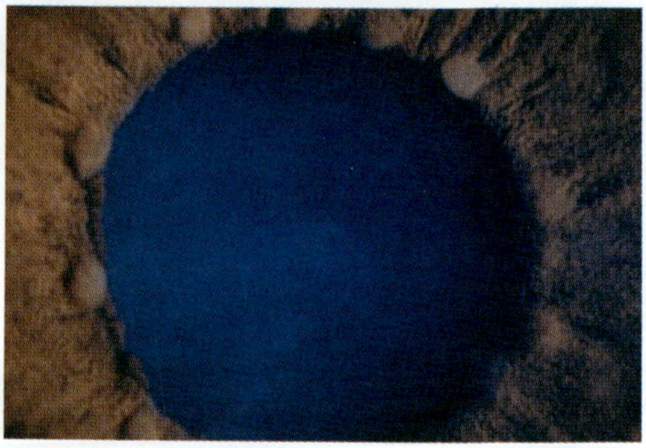

A. Bussaca nodule
B. Koeppe's nodule
C. Ectropion uveae
D. Iris melanoma

ANSWERS OF IMAGE-BASED QUESTIONS

1. a The slide shows occlusio pupillae which is a feature of anterior uveitis.
2. c The slide indicates 'sauce and cheese' retinopathy which is a feature of CMV retinitis.
3. c The first slide shows 'headlight-in-fog' appearance which is due to intense vitritis in patients of toxoplasmosis. The second slide is of healed lesion which is typically punched out and pigmented lesions involving the macular area.
4. a This is a slide of 'candle-wax drippings' which is thick venous sheathing in patients of sarcoidosis.

5. d The above slide shows snow-banking of intermediate uveitis which can only be seen by indirect ophthalmoscopy with scleral indentation.
6. c It is a slide of granulomatous anterior uveitis, showing mutton-fat KPs.
7. c This slide is showing iris neovascularisation, i.e., rubeosis iridis.
8. b These are Koeppe's nodules as they are at the pupillary margin and are a feature of granulomatous inflammation.

GUIDANCE

Pioneering takes steady dedicated efforts, it is advancing surely one step at a time.

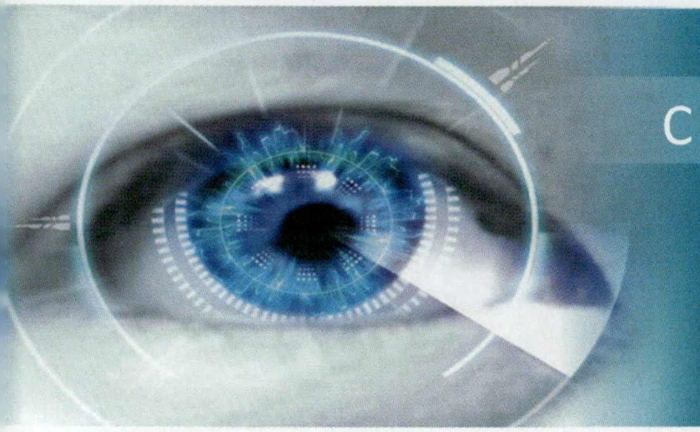

CHAPTER 7

Orbit

Anatomy

- Bony orbits are quadrangular, truncated pyramids with **volume of 30 cc.**
- **Medial wall: Thinnest,** and is formed by frontal process of maxilla, lacrimal bone, orbital plate of ethmoid, body of sphenoid.
- **Floor:** Orbital surface of maxillary bone, orbital surface of zygomatic bone and palatine bone.
- **Lateral wall:** Zygomatic bone and greater wing of sphenoid.
- **Superior wall (roof):** Orbital plate of frontal bone and lesser wing of sphenoid.
- **Inferior orbital fissure:** It is between floor and lateral wall.
- **Superior orbital fissure:** It is at orbital apex lateral to optic foramen. It is bounded by greater and lesser wing of sphenoid and frontal bone. It is divided into upper, middle and lower parts by a common tendinous ring for origin of recti.
- **Optic canal or Optic foramen: It is formed by two roots of lesser wing of sphenoid; at orbital apex.**
- **Suspensory ligament of Lockwood:** It is a thickened sling or hammock of facial sheath extending from the posterior lacrimal crest to the lateral orbital tubercle, on which rests the eyeball. It is formed by fusion of expansions from the muscular sheaths of medial rectus, inferior oblique, inferior rectus and lateral

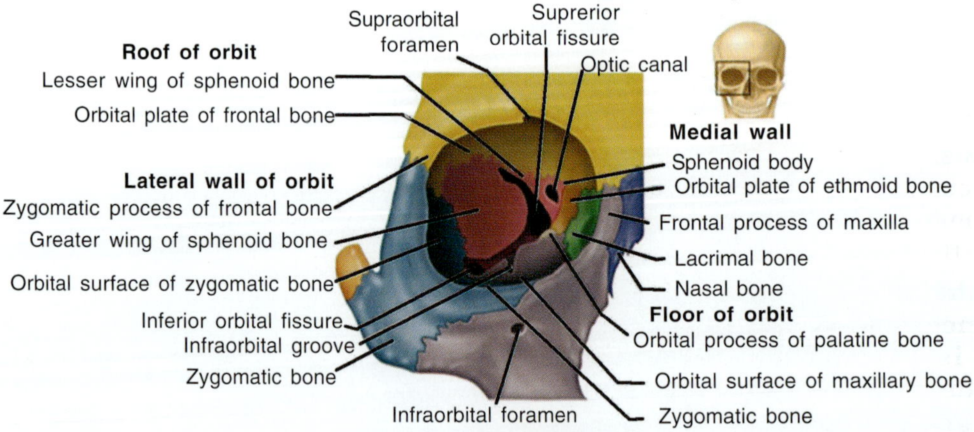

Fig. 7.1: Orbit

rectus muscle joined with a thickened inferior part of the tenons capsule.

- **Recti Muscles:** All four recti originate from Annulus of Zinn at the circumference of optic foramen at the apex of the orbit, run forward surrounding the optic nerve and posterior portion of the eyeball and are inserted into the sclera by means of flattened tendons, about 10 mm wide. The lines of insertion of these muscles are not equidistant from the cornea but have the form of spiral.

  The center of insertion of muscles from the cornea are as follows:

Medial rectus	5.5 mm
Inferior rectus	6.5 mm
Lateral rectus	6.9 mm
Superior rectus	7.7 mm

- **Inferior oblique:** The inferior oblique arises from the superior maxillary bone at the inner portion of lower border of the orbit, passes outward below the inferior rectus and is inserted into outer part of sclera *behind the equator.*
- **Superior oblique:** It arises from the bone at the upper and inner border of optic foramen and runs forward to the upper and inner angle of the orbit, at the anterior extremity of which it passes through a fibrous pulley; continues outward passing beneath superior rectus and is inserted into the outer part of sclera *behind the equator.*

Proptosis: Forward protrusion of normal-sized eyeball > 21 mm beyond the lateral orbital margin or difference of > 2 mm between the two eyes.

Exophthalmos: It denotes proptosis and hence the two terms are similar, but it is used in case of thyroid ophthalmopathy, i.e., Graves' disease.

Proptosis is measured by Hertels Exophthalmometer.

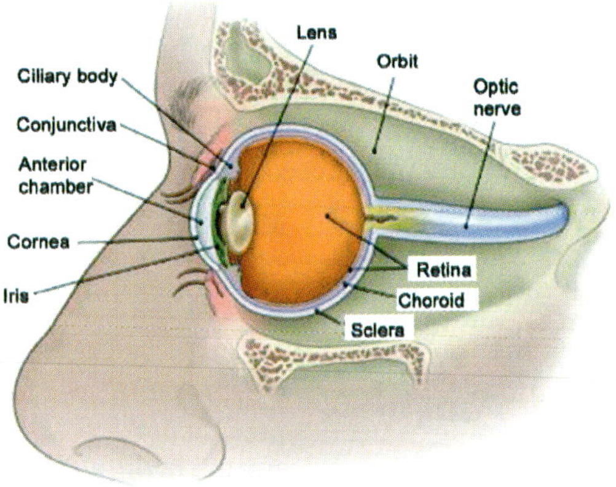

Fig. 7.2

CLASSIFICATION OF PROPTOSIS

A. Unilateral

1. Painful:

a. **Axial: It indicates that the protrusion of the eye is in a straight line with the AP axis.**
   - Orbital haemorrhage.
   - Orbital cellulitis.
   - Orbital mucocoele.
   - Cavernous sinus thrombosis.
   - Pseudotumor.

b. **Non Axial: Protrusion is not in line with the AP axis.**
   - Adenoid cystic carcinoma of lacrimal gland.
   - Nasopharyngeal carcinoma.
   - Metastasis.

2. Painless:

a. **Axial:**
   - Hemangioma.
   - Meningioma.
   - Glioma.
   - Schwannoma.
   - Metastatic.

b. Non Axial:

- *Down and medial* – Dermoid, lacrimal gland tumors.
- *Down and temporal* – Frontoethmoid mucocoele.
- *Superior* – Maxillary sinus tumor and mucocoele.

B. Bilateral

1. Painful:

- Cavernous sinus thrombosis.
- Graves' disease.

2. Painless:

- Graves' disease.
- Pseudotumor.
- Lymphoma.
- Caroticocavernous fistula.
- Leukemia.
- Metastasis.

Common Causes of Proptosis in Children

a. Orbital cellulitis.

b. Rhabdomyosarcoma.

c. Neuroblastoma.

d. Leukemia.

e. Retinoblastoma.

PULSATING PROPTOSIS

Causes

a. Caroticocavernous fistula.

b. Saccular aneurysm of ophthalmic artery.

c. Deficient orbital roof (leading to transmission of cerebral pulsation) as seen with:

1. Meningocele.
2. Neurofibromatosis type I.
3. Traumatic disruption of orbital roof.

Arteriovenous fistula is an abnormal communication between normal arteries and veins.

In Caroticocavernous fistula there is an abnormal communication between carotid artery and cavernous sinus.

It is of 2 main types:

A. Direct.

B. Indirect.

Clinical Features:

A. *Proptosis:*

- Pulsatile.
- Associated with bruit and thrill which are abolished by ipsilateral carotid compression.

B. *Ophthalmoplegia:*

Most commonly the sixth nerve is involved.

C. *Anterior segment:*

1. Chemosis.
2. Engorged episcleral and conjunctival blood vessels.
3. Secondary glaucoma, due to raised episcleral pressure.
4. *Anterior segment necrosis:*
   a. Corneal epithelial edema.
   b. Iritis leading to iris atrophy.
   c. Cataract.

D. *Posterior segment:*

- Vascular engorgement.
- CRVO.

Treatment: Current method involves interventional radiology with intravascular balloons via a catheter in the internal carotid artery.

Intermittent proptosis: It's a feature of **orbital varices** when in dependent position they fill up and lead to proptosis and otherwise the proptosis regresses back.

Varices or Orbital Venous Anomalies consists of congenital enlargements of one or more preexisting venous channels.

Clinical Features:

1. Generally unilateral and nasal.
2. Intermittent proptosis—It refers to non-pulsatile reversible proptosis (because orbital veins are devoid of valves).
3. Visible lesions in the eyelid and conjunctiva may be present.
4. Rarely acute orbital haemorrhage or thrombosis.
5. It enlarges progressively and is associated with recurrent episodes of haemorrhage and thrombosis.

Treatment: Surgery—It is difficult due to friability of the lesion and bleeding.

Note:

- Most common intraocular tumour in children is retinoblastoma.
- Most common intraorbital tumour in children is rhabdomyosarcoma.
- Most common intraocular tumour in adults is choroidal malignant melanoma.
- Most common intraorbital tumour in adults is a cavernous hemangioma.

DYSTHYROID OPHTHALMOPATHY

It is an autoimmune disease also called Graves' Ophthalmopathy. It may or may not be associated with hyperthyroidism. Patient may be euthyroid or hypothyroid. **It is the most common cause of proptosis in adults with any possible presentation, i.e., unilateral or bilateral, axial or non-axial and painful or painless proptosis.**

Pathophysiology

It occurs due to three processes in the orbit:

1. Infiltration of inflammatory cells in the orbit.
2. Multiplication of adipose tissue.
3. Enlargement of muscles due to fibrosis.

These three processes lead to increase in the intraorbital pressure causing proptosis and optic compression neuropathy.

Clinical Features:

Five main features are:

1. Eyelid retraction:

Lid signs in thyroid ophthalmopathy:

a. *Dalrymple's sign:* Lid retraction in primary gaze.
b. *von Graefe's sign:* Lid lag.
c. *Kocher's sign:* Staring appearance of eyes.
d. *Griffith sign:* Lid lag of lower lid in upgaze.
e. *Boston sign:* Jerky and uneven downward movement.
f. *Stellwags sign:* Decrease in frequency of blinking reflex.
g. *Enroth sign:* Puffy swelling of lids.
h. *Grifford sign:* Difficult eversion of upper lid.
i. *Jellinker sign:* Abnormal pigmentation of upper lid.

Treatment:

- *Surgical:* Recession of the LPS.
- *Medical treatment for lid retraction:*
  a. **Topical guanethidine:** It depletes sympathetic storage sites.
  b. Chemodenervation of LPS by botulinum toxin.

2. **Soft tissue involvement:**
   a. Conjunctival injection.
   b. Chemosis.
   c. Edema and fullness of eyelids.
   d. Superior limbic keratoconjunctivitis.

Treatment:

- Tear substitutes.
- For superior limbic keratoconjunctivitis—Adrenaline and Acetylcysteine. Acetylcysteine dissolves mucus.

3. **Proptosis:** Is most commonly axial.

Treatment:

If progressive and painful:

a. Steroids.
b. RTH.
c. Surgery.

4. **Dysthyroid optic neuropathy:**
   - It occurs due to compression of optic nerve at orbital apex by enlarged recti.
   - It presents with all features of optic nerve disease, i.e., decreased visual acuity,visual field defect and afferent pupillary defect.
   - Treatment is same as in proptosis. If there is sudden loss of vision with defective *afferent pupillary* response, it indicates optic nerve compression, hence, definitive treatment is optic canal decompression.

5. **Restrictive thyroid myopathy:**
   - Patient presents with diplopia and squint.
   - Ophthalmoplegia is due to muscle contraction and not palsy.
   - Sequence of involvement of muscle is:

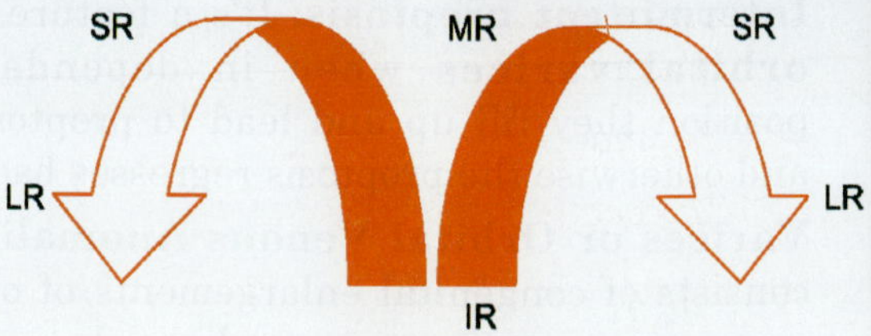

Fig. 7.3

- Forced duction test is positive.

Lacrimal Gland Tumor

Benign:

- **Most common tumour of lacrimal gland is – Pleomorphic adenoma (mixed cell tumor).**

Clinical Features:

1. It typically presents in the adult life as painless, smooth, firm swelling progressive swelling in the outer quadrant.
2. In most cases it arises from the orbital portion of the lacrimal gland causing non-axial proptosis, i.e., down and medial.

Investigations:

CT scan.

Treatment:

Surgical excision through lateral orbitotomy. Prognosis is excellent if tumour is excised completely without disruption of the capsule.

Malignant:

3 main types:

- *Adenoid cystic carcinoma:* It is a painful tumour. **It is the most dangerous malignant tumour as it spreads very fast due to perineural invasion.** The perineural invasion can lead to motor nerve palsies. It may extend into the cavernous sinus.

- *Pleomorphic adenocarcinoma.*
- *Mucoepidermoid carcinoma.*

Clinical Features:

1. History of presentation is shorter than with benign tumour.
2. There is bone destruction which is not seen with benign tumours.
3. It may present as a long-standing proptosis which may suddenly start increasing in size.

Investigations:

1. CT scan.
2. Biopsy to establish the histopathological diagnosis.
3. Neurological assessment to check for the involvement of the cavernous sinus.

Treatment:

1. Radical surgery in form of orbital exenteration or mid-facial resection can be tried, but in most patients the prognosis for life is very poor.
2. Radiotherapy and local resection may prolong life and reduce pain.

Optic Nerve Glioma

- Common in children.
- Female > males.
- 25%–50% patients have associated Neurofibromatosis-I.
- Presentation is generally with visual loss.
- **C/F:** It is a slow growing tumor hence proptosis is a late feature and generally eyeball is down and out or may be axial. In initial stages it presents with the signs of optic nerve involvement.
- **Investigations** CT Scan—**Fusiform enlargement** of nerve along with enlargement of optic canal.

Pathology:

- Common variety is Pilocytic **(Pilocytic astrocytoma).**
- Arises from Astrocytes.

Treatment:

1. Observation.
2. Radiotherapy.
3. Surgery.

Neuroblastoma

- Malignant tumour arising from primitive neuroblasts of sympathetic chain, most commonly in abdomen, followed by thorax and pelvis.
- Most common solid tumour in childhood.
- **Metastasis to orbit occurs in 40% of cases.**
- Deposits may be bilateral and typically present with an abrupt onset of proptosis accompanied by lid ecchymosis.

Other tumours causing orbital metastasis in children are:

1. Ewing's sarcoma.
2. Acute myeloid leukemia.

Cavernous Hemangioma

- It is the most common benign orbital tumour in adults.
- Most common site is in muscle cone just behind the globe.
- This is an hemangioma which is a well-encapsulated tumour.

Clinical Features:

1. Most common age of presentation is middle age.

2. Slowly progressive unilateral proptosis.
3. Optic disc oedema and chorioretinal folds.
4. Occasionally, tumour at the orbital apex causes compression of optic nerve without any proptosis.

Treatment:

Surgical excision.

Craniopharyngioma

They are slow-growing tumours arising from vestigial remnants of Rathke's pouch along the pituitary stalk. It can occur both in children and adults.

C/F: Presents with:

1. Interference in hypothalamic function leading to dwarfism, delayed sexual development and obesity.
2. Decreased visual acuity.
3. Suprasellar calcification.

D/D: A child, with **bitemporal** hemianopia (indicating chiasmal lesion) with CT scan showing suprasellar mass with **calcification**, the most probable diagnosis would be craniopharyngioma. **Pituitary adenoma** is found more commonly in adults and not in children. **Astrocytoma or optic nerve glioma** also presents in childhood but does not present with above field defect and the tumour is on the optic nerve and not suprasellar. Therefore on CT scan, it shows fusiform enlargement of optic nerve. Meningiomas are more common in middle-aged women.

Treatment:

Mainly surgical with post operative radiotherapy.

Meningioma

Presents commonly in middle aged women.

Clinical Features:

1. Visual loss.
2. Proptosis.
3. It causes sclerosis of the bony orbit.
4. *Visual field defects:* It depends upon the location of the tumour:

   A. *Tuberculum Sellae:* It compresses the junction of chiasma with optic nerve leading to ipsilateral central scotoma and a contralateral upper temporal defect **(Junctional scotoma of Traquair).**

   B. *Sphenoidal Ridge:*
   - Typically presents as fullness in temporal fossa due to reactive hyperostosis.
   - Compresses the optic nerve which initially causes central scotomas.

Rhabdomyosarcoma

- It is the most common primary malignant orbital tumour in children.
- It arises from pleuripotential mesenchymal precursors which differentiate into striated muscle cells.
- The four main histological types are:
  1. *Embryonal:* Most common.
  2. *Alveolar:* Most aggressive.
  3. *Botyroid.*
  4. *Pleomorphic:* Best prognosis but least common.

Clinical Features:

1. Presentation is usually in first decade of life.
2. Rapidly progressive proptosis which may be mistaken for an inflammatory process.
3. *On Examination:* Mass in the orbit.

4. Eyelid edema and proptosis.

Investigations:

1. CT scan–Irregular, well defined soft tissue mass.
2. Biopsy to confirm the diagnosis.
3. Systemic investigations for evidence of metastatic spread.

Treatment:

1. With high dose of local radiotherapy followed by chemotherapy. This tumour is very radiosensitive most of the times.

   Chemotherapy used is Vincristine, Cyclophosphamide, Actinomycin D.
2. Exenteration–For rare–occurring, radiotherapy resistant tumour.

Multiple myeloma: Hypergammaglobulinemia is diagnostic of multiple myeloma though it rarely presents as an orbital mass. The more common presentation is corneal crystals diffusely distributed in the corneal stroma.

Monoclonal Gammopathy occurs in association with:

1. Multiple myeloma.
2. Waldenstrom's macroglobulinemia.
3. Lymphoma.

Cavernous Sinus Thrombosis

Cavernous sinus is a large venous sinus situated in the middle cranial fossa on either side of the body of sphenoid bone. All the nerves, i.e., 3rd, 4th, 5th and 6th, are passing through cavernous sinus. Oculomotor, Trochlear and ophthalmic division of trigeminal pass through lateral wall whereas the abducent nerve passes through centre of the sinus alongwith internal carotid artery.

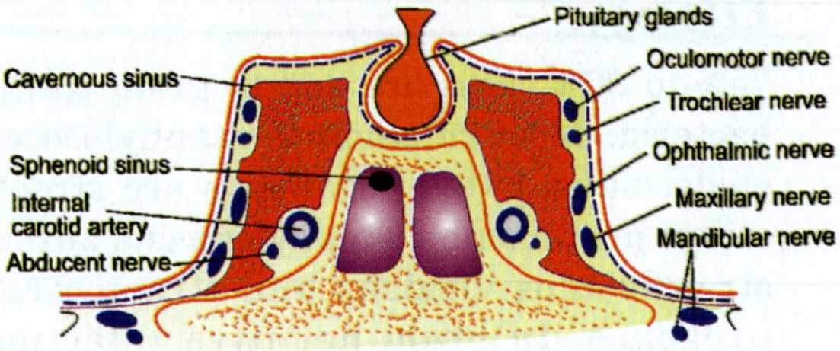

Fig. 7.4

Features of CST:

1. Mostly bilateral (> 50%).
2. Mastoid tenderness with swelling.
3. Cerebral symptoms with vomiting and rigor.
4. Late onset proptosis.
5. Decreased or absent corneal sensation due to the involvement of Vth nerve.
6. Complete limitation of eyeball movement due to involvement of IIIrd, IVth and VIth nerve. Involvement of opposite eye–**First sign being paralysis of VI nerve.**
7. Dilated and fixed pupil, due to internal ophthalmoplegia. Though it may not be fully dilated due to simultaneous oculosympathetic involvement.
8. Papilloedema may be present.
9. Engorgement of retinal veins—Superior ophthalmic vein is a tributary of cavernous sinus. Impaired venous drainage leads to engorged retinal veins.

Since all the nerves are affected, i.e., 3, 4, 5 and 6th, hence initially there is ptosis, but *at a later stage there is proptosis and hence ptosis not appreciated.*

Endophthalmitis

It is a rare devastating ocular infective condition characterized by inflammation of the inner coats of the eyeball.

Etiology:

75% to 90% cases are due to gram positive bacteria. Most common is staphylococcus epidermidis. Other organisms are streptococcus pneumoniae, staphylococcus aureus, streptococcus viridans and streptococcus pyogenes. In gram negative infections pseudomonas aeruginosa is the most common. Others are Proteus, E. coli, Haemophilus and Influenza. Fungi account for 3% to 8% of the infections and are caused by Aspergillus, Candida and Fusarium.

Clinical Features:

Majority of cases occur in first postoperative week. Late onset endophthalmitis may present in first six weeks and is due to fungal infections or infection due to low virulent organisms like Propionibacterium acne.

1. Increasing pain and redness.
2. Decrease in visual acuity.
3. Headache associated with drowsiness.
4. Lid edema with conjunctival congestion and chemosis.
5. Corneal edema.
6. Hypopyon.
7. Keratic precipitates.
8. Vitreous debris and decreased fundal glow.

Management:

The most reliable is to collect the vitreous specimen. Vitreous aspirate is taken for smear examination and culture in patients of endophthalmitis, hence should be stored at 4°C. But commonly done procedure is to inoculate it into transport medium, i.e., **Robertson cooked meat broth** which can be stored at room temperature.

Treatment:

The current approach relies on intravitreal antibiotics and vitrectomy. Gram positive infections are treated by Vancomycin injections (intravitreal) and for gram negative infections the preferred drug is ceftazidime (second generation). **Gentamycin and amikacin are avoided as they cause macular toxicity**. Corticosteroids (Dexamethasone) are given to curtail inflammation. Dexamethasone is given. If the infection is fungal then steroids are strictly contraindicated as it can cause aggravation of infection.

Surgical treatment: Vitrectomy, reduces the bulk of infection and clears the media.

Other Modalities:

Topical: Fortified antibiotics:
- Cefazolin and Gentamycin
- Natamycin
- Corticosteroids
- Cyclopentolate

Subconjunctival Injections:
- Cephazoline
- Gentamycin
- Amphotericin B

Systemic:
- Cephazoline
- Gentamycin
- Ciprofloxacin
- Ketaconazole

Panophthalmitis: It is the inflammation of all layers of the eyeball. The signs and symptoms are similar to endophthalmitis and in addition **there is restriction of ocular movements**. The initial management is conservative as mentioned above. If not controlled conservatively then surgical treatment is **evisceration with frill excision**. In this procedure a collar of sclera is left around the optic nerve. This method allows a more rapid healing and incidence of spread of infection is also less. But whenever there is risk of rupture of globe and hence escape of pus in the orbit, we prefer enucleation. This is because it will prevent the infection in the optic nerve which can be complicated by meningitis and intracranial infection.

INTRAOCULAR TUMORS

A. Retinoblastoma

- Majority of case become apparent in less than 3 years.
- Most common age of presentation is **18 months.**
- It is the second most common tumor of **all** age groups.
- Inheritance AD, but only 6% cases are familial.
- Familial cases have early onset, bilateral involvement and are predisposed to develop second non-ocular malignancy including pinealoblastoma and osteogenic sarcoma.
- Bilateral retinoblastoma with pinealoblastoma is termed as **trilateral retinoblastoma.**
- Benign counterpart of retinoblastoma—**Retinocytoma or Retinoma.**
- The specific area corresponding to retinoblastoma gene was identified on 14 band, on long arm of chromosome 13—**13 q 14.**
- It arises from primitive multipotent neuroectodermal cells of retina.
- **13 q syndrome**—Retinoblastoma when associated with other dysmorphic features like microcephaly, broad nasal bridge, hypertelorism and mental handicap, it is called 13 q syndrome.
- Patients with familial retinoblastoma have 50% risk of transmitting the disease to their progeny.

Clinical Features:

Mode of presentations are:

1. Leukocoria (60%).
2. Strabismus (20%).
3. Secondary glaucoma.
4. Pseudouveitis.
5. Orbital inflammation, mimicking orbital cellulitis.
6. Proptosis.
7. Heterochromia iridis, rubeosis iridis.
8. Microphthalmos in rare cases.
9. Indirect ophthalmoscopy with scleral indentation should be performed in both eyes.

   Growth may be:

   a. *Exophytic:* When the tumour grows towards the choroid.

   b. *Endophytic:* When the tumour grows towards the vitreous. It mimics Endophthalmitis.

   c. *Mixed.*
10. Lamina cribosa offers maximum resistance to the tumors and hence involvement of retrolaminar area indicates poor prognosis. To check systemic metastasis, section of optic nerve is done.
11. 1% cases may show spontaneous regression leading to pthisis bulbi.

Stages of the Disease

1. Quiescent stage.
2. Glaucomatous stage.
3. Stage of extraocular extension–It commonly bursts through limbus.
4. Distant metastasis.

Differential Diagnosis of Leukocoria (Pseudogliomas)

1. Persistent Hyperplastic Primary Vitreous (PHPV).
2. Retinopathy (ROP).
3. Toxocariasis.
4. Coats' disease.
5. Central colobomas.
6. Retinal astrocytoma/Retinoma.
7. Congenital cataract.
8. Fungal endophthalmitis.
9. Cyclitic membrane.
10. Retinal dysplasia.
11. TB of choroids.

In contrast to pseudogliomas, in retinoblastoma, there is increased intraocular pressure.

Pathology:

Gross:

1. Chalky white friable mass with dense foci of **calcification** and **necrosis.**
2. Seeding into vitreous cavity.
3. Extension to uvea, epibulbar structures, optic nerve and orbit.

Microscopic:

Basophillic mass with light eosinophillic areas due to necrosis.

Tumour cells may be:

A. *Well differentiated:* It has good prognosis.
   1. Flexner-Wintersteiner rosette.
   2. Homer-Wright rosette.
   3. Fleurettes.

B. *Poorly-differentiated:* It has poor prognosis.

Management of Retinoblastoma

A. *Ocular examination:* Examination under anesthesia provides an opportunity to detect early lesions in opposite eye or another tumour foci in the same eye.
   1. External examination for details in anterior segment.
   2. Measurement of corneal diameter to exclude microphthalmos or secondary buphthalmos.
   3. Measurement of intraocular pressure.
   4. Indirect ophthalmoscopy with scleral indentation—Denote the site and extent of tumour.

B. *Gross systemic examination.*

C. *Ancillary tests:* These are needed for confirmation when clinical picture is not so typical.
   1. *USG:* It helps in diagnosis of retinoblastoma, and can pick up lesions as small as 2 mm. It detects the **foci of calcification** (most diagnostic) and also reveals **orbital shadowing** (absence of normal soft tissue echoes in the orbit). Generally, the frequency used in ophthalmics is 8–10 MHZ. These high frequencies produce shorter wavelengths which allow good resolution of minute ocular and orbital structures.
   2. *CT scan:* It has the following advantages over USG:
      a. Can detect extraocular extension.
      b. Can detect presence of pinealoblastoma.
      c. Can detect intracranial metastasis.
   3. *MRI:* It detects extraocular extension better than CT scan.
   4. *Fundus fluorescein angiography:* Its only role in retinoblastoma is to differentiate a viable tumour from an

avascular residue, **following radiotherapy** or in case of **spontaneously regressed retinoblastoma.**

5. *Biochemical tests for aqueous enzymes:* It is not necessary for diagnosis but may be helpful in endophthalmitis like presentation. Following enzymes are found to be raised in aqueous compared to plasma:
   a. Lactic dehydrogenase (LDH).
   b. Phosphoglucoisomerase.
   c. Neuron specific enolase (NSE).
6. *Cytology—Fine needle aspiration biopsy (FNAB):* It helps in diagnosis in situations where retinoblastoma is not a strong possibility. It is done very rarely as it can lead to needle-track dissemination of tumour cells.

   Tumor cells are densely packed, deeply basophilic with hyperchromatic nuclei and scanty cytoplasm.
7. *Bone marrow biopsy and lumbar puncture:* These procedures may be needed in a metastatic workup of a case.
8. *X-ray–Rhese view:* It will show enlargement of optic foramen (if tumor spreads to the optic nerve).

STAGING OF RETINOBLASTOMA

Staging of Retinoblastoma for planning, treatment and prognostication.

Due to the increased risk of secondary tumors following radiation in patients with retinoblastoma, it was found that the Reese-Ellsworth classification system no longer accurately reflected prognosis with the newer treatment modalities. Thus, the International Classification of Retinoblastoma (ICRB) was developed to better predict those with intraocular retinoblastoma who are likely to be cured without the need for enucleation or external-beam radiation treatment.

We can stage retinoblastoma as:

I. Intraocular

II. Extraocular

  A. In orbit

  B. Distant metastasis

INTERNATIONAL CLASSIFICATION OF RETINOBLASTOMA (ICRB)

For Intraocular Tumours

Group A: Small intraretinal tumors (< 3 mm) away from foveola and disc.

Group B: Tumors > 3 mm, macular or juxtapapillary location, or with subretinal fluid.

Group C: Tumor with focal subretinal or vitreous seeding within 3 mm of tumor.

Group D: Tumor with diffuse subretinal or vitreous seeding > 3 mm from tumor.

Group E: Extensive retinoblastoma occupying > 50% of the globe with or without neovascular glaucoma, hemorrhage, extension of tumor to optic nerve or anterior chamber.

Treatment:

A. Focal Treatment:

1. **Cryotherapy:** By triple freeze and thaw method, the vascular supply of the tumour is destroyed.
2. **Laser therapy:** By Argon, diode or xenon arc. Double row of contagious laser spots are applied around the lesion to cut off the vascular supply.

3. **Thermotherapy and Thermochemotherapy:** In thermotherapy the tumour is destroyed by heating with a laser to temperatures which are **less than that for photocoagulation.** This may be performed with diode, argon or double frequency Yag. The effect can be enhanced by **platinum based chemotherapeutic** agents, method called Thermochemotherapy.

B. **Radiotherapy:**

Brachytherapy:

In this procedure, a radioactive plaque is placed over the sclera corresponding to the location of the tumour and then radiations are given in a localized manner over the plaque. The advantage over EBRT (External Beam Radiotherapy) is that the rest of the eye receives a lower dose of radiations and thus the complications are less.

C. **Chemotherapy:**

i. ***Primary neoadjuvant chemotherapy:***

- It plays role of chemoreduction, where the size of tumour is decreased making it amenable to direct local therapy.
- Drugs used are:

Etopside	Very good
Carboplatin	Ocular penetration
Vincristine	
Teniposide	
Cyclosporin	
Cyclophosphamides	

ii. ***Adjuvant chemotherapy:***

- It has a role in cases with extensive disease and in preventing metastasis (in cases with risk factors).
- Drugs used are:

  Etopside, carboplatin, vincristine, cyclophosphamide, cyclosporin.

iii. ***Local chemotherapy:***

Studies with subconjunctival carboplatin and intraocular chemotherapeutic agents are being conducted and results awaited.

D. **Surgical**

1. ***Enucleation:*** Removal of the eyeball with section of maximum part of the optic nerve is termed as enucleation. After the procedure orbital implants are put. These can be made up of: Medpor, hydroxyapatite, PMMA.
2. ***Exenteration:*** In orbital retinoblastoma, exenteration (Removal of all the orbital contents along with section of the lids) is done followed by radiotherapy. Once tumour breaches the sclera and extends to the orbit, prognosis for life is very dismal in spite of aggressive treatment.

Treatment:

Intraocular Tumor:

Group A:	Focal thearpy with laser photocoagulation or cryotherapy.
Group B/C/D:	We give chemotherapy for chemoreduction followed by either laser photocoagulation or cryotherapy.
Group E:	Enucleation.

Extraocular Tumor:

In orbit:	Exenteration
Distant metastasis:	HDC (High dose of chemotherapy) specially in CNS involvement with ASCR (Autologous stem cell rescue).

B. Retinal Astrocytoma

1. It is the benign counterpart of retinoblastoma. It is also known as Retinoma or Retinocytoma.

2. Lesions arise from inner retinal layers frequently situated at or near optic nerve head.
3. During early life they are semi-translucent but later assume more dense white colour with multiple areas of calcification giving rise to mulberry-like appearance.
4. Treatment is not needed as these lesions are asymptomatic and show minimal tendency to grow.

C. Malignant Melanoma (Choroidal)

- *Most common intraocular tumour in adults is choroidal malignant melanoma.*
- Presents during sixth decade.
- **Signs and Symptoms:**
  1. Decreased visual acuity.
  2. Visual field defect.
  3. Asymptomatic.
  4. If metastasis, can cause death.
- **On examination:** Pigmented and elevated oval shaped mass, which may break through Bruch's membrane causing exudative retinal detachment.
- **Investigations:**
  A. Medical examination.
  B. Ocular examination:
    1. Indirect ophthalmoscopy.
    2. Slit lamp bimicroscopy.
    3. Transillumination.
    4. Fluorescein angiography.
    5. CT scan.
    6. MRI.
    7. Color Doppler.
    8. FNAB—Fine Needle Aspiration Biopsy.
- **Treatment:** Depends upon the size of tumour and the degree of involvement.

1. *Enucleation:* For very large tumour and if all useful vision lost.
2. *Radioactive plaques* (Brachy-therapy): For small tumours.
3. *Cyclotron—Generated Charged Particle Irradiation:* It is a very promising approach which may prove to be an alternative to enucleation. Tumour is marked by transillumination and *tantalum clips*, and radiation is given over several sessions.
4. *Photocoagulation (with xenon arc or argon laser):* For small tumours.
5. *Partial lamellar sclerouveactomy:* For certain selected tumours anterior to equator and less than 15 mm in diameter.
6. *Exenteration:* For melanomas with extensive extraocular extension.If small extraocular extension, we can do radiotherapy.
7. *Palliation:* CTh and Immuno-therapy.

Spread of Tumour

- Local invasion is less common compared to retinoblastoma.
- No lymphatic spread.
- **Hematogenous spread specially to liver.**

Trauma

1. **Blunt/Concussion Injury.**
2. **Perforating Injury.**

Features of Concussion Injury

1. *Conjunctiva:* Subconjunctival haemorrhage, chemosis, emphysema.
2. *Cornea:* Corneal edema, corneal abrasions, blood staining due to long standing hyphema.

3. *Iris trauma:* Sphincteric tear, transient iritis, iridodialysis.
4. Traumatic **hyphema.**
5. *Glaucoma:* Hemolytic, Hemosiderotic, Ghost cell, Angle-recession.
6. *Lens:* Opacity, Vossius ring, lens subluxation.
7. *Commotio retinae* (Berlin's edema).
8. Choroidal rupture.
9. Macular hole.
10. Optic nerve avulsion.
11. Retinal dialysis.
12. *Chorioretinitis sclopeteria:* Chorioretinal rupture with retinal haemorrhage.
13. Vitreous base avulsion, Vitreous haemorrhage.
14. Giant retinal tears.

Features of Perforating Injury

1. Conjunctival laceration.
2. Corneal, corneoscleral and posterior scleral laceration.
3. Intraocular F.B.
4. Corneal laceration with iris or vitreous prolapse.
5. Sympathetic ophthalmitis.
6. Vitreous haemorrhage.
7. Globe rupture.

Blow-Out Fractures

It is the fracture of orbital floor which typically occurs by a sudden increase in the orbital pressure by a striking object > 5 cm in diameter such as a fist or tennis ball.

Two Types:

a. Pure blow-out fracture: Does not involve the orbital rim.

b. Impure blow-out fracture: Involves the rim.

Clinical Features:

1. Ecchymosis, edema, subcutaneous emphysema.
2. Enophthalmos.
3. Infraorbital nerve anesthesia, leads to decreased sensations on the affected cheek.
4. Diplopia.

Treatment:

1. Initially one should start anti-inflammatory drugs and antibiotics for ten days. If the muscle is not entrapped in the fracture site then there will be improvement of symptoms and the fracture will heal by itself.
2. If there is no improvement of symptoms in first ten days then surgery is needed. We dislodge the muscle from the fracture site and do a microplating of the fracture site.

Note:

If a patient presents with a history of trauma, proptosis and scleral hyperaemia, there can be two possibilities:

a. Carotico-cavernous fistula (CC fistula).

b. Retrobulbar hematoma.

If the presentation is late, diagnosis is in favour of retrobulbar hematoma. In carotico-cavernous fistula, the presentation is of abrupt onset and almost immediately. Also the proptosis is pulsatile in CC fistula.

OCULAR FOREIGN BODY

- Foreign body in the eye can either be extraocular, intraocular and intraorbital. Extraocular foreign body is the most common presentation found in daily practice. The FB may be in the conjunc-tiva, in fornix, subconjunctival space, over the cornea (superficial or deep).

- Common FBs are the chips of iron and steel (90%). Rest 10% includes—glass, stone, lead pellets, copper, aluminium, plastic and wood. The most common mode of foreign body in eye is chisel and hammer.
- **Modes of Damage:**
  1. Mechanical effects (specially if > 2 mm in size).
  2. Introduction of infection.
  3. Reaction of foreign body.
  4. Post traumatic iridocyclitis.
  5. Sympathetic ophthalmitis.
- **Reactions of Foreign Body (Intraocular):**

  Depends whether the FB is organic or inorganic.

Inorganic FB:

Four types of reactions can be noted:

A. *No reaction:* By glass, plastic, gold, silver, platinum.

B. *Local irritative reaction:*

  i. Leads to encapsulation of FB.

  ii. By lead and aluminium.

C. *Suppurative reaction* by pure copper, zinc, nickel and mercury particles.

D. *Specific reactions:* By iron and copper alloy.

These specific reactions are:

1. Siderosis bulbi:

- Produce degenerative changes.
- Epithelial structures of eye are most involved.
- Occurs generally after 2 months to 2 years of injury.

2. Chalcosis:

- No degenerative changes.
- Deposited under membranous structures of eye.

Clinical Features:

a. KF ring.

b. Sunflower cataract.

c. Retina—Golden plaques at posterior pole.

Organic FB (Wood, other vegetable matter):

They produce proliferative reaction characterized by formation of giant cells.

WAARDENBURG'S SYNDROME

Systemic Features:

1. Sensorineural hearing loss.
2. Vestibular hypofunction.
3. Broad, flat, nasal bridge.
4. Impaired speech with or without cleft palate.
5. Prominent white forelock.
6. Cutaneous vitiligo.
7. Confluent eyebrows.
8. EEG abnormalities.

Ocular Features:

1. Telecanthus.
2. Heterochromia iridis.
3. Poliosis.
4. Lateral displacement of lacrimal punctum.
5. Increased susceptibility to dacryocystitis.
6. Hypopigmentation of fundus or mottled fundus.
7. Bilateral anterior lenticonus.

NEUROFIBROMATOSIS–I

Ocular Features:

1. Optic nerve glioma.
2. Other neural tumours.
3. Spheno–orbital encephalocele.
4. Eyelid plexiform neurofibromas.
5. Prominent corneal nerves.
6. Congenital ectropion uveae.
7. Congenital glaucoma (rare).
8. Choroidal hematomas.
9. Lisch nodules.

NEUROFIBROMATOSIS–II

1. Juvenile posterior subcapsular cataract.
2. Combined hamartomas of the retina and retinal pigment epithelium.

X-RAY VIEWS OF ORBIT

A. Caldwell-luc View

- PA view.
- Occipitofrontal.
- Structures seen:
  a. **Superior orbital fissure.**
  b. Greater and lesser wing of sphenoid.
  c. Ethmoid and frontal sinus.
  d. Floor of sella.

B. Town's View

- AP view.
- Frontooccipital.
- Structures seen:
  a. Dorsum sellae of sphenoid bone.
  b. Inferior orbital fissure.

C. Water's View

- **Occipitomeatal**
  – Structure seen: Floor of orbit (Important in blow-out fractures).
- **Occipitomental**
  – Maxillary sinus and floor of orbit are seen.

D. Rhese View

For optic foramen.

SURGERIES FOR REMOVAL OF EYE

Enucleation

Procedure—Removal of eyeball with stump of optic nerve leaving behind the extraocular muscles. It is then replaced by **implants: Generally after enucleation, the orbital implant is placed during the same sitting.**

1. PMMA implant.
2. Hydroxyapatite implant.

Indications:

1. Blind painful eye.
2. Intraocular tumor.
3. Severe trauma with risk of sympathetic ophthalmia.
4. Phthisis bulbi.
5. Microphthalmia.
6. Endophthalmitis/Panophthalmitis.
7. Cosmetic deformity.

Evisceration

Procedure: Removal of entire intraocular contents of the eye, leaving the scleral shell and extraocular muscle attachments intact. After this procedure, artificial eye is implanted.

Indications:

Same as enucleation.

Except in the following two conditions where it is absolutely contraindicated:

1. Intraocular tumors.
2. Severe trauma with risk of sympathetic ophthalmitis.

Exenteration

Procedure: Complete removal of eyeball, the retrobulbar orbital soft tissues including the periosteum of bone, and most or all of the eyelids.

Indications:

1. Malignancies.
2. Mucormycosis.
3. Chronic orbital pain.
4. Orbital deformities.

CRANIOFACIAL SYNOSTOSIS

This is a group of rare, hereditary disorders characterized by synostosis of the sutures of upper part of the skull leading to limited expansion of skull, accompanied by severe orbital abnormalities.

The skulls show various shapes due to difference in time, extent and number of suture closures.

1. **Brachyccphaly:** Wide skull due to involvement of coronal or lambdoidal suture leading to a wide skull.
2. **Oxycephaly or Acrocephaly:** High skull, due to closure of coronal suture associated with other sutures.
3. **Scaphocephaly:** Long and narrow skull due to premature closure of sagittal sutures.
4. **Plagiocephaly:** Due to asymmetric involvement of sutures. **Clover leaf skull** is a type of plagiocephaly leading to trilobed skull.

Most Common Examples are:

A. Crouzons Syndrome

- It is also known as **Craniofacial dysostosis or Parrot head.**
- It is characterized by developmental cranial deformity, a beaknose, hypoplastic maxilla, marked prognathism and number of ocular defects.
- **Pathophysiology:** Premature closure of cranial and facial sutures causing arrested growth of maxilla and zygoma leading to decreased orbital volume.

Clinical Features:

1. *Proptosis:* It may cause corneal exposure leading to exposure keratitis.
2. *Hyperteleorism:* It is increased distance of medial canthus due to extra bony tissue and hence with increased interpupillary distance.
3. *Exotropia* which may lead to amblyopia.
4. *Optic atrophy.*

B. Apert's Syndrome

- **Also called Acrocephalosyndactyly.**
- It is the most severe form of craniostenosis involving all sutures.

Clinical Features:

1. Mentally handicapped.
2. Contracted orbital volume leading to **Proptosis.**
3. Hypertelorism.
4. Exotropia which can lead to amblyopia.
5. Anti-mongoloid slant.
6. Optic atrophy.

LATERAL FACIAL MICROSTOMIAS

It constitutes a spectrum of anomaly involving structures derived from **first and second branchial arches** leading to asymmetrical underdevelopment of face.

A. Treacher Collins Syndrome

There is a generalized rotation of orbital content; with associated malar, zygomatic and mandibular hypoplasia.

Clinical Features:

1. Anti-mongoloid slant.
2. Eyelid coloboma.
3. Strabismus which may lead to amblyopia.

B. Goldenhar's Syndrome

Also called **Oculo-Auricular-Vertebral Syndrome.**

Clinical Features:

Depressed lateral orbital rim, with wide mouth, *preauricular skin tags, deafness, vertebral malformations.*

Ocular Features:

a. Epibulbar dermoids.

b. Microphthalmos, Microcornea.

c. Anophthalmos.

d. Hypoplasia of optic nerve and macula.

e. Strabismus.

NEET DRILL

1. Capacity of the orbit is 30 cc.
2. Shape of the orbit is quadrilateral or pyramidal in shape.
3. Proptosis is distance between the lateral orbital margin and the apex of the cornea of > 21 mm.
4. Weakest wall of the orbit is medial wall due to cribiform plate of the ethmoid sinus.
5. Blow-out fractures are fracture floor of the orbit due to blunt trauma.
6. Most common type of lacrimal gland tumour is benign mixed tumour, i.e., pleomorphic adenoma.
7. The nerve passing through the body of the cavernous sinus is 6th nerve.
8. Most common intraorbital malignant tumour of children is rhabdomyosarcoma.
9. Most common intraorbital benign tumour of children is dermoid.
10. Most common primary neoplasm of orbit is non-Hodgkin's lymphoma commonly the B cell type.
11. Cause of intermittent proptosis is orbital varices.
12. First muscle to be involved in thyroid ophthalmopathy is IR, i.e., inferior rectus.
13. Most common mode of spread of retinoblastoma is through the optic nerve.
14. Most common non-ocular malignancy in retinoblastoma is osteosarcoma.
15. Mutation in retinoblastoma is 13q14.
16. X-ray finding of blow-out fracture is "Tear-drop sign".
17. Part of the muscle involved in thyroid myopathy is belly of the muscle.
18. First movement to be affected in thyroid ophthalmopathy is Elevation.
19. Most common mode of presentation of retinoblastoma is leukocoria and the second most common mode is strabismus.
20. Optic nerve glioma is a feature of both NF1 and NF2 but more common in NF1.
21. Familial cases of retinoblastoma are 6% and sporadic cases are 94%.
22. In retinoblastoma, 60% are unilateral and 40% are bilateral.
23. Anti-fungals that can be given intra-vitreally are Amphotericin B and Voriconazole.

24. Most common source of metastasis in the orbit: Breasts in females and lungs in males.

25. Most common source of metastasis in children is Neuroblastoma.

MULTIPLE CHOICE QUESTIONS

1. **A child presents with unilateral proptosis which is compressible and increases on bending forwards. It is non-pulsatile and has no thrill or bruit. MRI shows retroorbital mass with echogenic shadows. The most probable diagnosis is:**
   A. Orbital mass
   B. Orbital encephalocele
   C. Orbital A-V malformation
   D. Neurofibromatosis

2. **Which one of the following statements is incorrect about optic nerve glioma?**
   A. Has a peak incidence in first decade
   B. Arises from oligodendrocytes
   C. Causes meningeal hyperplasia
   D. Is associated with type I neurofibromatosis

3. **The most common second malignant in survivals of retinoblastoma:**
   A. Thyroid cancer
   B. Nasopharyngeal carcinoma
   C. Optic glioma
   D. Osteosarcoma

4. **The most common retrobulbar mass in adults is:**
   A. Neurofibroma
   B. Meningioma
   C. Cavernous hemangioma
   D. Schwannoma

5. **The mother of a one-and-a-half-year old child gives history of a white reflex from one eye for the past 1 month. On computed tomography scan of the orbit there is calcification seen within the globe. The most likely diagnosis is:**
   A. Congenital cataract
   B. Retinoblastoma
   C. Endophthalmitis
   D. Coats' disease

6. **Vortex vein invasion is commonly seen in:**
   A. Retinoblastoma
   B. Malignant melanoma
   C. Optic nerve gliomas
   D. Medullo-epitheliomas

7. **Hereditary retinoblastomas develop from the following chromosomal deletions:**
   A. 13 q 14 B. 13 p 14
   C. 14 p 13 D. 14 q 13

8. **A one year old child having leukocoria was detected to be having a unilateral, large, retinoblastoma filling half the globe. Current therapy would involve:**
   A. Enucleation
   B. Chemotherapy followed by local dyes
   C. Direct laser ablation using photodynamic cryotherapy
   D. Scleral radiotherapy followed by chemotherapy

9. **A patient is on follow-up with you, after enucleating of a painful blind eye. After enucleating of the eyeball, a proper sized artificial prosthetic**

eye is advised after a postoperative period of:

A. About 10 days

B. About 20 days

C. 6–8 weeks

D. 12–24 weeks

10. All of the following is associated with weakness of extraocular muscle except:

A. Fisher syndrome

B. Myasthenia gravis

C. Eaton Lambert syndrome

D. Thyrotoxicosis

11. Most common ocular foreign body is:

A. Chisel and Hammer

B. Glass

C. Plastic

D. Stone

12. Retinoblastoma differs from pseudoglioma by:

A. Decrease IOT

B. Blurring of vision

C. Enlargement of optic foramen

D. All of the above

13. A mass present in muscle cone, encapsulated, presentation in 3rd to 4th decade with gradually increasing proptosis:

A. Capillary hemangioma

B. Cavernous hemangioma

C. Dermoid

D. Hemangioendothelioma

14. True about telecanthus is:

A. Increase in intercanthal distance with normal interpupillary distance

B. Widely separated medial wall of orbits

C. Increased intercanthal distance with increased interpupillary distance

D. None of the above

15. In Neurofibromatosis-1 most common tumor is:

A. Optic nerve glioma

B. Cerebral astrocytoma

C. Glioblastoma multiforme

D. Meningioma

16. In regard to intraocular retinoblastoma, which of the following statements is false?

A. 94% of cases are sporadic

B. Patients with sporadic retinoblastoma do not pass their genes to their offsprings

C. Calcification in the tumour can be detected on USG

D. Reese-Ellsworth classification is useful in predicting visual prognosis following radiotherapy

17. A 6-year-old boy has been complaining of headache, ignoring to see the objects on the sides for four months. On examination, he is not mentally retarded, his grades at school are good and visual acuity is diminished in both the eyes. Visual charting showed significant field defect. CT scan of the head showed supraseller mass with calcification. Which of the following is the most probable diagnosis?

A. Astrocytoma

B. Craniopharyngioma

C. Pituitary adenoma

D. Meningioma

18. A 50-year-old man presented with orbital mass. Systemic examination revealed anaemia and investigations

revealed hypergammaglobulinema. The patient should be investigated to rule out:

A. Squamous cell carcinoma

B. Optic nerve glioma

C. Multiple myeloma

D. Malignant melanoma

19. All the following signs could result from infection within the right cavernosus sinus, except:

A. Loss of pupillary light reflex

B. Loss of corneal blink reflex

C. Ptosis

D. Right ophthalmoplegia

20. Sclerosis of bony orbit is seen in:

A. Neurofibroma

B. Retinoblastoma

C. Meningioma

D. Glioma

21. Common ocular manifestation in Trisomy 13 is:

A. Capillary hemangioma

B. Bilateral microphthalmos

C. Neurofibroma

D. Dermoid cyst

22. The differential diagnosis of retinoblastoma would include all except:

A. Persistent hyperplastic primary vitreous

B. Coats' disease

C. Retinal astrocytoma

D. Retinal detachment

23. Enucleation of the eyeball is contraindicated in:

A. Endophthalmitis

B. Panophthalmitis

C. Intraocular tumours

D. Painful blind eye

24. 8-year-old boy presented with swelling in left eye of 3 months duration. Examination revealed proptosis of left eye with preserved vision. Right eye is normal. CT scan revealed intra orbital extraconal mass lesion. Biopsy revealed embryonal rhabdomyosarcoma. Metastatic work up was normal. The standard line of treatment is:

A. Chemotherapy only

B. Wide local excision

C. Enucleation

D. Chemotherapy and radiation therapy

25. A 23-year-old child presented with leukocoria in the right eye since 2 months. On examination, a total retinal detachment was present in the same eye. Ultrasound B scan revealed a heterogenous subretinal mass with calcification, associated with retinal detachment. The most likely clinical diagnosis is:

A. Coats' disease

B. Retinoblastoma

C. Toxocariasis

D. Retinal tuberculoma

26. Which wall is most often fractured in a blow-out fracture of the orbit due to fisticuff injury?

A. Superior wall B. Inferior wall

C. Medial wall D. Lateral wall

27. Leukocoria is seen in all except:

A. Retinoblastoma

B. Congenital glaucoma

C. Persistent primary hyperplastic vitreous

D. Fungal endophthalmitis

28. A five-year-old child presents with mild proptosis and loss of vision of one eye. On examination direct pupillary reflex is absent and consensual reflex is present. What is the most probable diagnosis?

A. Retinoblastoma

B. Optic disc angioma

C. Optic nerve glioma

D. Optic sheath meningioma

29. A 48-year-old lady presents with unilateral mild axial proptosis. There is no history of redness or pain. Which of the following is the most appropriate investigation?

A. CT scan to rule out meningioma

B. USG to rule out orbital pseudotumor

C. T3 and T4 measurement to rule out thyrotoxicosis

D. Doppler to rule out hemangioma

30. Traumatic eye with late presentation of unilateral proptosis and scleral hyperaemia is seen in:

A. Retrobulbar hematoma

B. Retrobulbar cellulitis

C. Caroticocavernous fistula

D. Pneumo orbit

31. Concussion injuries to the eye will cause all of the following except:

A. Subluxation of lens

B. Soft exudate

C. Macular hole

D. Berlin's oedema

32. Best X-ray view to visualize superior orbital fissure is:

A. Anteroposterior

B. Basal

C. Towne's

D. Caldwell Luc's view

33. Most common orbital tumour in children is:

A. Retinoblastoma

B. Rhabdomyosarcoma

C. Melanoma

D. Chloroma

34. Retinoblastoma can present with all, except:

A. Leukocoria

B. Squint

C. Microphthalmos

D. Cataract

35. Which is not a complication of blunt trauma to eye?

A. Hyphema

B. Retinal detachment

C. Double perforation of iris

D. Iridodialysis

36. Which of the following is not prognostic significance in choroidal melanoma?

A. Presence of retinal detachment

B. Size of the tumor

C. Cytology of the tumor cells

D. Presence of extraocular extension

37. Berlin's edema occurs due to:

A. Penetrating injury to eye

B. Blunt trauma to eye

C. Radiation injury to eye

D. Chemical injury to eye

38. Most common type of optic nerve glioma is:

A. Protoplasmic B. Pilocytic

C. Gemistocytic D. Fibrous

39. A child with a unilateral white reflex and raised intraocular pressure. The required investigations are:

A. USG
B. Observation under anesthesia
C. Tonometry
D. X-ray

40. Bilateral retinoblastoma ideally is managed by:
A. Radiation
B. Laser excision
C. Enucleation
D. Adjuvant chemotherapy
E. Thermotherapy

41. Thyroid ophthalmopathy associated with:
A. External ophthalmoplegia
B. Internal ophthalmoplegia
C. Proptosis
D. Large extraocular muscle
E. Lid lag

42. Management of retinoblastoma:
A. Enucleation
B. Chemotherapy
C. Radiotherapy
D. USG
E. Fluorescein angiography

43. Blow-out fracture orbit involve:
A. Floor
B. Medial wall
C. Lateral wall
D. Roof
E. Apex

44. Familial retinoblastoma:
A. Has autosomal recessive inheritance
B. More commonly bilateral
C. Due to mutation
D. More common than sporadic retinoblastoma

45. Enucleation is done for:
A. Retinoblastoma
B. Malignant melanoma
C. Glaucoma
D. Pthisis bulbi
E. Vitreous hemorrhage

46. Blow-out fracture orbit is characterized by:
A. Diplopia
B. "Tear drop" sign
C. Forced duction test
D. Exophthalmos

47. One year old male child with cat's eye reflex and raised IOT:
A. Toxoplasma gondi infection
B. Toxocara canis
C. Retinoblastoma
D. Retinopathy of prematurity
E. Noorie's disease

48. Knudson's two hit hypothesis is for:
A. Glaucoma
B. Retinoblastoma
C. Optic glioma
D. Meningioma

49. In Waardenburg's syndrome, following are seen except:
A. Widening of the eyebrow
B. Short palpebral fissure
C. Interstitial keratitis
D. Heterochromia iridis

50. Dysthyroid ophthalmopathy, all are true except:
A. Proptosis
B. Myopathy
C. Exophthalmos
D. Optic neuritis

51. Peribulbar injection is given in:
A. Subtenon space
B. Muscle space
C. Periorbital space
D. Subperiorbital space

52. Raised LDH levels in aqueous is seen in:
A. Galactosemia
B. Glaucoma
C. Hemangioblastoma
D. Retinoblastoma

53. Pseudorossettes are seen in:
A. Retinoblastoma
B. Ophthalmia nodosa
C. Phacolytic glaucoma
D. Trachoma

54. Proptosis is seen in:
A. Neuroblastoma
B. Meningioma
C. Sympathetic ophthalmia
D. Injuries

55. Enucleation means:
A. Removal of the contents of globe
B. Removal of the contents of globe and sclera except a frill around the optic nerve
C. Removal of entire globe along with portion of optic nerve
D. Removal of the entire contents of orbit

56. A 16-year-old male comes with injury to the eye with tennis ball. The following can be seen:
A. Hyphema
B. Subluxation of lens
C. Subconjunctival haemorrhage
D. Hypopyon

57. Anteroposterior stability of eyeball is provided by all except:
A. Orbital fat
B. S.O.
C. S.R.
D. Suspensory ligament of eyeball

58. Most common cause of bilateral proptosis is:
A. Thyrotoxicosis
B. Cavernous sinus thrombosis
C. Retinoblastoma
D. Pseudotumors

59. Safe and effective method of sterilization of surgical eye instrument is:
A. Acetone B. Formalin
C. Autoclaving D. Boiling

60. Bilateral congenital exophthalmos is seen in:
A. Goldenhar's syndrome
B. Clover leaf skull
C. Horner's syndrome
D. Neurofibromatosis

61. Most common intraorbital metastatic tumor in children is:
A. Non-Hodgkin's lymphoma
B. Neuroblastoma
C. CA nasopharynx
D. Malignant melanoma

62. Muscle earliest involved in thyroid ophthalmopathy:
A. Lateral rectus
B. Medial rectus
C. Inferior rectus
D. Superior oblique

63. Intermittent exophthalmos is seen in:

A. Varicosity of ophthalmic vein
B. Cavernous sinus thrombosis
C. Cavernous carotid fistula
D. Severe thyrotoxicosis

64. Ciliary ganglion lies between:

A. Optic nerve and lateral rectus
B. Lateral rectus and inferior oblique
C. Lateral and inferior recti
D. Orbit and superior oblique

65. True about ligament of lockwood:

A. Suspensory ligament of eyeball
B. Forms sheath of extraocular surface
C. Forms tendinous ring
D. All of the above

66. Which of the following cause leukocoria?

A. Eales' disease
B. Coats' disease
C. Central serous retinopathy
D. Retinitis pigmentosa

67. Blow-out fracture of zygomatic arch causes:

A. Anosmia
B. Diplopia
C. Exophthalmos
D. Epistaxis

68. Frequency of USG used in ophthalmics is:

A. 8 B. 18
C. 15 D. 12

69. Pulsatile exophthalmos is not seen in:

A. Neurofibromatosis
B. Varicose vein
C. Blow-out fracture of roof
D. Cavernous fistula

70. Depth of anterior chamber in normal person is:

A. 1–2 mm B. 3–4 mm
C. 0.5–0.9 mm D. 2–3 mm

71. All are true about orbit, except:

A. Maxillary nerve runs through inferior orbital fissure
B. Superior orbital fissure is bounded by sphenoid wings and ethmoid bone
C. Volume = 30 ml
D. Inferior oblique arises from floor

72. The retinoblastoma stage III is treated by:

A. Enucleation
B. Exenteration
C. Radiotherapy
D. None of the above

73. Following muscles originate from ring of zinn except:

A. Superior rectus
B. Medial rectus
C. Inferior rectus
D. Inferior oblique

74. The most common clinical presentation of retinoblastoma:

A. Leukocoria
B. Endophthalmitis
C. Metastatic spread
D. Strabismus

75. Medial wall of orbit is formed by:

A. Body of sphenoid
B. Maxillary
C. Ethmoid
D. All of the above

76. Contracted socket occurs because of all the following except:

A. Chronic low grade infection

B. Chronic mechanical irritation

C. Irradiation

D. Loss of fatty tissue during surgery of enucleation

77. Which of the following conditions does not cause pseudoexophthalmos?

A. High myopia

B. Lid retraction

C. Optic nerve glioma

D. Facial nerve palsy

78. Amaurotic cats eye reflex is seen in:

A. Congenital glaucoma

B. Toxoplasmosis

C. Complete retinal detachment

D. None of the above

79. Hereditary retinoblastoma occurs in what percentage of cases?

A. 10% B. 6%

C. 20% D. 8%

80. In a child with retinoblastoma, which of the following is not a common finding?

A. Intraocular calcification

B. Intracerebral calcification

C. Multiple cranial deposits

D. Widening of the optic foramen

81. D shaped pupil is seen in:

A. Glaucoma

B. Dislocation of lens

C. Iridodialysis

D. Iridocyclitis

82. The most serious danger to vision is:

A. Fracture of cribiform plate

B. Fracture through optic foramen

C. Fracture roof of the orbit

D. Blow-out fracture

83. In retinoblastoma after enucleation, which tissue needs critical evaluation for systemic metastasis?

A. Optic nerve

B. Retinal artery

C. Vortex vein

D. Sclera and episclera

84. A person sustained blunt trauma with immediate loss of vision. On examination the anterior chamber of the eye is deep. The cause could be:

A. Vitreous haemorrhage

B. Retinal detachment

C. Subluxation of lens

D. Hyphema

85. A person with history of blunt trauma to the right eye 6 months back developed pain and circumcorneal congestion of the eye. The most important immediate investigation in this case is:

A. Intraocular tension

B. Indirect ophthalmoscopy

C. B scan

D. Gonioscopy

86. In concussion injury to eye all are seen except:

A. Berlin's edema

B. Macular hole

C. Lens subluxation

D. Retinal exudates

87. Goldenhar's syndrome is associated with what prominent ocular manifestation?

A. Microcornea

B. Megalocornea

C. Epibulbar dermoids

D. Sclerocornea

E. Nystagmus

88. Difficulty in convergence of the eyes in thyrotoxicosis is denoted by:

A. Stellwag's sign

B. Mobius sign

C. von Graefe's sign

D. Joffroy's sign

89. Which part of orbicularis oculi is known as Horner's muscle?

A Orbital B. Lacrimal

C. Temporal D. Muller's muscle

90. Following are inert foreign bodies in eye except:

A. Gold B. Silver

C. Copper D. Platinum

91. Panophthalmitis occurs following:

A. Perforated corneal ulcer

B. Blunt injury

C. Orbital cellulitis

D. Cavernous sinus thrombosis

92. Most common cause of fracture of roof of orbit:

A. Blow on forehead

B. Blow on lower jaw

C. Blow on parietal bone

D. Fall on back of the head

93. A patient had running nose and pain over medical aspect of eye being treated with decongestants for many days. He later developed chemosis, protosis and diplopia on abduction of right eye with congestion of optic disc. What is the probable diagnosis?

A. Acute ethmoidal sinusitis

B. Orbital cellulitis

C. Cavernous sinus thrombosis

D. Orbital apex syndrome

94. A 5 years old boy presented with leukocoria in right eyeball, while other eye had 2–3 small lesions in the periphery. What will be the ideal management for this patient?

A. Enucleation of both eyes

B. Enucleation of right eye and conservative management for the other eye

C. Enucleation for right eye and radiotherapy for the other eye

D. 6 cycles of chemotherapy

95. A tennis player gets hit by a ball in the face following which he has complaints of decreased vision. Which of the following tells that injury is due to trauma?

A. Optic neuritis

B. Pars planitis

C. Vitreous base detachment

D. Equatorial edema

96. Most common cause for bilateral proptosis in children:

A. Cavernous haemangioma

B. Rhabdomyosarcoma

C. ALL

D. AML

97. 40 years male give past history of repeated pain over medial canthus and is on use of decongestants. Now presents with intense chills, rigor with diplopia on lateral gaze optic disc is found to be congested diagnosis may be:

A. Ethmoidal sinusitis

B. Orbital cellulitis

C. Cavernous sinus thrombosis

D. Orbital apex syndrome

98. Blow-out fracture of orbit leads to involvement of:

A. Posterior medial wall

B. Lateral wall

C. Medial wall

D. Roof

99. Panophthalmitis occurs following:

A. Perforated corneal ulcer

B. Blunt injury

C. Orbital cellulitis

D. Cavernous sinus thrombosis

100. von-Graefe's sign:

A. Lagging behind of the upper lid

B. Retraction of the upper eyelid within frequent blinking

C. Absence of wrinkling of the forehead

D. Convergence of the eye is difficult

101. A man presents 6 hours after the head injury complaining of mild proptosis and scleral hyperaemia. The most probable diagnosis is:

A. Pneumo-orbit

B. Caroticocavernous fistula

C. Retro-orbital hematoma

D. Orbital cellulitis

102. A case of injury to the right brow due to fall from a scooter presents with sudden loss of vision in the right eye. The pupil shows absent direct reflex but a normal consensual papillary reflex is present. The fundus is normal. The treatment of choice is:

A. Intensive I/V corticosteroids as prescribed for spinal injuries to be instituted within six hours

B. Pulse methylprednisolone 250 mg four times daily for three days

C. Oral prednisolone 1.5 mg/kg body weight

D. Emergency optic canal decompression

103. A 23-year-old male presents with progressive proptosis of his right eye. The proptosis increases on bending forward and is compressible. No thrill or bruit was present. Orbital ultrasound revealed an echogenic mass with foci of echo shadows. The most likely diagnosis is:

A. Orbital A-V fistula

B. Orbital varix

C. Neurofibromatosis

D. Orbital encephalocele

104. The most common mode of spread of retinoblastoma is:

A. Haematogenous

B. Lymphatic

C. Optic nerve

D. Trans-scleral

105. An elderly diabetic patient presents with severe panophthalmitis with orbital cellulitis. A sample was collected from periorbital region, which on gram staining shows irregularly branching, aseptate and broad hyphae. The most likely etiological agent is:

A. Penicillium

B. Aspergillus

C. Candida

D. Apophysomyces

106. Bilateral proptosis is seen in:

A. Leukemia

B. Neuroblastoma

C. Fibrous histiocytoma

D. Cavernous hemangioma

107. The common ocular pathology associated with trisomy 13 is:

A. Capillary hemangioma
B. Bilateral micro-ophthalmia
C. Dermoid cyst
D. Neurofibroma

108. The most common presentation of retinoblastoma is:

A. Leukocoria and strabismus
B. Leukocoria and pseudohypopyon
C. Leukocoria and heterochromia irides
D. Leukocoria and hyphaema

109. Second common malignancy in patient of retinoblastoma is:

A. Osteosarcoma
B. Ewing's sarcoma
C. Medulloblastoma
D. Osteoblastoma

110. Most common intracranial tumor encroaching the orbit is:

A. Astrocytoma
B. Glioblastoma multiforme
C. Sphenoid wing meningioma
D. Medulloblastoma

111. A hectic bout of fever with bilateral proptosis in a 25 years old diabetic following an injury to face is most diagnostic of:

A. Cavernous sinus thrombosis
B. Thyrotoxicosis
C. Intracranial neoplasm
D. Orbital tumor

112. Regarding retinoblastoma all are the true except:

A. 13q4p mutation
B. Autosomal dominant
C. 25% bilateral
D. 40% heritable forms

113. Calcification is seen in all of the following except:

A. Optic drusen
B. Retinoblastoma
C. Choroidal osteoma
D. PHPV

114. All of the following bones are a part of the inferior wall of the orbit except:

A. Ethmoid B. Palatine
C. Zygomatic D. Maxilla

115. Thc most common mode of spread of retinoblastoma:

A. Lymphatics
B. Optic nerve
C. Direct invasion
D. Vascular

ANSWER AND EXPLANATION

1.	c	Encephalocele and Neurofibromatosis presents as pulsatile proptosis. Orbital mass will not present as compressible proptosis, hence the answer is A-V malformations.
2.	b	It arises from astrocytes, it's an astrocytoma.
3.	d	Osteogenic sarcoma is the most common non-ocular malignancy in retinoblastoma. It mainly occurs in hereditary cases.
4.	c	Cavernous hemangioma is an encapsulated hemangioma seen most commonly inside the muscle cone.

5.	b	Most common intraocular tumour in children of this age group is retinoblastoma. Also the tumour is characterized by calcification and necrosis.
6.	b	Vortex vein invasion is common in malignant melanoma whereas optic nerve invasion is common in retinoblastoma.
7.	a	Most commonly retinoblastoma is sporadic. Most common mode of inheritance in hereditary retinoblastoma is autosomal dominant.
8.	a	Conservative mode of treatment is indicated only in tumours of small size.
9.	a	After enucleation, we put orbital implants. We wait for the inflammation to subside, i.e., around 10 days. If hydroxyapatite implant is to be put, it can even be done in the same sitting.
10.	d	In thyrotoxicosis there is fibrosis of the muscle, i.e., restrictive myopathy.
11.	a	Most common ocular FB is iron and the most common mode is chisel and hammer.
12.	c	There is increased IOP in retinoblastoma. Blurring of vision can be seen in pseudoglioma also.
13.	b	An encapsulated intraconal mass in the middle age patient is most commonly cavernous hemangioma.
14.	a	In telecanthus the IPD is normal whereas in hyperteleorism IPD is more.
15.	a	Optic nerve glioma is an astrocytoma common in patients of NF-1. It is a tumour of children more common in girls.
16.	b	If the sporadic case has involved the germ cell alongwith the somatic cell, then it will lead to hereditary case.
17.	b	Any suprasellar mass with calcification in a child, first diagnosis is craniopharyngioma.
18.	c	A middle aged patient with hyperglobulinemia, the most probable diagnosis is multiple myeloma.
19.	c	Ptosis should be a feature as there is third nerve palsy, but due to proptosis ptosis is not appreciated.
20.	c	Meningiomas are tumours more common in women, arising from the meningoendothelial cells of the arachnoid villi. It is characterized by opticociliary shunts if it involves the optic nerve sheath and in intracranial meningiomas it causes sclerosis of the bony orbit.
21.	b	Trisomy-13 is called Patau syndrome and is characterized by microphthalmos, cataract, corneal opacity and retinal dysplasias.
22.	d	Only central retinal detachment presence as leukocoria, i.e., white eye reflex.
23.	a	Endophthalmitis is treated by intravitreal injections of antibiotics. If not managed and removal of the eye is indicated, we should go for evisceration. This is because the outer coats of the eyeball are not involved and hence we should not remove it.
24.	d	Rhabdomyosarcoma is very responsive to radiotherapy.
25.	b	It indicates an exophytic retinoblastoma where there is exudative retinal detachment.
26.	b	Blow-out fracture is the floor fracture occurring due to blunt trauma.

27. b In congenital glaucoma the cornea is white due to edema as a result of increased IOP, but leukocoria is not seen.

28. c Optic nerve glioma initially presents with all the signs of optic nerve disease and proptosis is a late feature.

29. c Most common cause of proptosis in adults is thyroid ophthalmopathy. The proptosis can be axial or non-axial, painful or painless and unilateral or bilateral.

30. a Proptosis after trauma, late presentation, scleral hyperaemia, most probable diagnosis is retrobulbar hematoma.

31. b Soft exudates are axonal debris and seen mostly as result of hypoxia in the retina.

32. d Caldwell-Luc view is the PA view.

33. b Rhabdomyosarcoma is a tumour arising from the pleuropotential mesenchymal cells which later develop in striated muscles.

34. d Some cases of retinoblastoma have been documented to be associated with microphthalmos.

35. c Perforation of iris can only occur after perforating injuries. Blunt trauma can cause disinsertion of iris, i.e., iridodialysis.

36. a Commonly choroidal melanomas break through the Bruch's membrane and lead to exudative retinal detachment. Hence it is not considered as a prognostic factor.

37. b Also called Commotio Retinae is edema at the macula due to blunt trauma. It presents as cherry-red spot at the macula.

38. b Pilocytic means that the tumour cells are hair-like. Pilocytic astrocytoma is the most common type.

39. a,b, c,d In a child, a detailed retinal examination, tonometry, corneal diameter, gonioscopy etc can only be done under anesthesia.

40. a,c, d,e Any modality of treatment in each eye will depend upon the extent of the tumour. Generally in bilateral cases, every effort is made to save at least one eye. We do laser photocoagulation to damage the blood supply of the tumour and not laser excision.

41. c,d, e Internal muscles are not involved in thyroid ophthalmopathy.

42. a,b, c,d, e Fluorescein angiography in retinoblastoma helps to know the viability of the tumour after a conservative treatment like laser, cryo or radiotherapy.

43. a,b Since medial wall is the weakest wall, it can be involved in blow-out fractures alongwith the floo. Such patients present with subcutaneous emphysema.

44. b,c Familial retinoblastomas are autosomal dominant and are less common (6%) than sporadic cases (94%).

45. a,b, c,d Vitreous haemorrhage is treated by vitrectomy; we never go for removal of the eye. Enucleation is a modality of treatment for absolute glaucoma which is a painful blind eye.

46. a,b c There is enophthalmos in blow-out fractures and not exophthalmos.

47. c Most common age of presentation in retinoblastoma is within 18 months.

48. b Knudson gave the hypothesis that there are two mutations needed for

a retinoblastoma to manifest. Either both hits are on somatic cells or one is at the somatic cell and one at the germ cell. Respectively it can be a non-hereditary or a hereditary case.

49. c Interstitial keratitis is a feature of granulomatous inflammations like syphilis, leprosy, TB etc.

50. d Optic nerve involvement in thyroid disease is compression optic neuropathy and not optic neuritis.

51. c Surgical spaces of the orbit are: subperiosteal space, peripheral orbital space, central space (i.e., the muscular cone or retrobulbar space) and subtenons space.

52. d All the three enzymes, i.e., LDH (Lactose dehydrogenase), NSE (Neuron specific enolase) and PGI (Phosphoglucoisomerase) are raised in patients of retinoblastoma.

53. a Microscopic pathological study in retinoblastoma shows various patterns like Homer-Wright, Flexner-Wintersteiner and Fleurettes.

54. a,b Neuroblastoma metastasizes in the orbit causing proptosis.

55. c In evisceration the scleral coat alongwith the muscles attached is not removed, whereas in enucleation there is removal of the whole eyeball with maximum part of the optic nerve.

56. a,b, c Hypopyon is pus cells in the anterior chamber and is a feature of infection. All other features can be seen in patients of blunt trauma.

57. a Suspensory ligament extends from the posterior lacrimal crest to lateral orbital tubercle. The anteroposterior stability to the eyeball is provided by the tenons capsule or fascia bulbi which is an envelope of elastic connective tissue that fuses posteriorly with the optic nerve sheath and anteriorly with a thin layer of tissue called the intermuscular septum, 3 mm posterior to the limbus. Connections between the tenons capsule and the periorbital tissues help suspend the globe in the orbit.

58. a Most common cause of either bilateral or unilateral proptosis in adults is thyroid ophthalmopathy.

59. c Autoclaving is the safest method of sterilisation.

60. b Clover-leaf skull is a craniofacial synostosis leading to limited expansion of the skull alongwith severe orbital malformations.

61. b Most common intraorbital tumour in children is rhabdomyosarcoma and the most common intraorbital metastatic tumour is neuroblastoma.

62. c Sequence of involvement of muscles is inferior rectus, medial rectus, superior rectus and at the last lateral rectus.

63. a Intermittent is when proptosis occurs at a particular posture and then at other times the position of the eye is normal. Hence, it occurs when there are varicose veins in the orbit.

64. a Ciliary ganglion is a peripheral parasympathetic ganglion lying near the apex of the orbit between the tendon of the lateral rectus and the optic nerve.

65. a Suspensory ligament of the eyeball is formed by the sheath of extraocular muscles, i.e., medial rectus, inferior oblique, inferior rectus and lateral rectus muscle formed by the thickened part of the tenon's capsule.

66. b Leukocoria is white eye reflex also called Amaurotic Cat's eye reflex. Coats' disease is a severe form of retinal telangiectasia commonly seen in small boys.
67. b Blow-out fracture is fracture floor due to blunt trauma. Floor is formed of Zygomatic arch, maxillary bone and a small palantine bone.
68. a Ultrasonic frequencies in the range of 10 MHz are used for ophthalmic diagnosis.
69. b Varicose veins present as intermittent proptosis.
70. d Depth of anterior chamber is 2.4–2.5 mm.
71. b SOF is bounded by lesser and greater wing of sphenoid, situated lateral to the orbital foramen at the orbital apex.
72. b Stage III is extraocular extension (i.e., the tumour has spread to the orbit) and is thus treated by exenteration (all the orbital contents alongwith the periosteum of the bone is removed).
73. d All the recti originate from Annulus of Zinn.
74. a Most common mode of presentation is leukocoria and the second most common mode is strabismus, i.e., squint.
75. d Medial wall is formed by four bones, i.e., frontal process of maxillary bone, lacrimal bone, cribiform plate of ethmoid and body of the sphenoid.
76. d Contracted socket is a condition where the volume of the socket is reduced.
77. c Optic nerve glioma causes true exophthalmos.
78. c Leukocoria occurs in toxocariasis and not in toxoplasmosis.
79. b 94% of cases are sporadic and 6% are familial.
80. b Intracerebral calcification is not a feature of retinoblastoma.
81. c Iridodialysis is disinsertion of the iris and leads to D-shaped pupil.
82. b Optic nerve passes through the optic foramen. The other structure passing through it is ophthalmic artery.
83. a Retinoblastoma spreads through the optic nerve.
84. c Immediate loss of vision with a deep anterior chamber the most probable cause is subluxation of lens.
85. a The patient may be developing angle-recession glaucoma. It occurs after blunt trauma due to trauma to the trabecular meshwork. There is tearing in the ciliary body leading to the recession of the angle.
86. d Retinal exudates occur due to hypoxia and are not a feature of trauma.
87. c Goldenhar's syndrome is Oculo-Auricular-Vertebral syndrome.
88. b Mobius sign occurs due to restrictive myopathy involving the medial rectus.
89. b Horner's muscle is the part of orbicularis oculi attached to the lacrimal sac.
90. c Copper in eye, i.e., chalcosis is characterized by deposition of copper under the membranous structures of the eye. It causes KF ring, sunflower cataract and golden plaques at the posterior pole.

91. a Panophthalmitis is inflammation of all the three coats of the eyeball.

92. a Fracture roof of the orbit is a rare condition and occurs most commonly after accidents due to blow on the forehead.

93. c First sign of cavernous sinus thrombosis is sixth nerve palsy. History suggests that the patient had sinusitis which leads to orbital cellulitis, later complicating into cavernous sinus thrombosis.

94. b Management depends upon the size of the tumour.

95. c All other options are not a feature of blunt trauma.

96. c The best option is ALL as it is more common in children. Leukaemia commonly presents as unilateral proptosis, but may present as bilaterally.

97. c History suggests that the patient suffers from CST.

98. c Since medial wall is the weakest wall of the orbit, hence it may be involved in blow-out fractures.

99. a Panophthalmitis is the inflammation of the all the three coats of the eyeball.

100. a Lid retraction is called Dalrymple's sign, limited convergence is Mobius sign.

101. c Most probable cause is retrobulbar hematoma. C-C fistula will present as pulsating proptosis.

102. d Since the history indicates that optic nerve is getting involved, hence drastic step has to be taken to save the nerve.

103. b Intermittent proptosis changing with the posture of the head is due to orbital varices.

104. c The most common mode of spread is by direct extension through optic nerve and is diagnosed by seeing the enlargement of optic foramen on X-ray, Rhese view.

105. d Aspergillus and candida are the most common fungal cause of orbital cellulitis. But both penicillium and aspergillus are septate fungi. Apophysomyces elegans is an emerging zygomycete that has been reported to cause invasive cutaneous and rhino-orbito-cerebral infections.

106. b Neuroblastoma is the most common metastatic tumour of the orbit in children and around 40% of the cases are bilateral. Leukemia can also cause proptosis in advanced cases due to infilteration of the orbital tissues, but most commonly presents as unilateral proptosis. Fibrous histiocytoma is the most common mesenchymal orbital tumour of adults. It can be benign or malignant. In children it commonly occurs after radiotherapy treatment for retinoblastoma or any cause of orbital radiotherapy. Cavernous hemangioma is the most common benign orbital tumour in adults and presents unilaterally.

107. b Trisomy-13 is called Patau syndrome.

Features are:

Ocular Features:

a. Microphthalmos.

b. Corneal opacity.

c. Peter's anomaly.

d. Cataract.

e. Retinal dysplasia.

Systemic Features:

a. Microcephaly.

b. Cleft lip and palate.

c. Low–set ears.

108. a Most common mode of presentation is leukocoria and the second most common mode is strabismus.

109. a It is the most common non-ocular malignancy particularly seen in hereditary cases.

110. c Meningioma is a benign brain tumour arising from the arachnoid. It is more common in females after the age of 50 years. 20% of meningiomas are sphenoid wing meningiomas.

111. a Bilateral proptosis with fever after trauma to the face, most probable diagnosis is cavernous sinus thrombosis.

112. d 94% cases are sporadic and only 6% are familial.

113. d Optic disc drusen (ODD) or optic nerve head drusen (ONHD) are globules of mucoproteins and mucopolysaccharides that progressively calcify in the optic disc. They are thought to be the remnants of the axonal transport system of degenerated retinal ganglion cells.

Choroidal osteoma is a benign ossifying tumor characterized by mature bone replacing choroid.

Retinoblastoma is known to have calcification.

114. a The roof (superior wall) is formed primarily by the orbital plate frontal bone, and also the lesser wing of sphenoid near the apex of the orbit.

The floor (inferior wall) is formed by the orbital surface of *maxilla*, the orbital surface of *zygomatic bone* and the minute orbital process of *palatine bone.*

The medial wall is formed primarily by the orbital plate of *ethmoid*, as well as contributions from the frontal process of maxilla, the *lacrimal bone*, and a small part of the body of the sphenoid. It is the thinnest wall of the orbit, evidenced by pneumatized ethmoidal cells.

The lateral wall is formed by the frontal process of zygomatic and more posteriorly by the orbital plate of the greater wing of sphenoid. The lateral wall is the thickest wall of the orbit, important because it is the most exposed surface, highly vulnerable to blunt force trauma.

115. b Most common mode of spread is through the optic nerve, and hence we do X-ray Rhese view to check for any enlargement of optic foramen.

RECENTLY ADDED QUESTIONS

1. **Common cause of fungal orbital cellulitis in patient of diabetic ketoacidosis is:**

A. Aspergillus B. Mucor

C. Candida D. Cryptococcus

2. **Most common orbital wall fractured in blow-out fracture orbit is:**

A. Medial wall B. Lateral wall

C. Floor D. Roof

3. **A diabetic patient came two days after cataract surgery with following presentation. He also has severe pain and redness in eyes. Which of**

the following is the first step in the management of this patient?

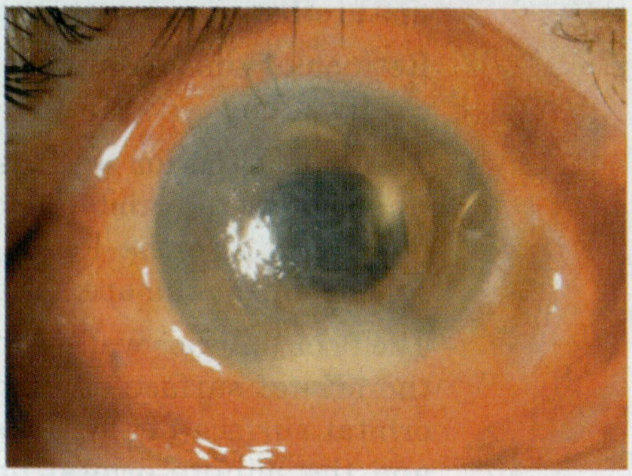

A. Intravitreal antibiotic

B. Intravitreal steroids

C. Intravenous mannitol

D. Intravenous antibiotics

4. **Evisceration of eye is not done in:**

A. Malignancy

B. Panophthalmitis

C. Severe globe trauma

D. Expulsive hemorrhage

5. **Which is not done in endophthalmitis?**

A. Intravenous antibiotics

B. Topical antibiotics

C. Intravitreal antibiotics

D. Parsplana vitrectomy

ANSWERS OF RECENTLY ADDED QUESTIONS

1. b Most common cause of fungal endophthalmitis is Candida albicans.

Most common cause of fungal orbital cellulitis is mucormycosis.

2. c Blow-out fracture is floor fracture due to blunt trauma. Weakest area of floor is posteromedial part.

3. a The above is a case of endophthalmitis and hence treatment will be intravitreal antibiotics.

4. a Two major contraindications of evisceration are :

1. Malignancy.
2. Risk of sympathetic ophthalmitis.

Rest indications of both enucleation and evisceration are same.

Indications of ENUCLEATION:

Blind painful eye.

Intraocular tumor.

Severe trauma with risk of sympathetic ophthalmia.

Pthisis bulbi.

Microphthalmia.

Endophthalmitis/panophthalmitis.

Cosmetic deformity.

EXENTERATION

Cutaneous tumors with orbital invasion.

Lacrimal gland malignancies.

Extensive conjunctival malignancies.

Other orbital malignancies:

Mucormycosis.

Chronic orbital pain.

Orbital deformities.

5. a Endophthalmitis is a true ophthalmic emergency and mandates prompt therapy if visual acuity is to be preserved.

Empirical Medical Therapy for Endophthalmitis:

Acute onset postcataract extraction (as used by Endophthalmitis Vitrectomy Study).

Intravitreal:

Vancomycin hydrochloride 1.0 mg in 0.1 mL (normal saline) and Ceftazidime 2.25 mg in 0.1 mL (normal saline) or Amikacin 200–400 μg in 0.1 mL (normal saline)

Dexamethasone 400 μg in 0.1 mL (optional)

Subconjunctival:

Vancomycin hydrochloride 25 mg in 0.5 mL (normal saline) and Ceftazidime 100 mg in 0.5 mL (normal saline) or amikacin 25 mg in 0.5 mL (normal saline) if β-lactam allergy exists and Dexamethasone 6 mg in 0.25 mL (normal saline).

Topical:

Vancomycin hydrochloride 50 mg/mL and Amikacin 20 mg/mL and

Atropine sulfate 1% or scopolamine hydrobromide 0.25% and

Prednisolone acetate 1%

IMAGE-BASED QUESTIONS

1. Most common cause of leukocoria:

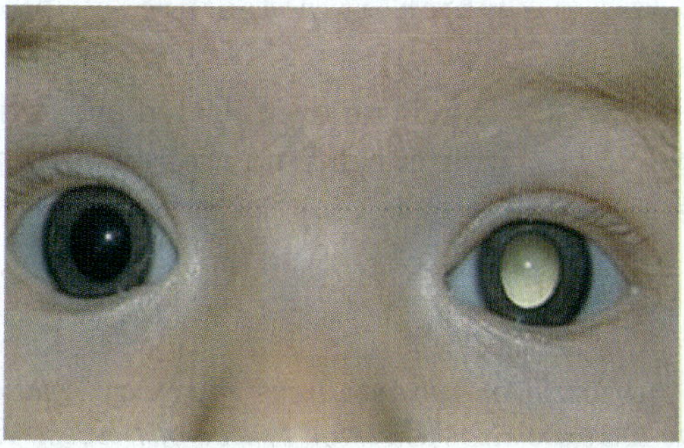

A. Retinoblastoma

B. Cyclitic membrane

C. Congenital cataract

D. Fungal endophthalmitis

2. In the following patient, prosthetic eye is put after:

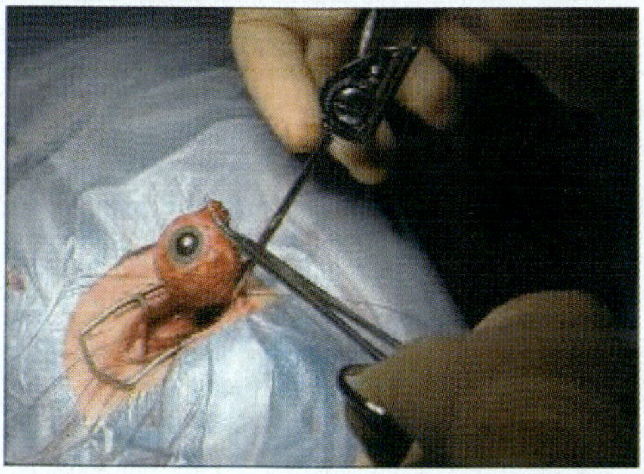

A. 2–3 weeks B. 1–3 weeks

C. 4–8 weeks D. 6–8 weeks

3. The diagnosis is:

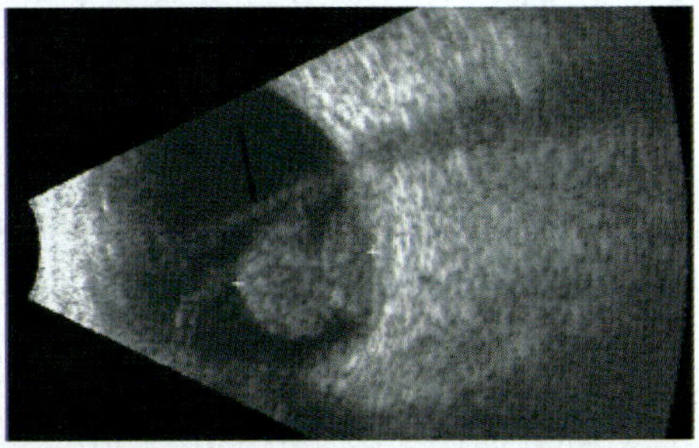

A. Retinoblastoma

B. Choroidal melanoma

C. Astrocytoma

D. Vitreous haemorrhage

4. The diagnosis is:

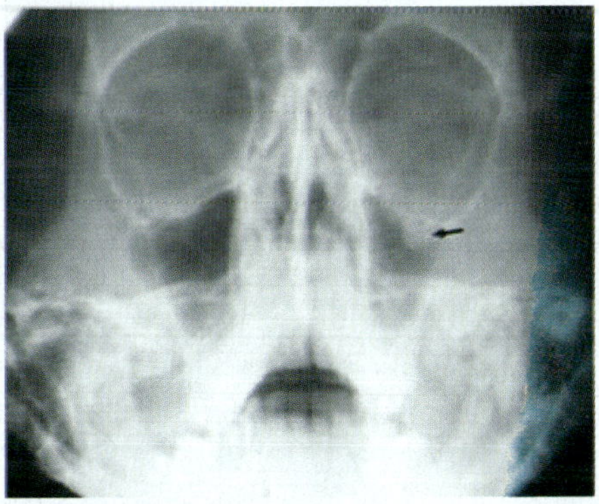

A. Maxillary tumour

B. Blow-out fracture

C. Maxillary sinusitis

D. Ethmoidal sinusitis

5. The diagnosis is:

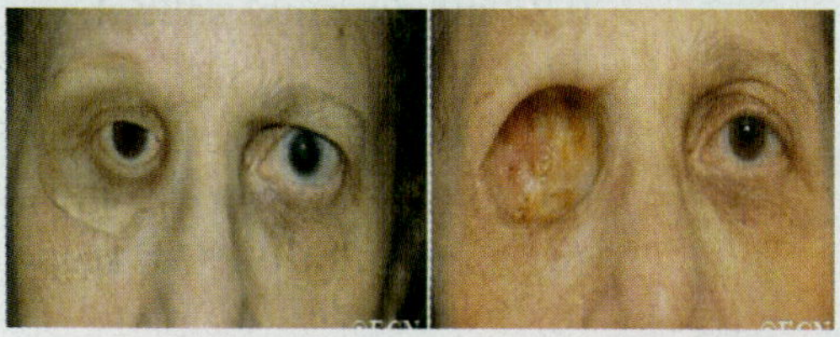

A. Enucleation

B. Evisceration

C. Exenteration

D. Congenital anomaly

ANSWERS OF IMAGE-BASED QUESTIONS

1. c The above slide shows white eye reflex also called leukocoria, and the most common cause is congenital cataract.
2. d The prosthetic eye is placed after complete healing after surgery, i.e., after 6–8 weeks.
3. b The above is a slide of USG B scan showing 'collar-button' appearance which is diagnostic of choroidal melanoma.
4. b The above slide shows 'tear-drop sign' which is a feature of blow-out fractures.
5. c This is an exenterated eye, where all orbital contents are removed, periosteum is removed and lids are cut.

GUIDANCE

NEVER BE SHAKEN, no matter what happens or what others may say. Never be flustered, never lose confidence. This is the way we should strive to live our lives. Being able to do so is a sign of genuine character.

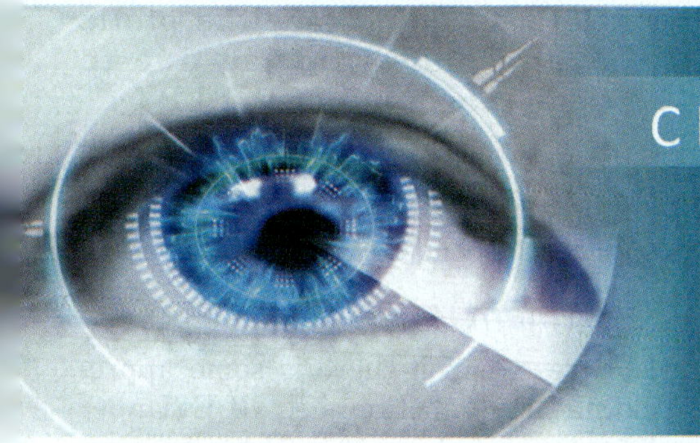

CHAPTER 8

Ocular Adenexae

ANATOMY

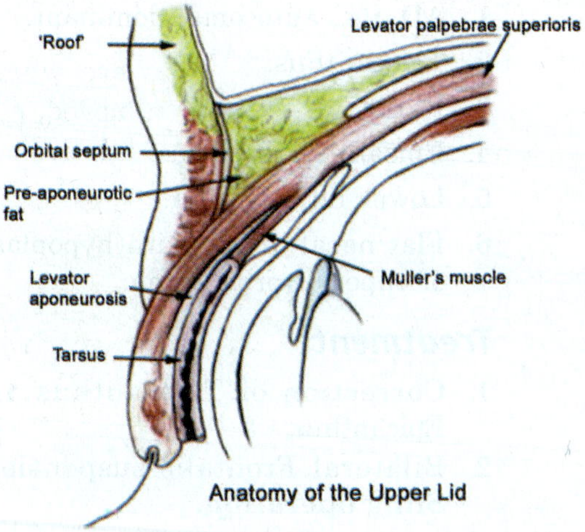

Fig. 8.1

The structure of eye lid margin

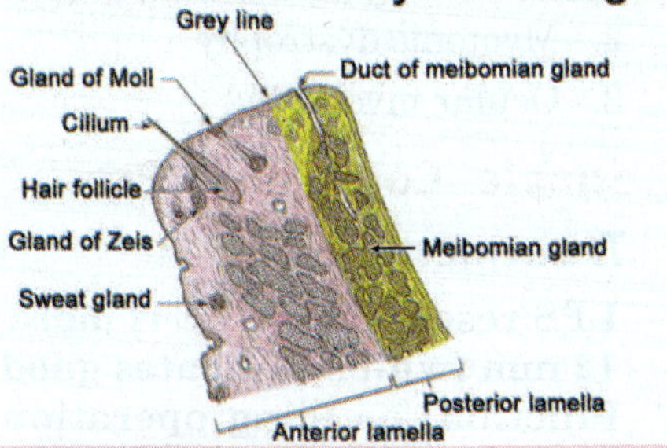

- The gray line divides eye lid margin into anterior and posterior part.
- Eye lashes, moll and zeis glands orifices takes place at the front part.
- Meibomian gland orifices are placed behind the gray line.

Fig. 8.2

Ptosis: It is the drooping of upper eyelid in relation to the globe.

Causes

a. Neurogenic.
b. Aponeurotic.
c. Mechanical.
d. Myogenic.

A. Neurogenic Ptosis (Acquired or Congenital)

1. Third nerve palsy.
2. Horner's syndrome (due to lesion of the sympathetic chain).
3. Marcus-Gunn jaw-winking syndrome.
4. Misdirection of third nerve: It occurs due to aberrant regeneration of the nerve due to surgical palsy.

Marcus-Gunn Jaw-Winking Syndrome

- It occurs due to nuclear or infranuclear connection between 3rd and 5th nerve.
- There is retraction of ptotic lid with stimulation of ipsilateral pterygoid muscle.

Treatment:

1. Levator resection for third nerve pals, if the function of LPS is appreciable.

2. Levator disinsertion (excision) combined with sling operation in case of Marcus-Gunn Jaw-Winking phenomenon.
3. Fasanella Servat operation for Horner's syndrome.

B. Aponeurotic Ptosis

There is localized dehiscence, disinsertion of aponeurosis or generalised attenuation or stretching.

- **Involutional or Senile ptosis:** It is an aponeurotic ptosis.

Treatment:

Mild case is treated by **Fasanella-Servat operation and severe cases require aponeurosis strengthening procedure.**

- **Post operative ptosis:** It is due to disinsertion or dehiscence of levator aponeurosis by manipulative trauma.

Treatment:

Fasanella-Servat operation.

C. Mechanical Ptosis

1. Scarring of upper palpebral conjunctiva.
2. Increased weight on the upper lid due to tumor, oedema, dermatochalasia.

Treatment:

Depends upon the cause.

D. Myogenic Ptosis

a. *Congenital:*
   1. Simple.
   2. Blepharophimosis syndrome.

Simple Congenital Ptosis

C/F:

- It occurs due to developmental dystrophy of levator muscle.
- It may be Unilateral or Bilateral.
- **Note: In down gaze the ptotic eyelid shows lid lag due to poor relaxation of the LPS.**
- It may be associated with weak-ness of SR muscle.
- There is head tilt with chin elevation.

Treatment:

LPS resection if there is some appreciable LPS function, i.e., ULE (Upper lid excursion) is more than 12 mm, otherwise Sling operation is done.

Blepharophimosis Syndrome

1. AD, i.e., autosomal dominant.
2. Telecanthus.
3. Ptosis.
4. Epicanthus inversus.
5. Lower lid ectropion.
6. Flat nasal bridge with hypoplasia of superior orbital rim.

Treatment:

1. Correction of Telecanthus and Epicanthus.
2. Bilateral Frontalis suspension–**Sling operation.**

b. *Acquired:*
   1. Myasthenia gravis.
   2. Myotonic dystrophy.
   3. Ocular myopathy.

Simple Congenital Ptosis

Treatment:

LPS resection if ULE is more than 12 mm (which indicates good LPS function) or Sling operation.

Measurements in Ptosis

1. **MRD: Marginal reflex distance:** Between upper lid margin and light reflex in primary gaze.

   Normal: 4–4.5 mm.

2. **Vertical fissure height:**
   Males: 7–10 mm.
   Females: 8–12 mm.
3. **ULE: Upper lid excursion:**
   Normal: 12 mm or more.
4. **Upper lid crease:**
   - Females: 10 mm.
   - Males: 8 mm.

SURGICAL PROCEDURES

1. **Fasanella: Servat Procedure**

   Excision of upper border of tarsus together with lower border of Muller's muscle and overlying conjunctiva.

   Indications:

   a. Horner's syndrome.

   b. Mild post-operative ptosis, not associated with a significant aponeurotic defect.

   c. Mild congenital myogenic ptosis, with good levator function.

2. **Levator Resection:**

   a. *Blaskovics operation:* Conjunctival route.

   b. *Everbusch's:* Cutaneous route.

3. **Frontalis Brow Suspension:** Sling operation **(Material of choice is fascia lata).**
4. **Aponeurosis strengthening:** It is done in case of aponeurotic ptosis.

Entropion

Inversion of eyelid margin is known as entropion.

Four main types are:

1. **Involutional:** It occurs due to old age. It **affects only lower lids.**

   It occurs due to:

   a. Over-riding of pre-septal over pretarsal part of orbicularis muscle during eyelid closure.

   b. Thinning and atrophy of tarsus and canthal tendons leading to horizontal lid laxity.

   c. Weakness of lower lid retractors.

2. **Cicatrical:** It occurs in cases of Cicatrical pemphigoid, Stevens-Johnson syndrome, Trachoma, Chemical burns.
3. **Congenital:** It occurs in cases where, lower eyelid retractors are not well developed.
4. **Acute spastic entropion:** It affects the lower lid.

Treatment

Involutional Entropion:

1. Cautery.
2. Transverse lid-everting sutures.
3. *Fox procedures:* Excision of base down triangle of conjunctiva and tarsal plate.
4. Shortening of lower lid retractors–*Lester-Jones operation.*
5. *Modified Wheelers operation:* Preseptal orbicularis bracing.
6. *Weis Procedure:* Full thickness horizontal splitting with marginal rotation.

Cicatrical Entropion:

1. Epilation.
2. Surgical correction of deformity.
3. Tarsal fracture.
4. Mucus membrane grafts.

Congenital Entropion:

1. Taping.
2. Lid everting sutures.
3. Injection of 1 ml of 80% alchohol s/c along edge of lid.
4. Painting collondion on skin.

Ectropion

Outward turning of eyelid margin is known as ectropion.

Four main types are:

1. Involutional.
2. Cicatrical.
3. Congenital.
4. Paralytic.

Involutional Ectropion:

- **Affects only lower lid.**
- **Treatment:**

  a. *Medial Ectropion*

     1. Ziegler cautery punctures.
     2. Medial conjunctivoplasty.
     3. Lazy-T procedure.

  b. *Extensive Ectropion*

     1. *Bick procedure.*
     2. *Modified Kuhnt-Szymanowski procedure.*

Cicatrical Ectropion:

- Due to tumor, trauma, burns.
- **Treatment:** Excision of scar with Z-plasty, transposition flaps, or free skin grafts.

Congenital Ectropion:

- Associated with Blepharophimosis syndrome.
- Affects lower lid.
- **Treatment:** Replacement of vertical skin defect with full-thickness skin graft.

Paralytic Ectropion:

- Due to facial nerve palsy.
- **Treatment:**

  a. Temporary Treatment

  1. Artificial tears, ointment and strapping of lids during night.
  2. If very poor Bells phenomenon, then treatment of choice is – Tarsorrhaphy, to prevent exposure keratitis.

  b. Permanent Treatment

  1. Medial canthoplasty.
  2. Graded levator recession.
  3. Prosthetic devices–Silicone rings.

External Hordeolum (Stye)

Stye is a small abscess caused by an acute staphylococcal infection of a lash follicle and its associated gland of Zeis or Moll.

C/F: It presents as a painful swelling on the lid margin.

Treatment:

1. Hot fomentation.
2. Oral anti-inflammatory.
3. Epilation of the affected lash.

Internum Hordeolum

It is a small abscess caused by an acute staphylococcal infection of Meibomian gland.

C/F: It presents as a painful swelling of the lid on the tarsal plate. It is more painful than a stye.

Treatment:

1. Hot fomentation.
2. Oral anti-inflammatory.
3. Oral antibiotics.

Chalazion (Meibomian Cyst)

It is a chronic inflammatory lesion caused by blockage of meibomian gland orifices and stagnation of sebaceous secretions.

C/F: It presents as a painless swelling on the lid. If multiple, it can lead to mechanical ptosis. Sebaceous cell carcinoma can present as a recurrent chalazion.

Treatment:

1. Incision and drainage.
2. Intralesional injections of Triamcilone acetate.

Madarosis

Loss of eyelashes or loss of eyebrows, both are termed as *madarosis.*

Loss of eyebrows occur due to leprosy and myxoedema.

Causes:

a. *Local:*

   1. Anterior lid margin disease: Blepharitis, Trachoma, S.J. syndrome.
   2. Infiltrating tumors.
   3. Burns.
   4. Radiotherapy or Cryotherapy of lid tumors.

b. *Skin:*

   1. Psoriasis.
   2. Generalized alopecia.

c. *Systemic:*

   1. Myxoedema.
   2. Leprosy.
   3. Syphilis.
   4. SLE.

d. *Following Removal:*

   1. Iatrogenic trichiasis.
   2. Trichotillomania.

Poliosis

Whitening of eye lashes is known as poliosis.

Causes:

a. *Local:*

   1. Chronic blepharitis.
   2. Sympathetic uveitis.

b. *Systemic:*

   1. VKH syndrome.
   2. Waardenburg's syndrome.

Chronic Blepharitis

It is an inflammation of the lid margin.

The two main types of chronic blepharitis are:

1. **Anterior**
   – Staphylococcal.
   – Seborrhoeic.
2. **Posterior, i.e., meibomitis.**

Staphylococcal Anterior Blepharitis

It is caused by chronic infection of the base of the lashes which results in formation of tiny intrafollicular abscesses. This leads to secondary dermal and epidermal ulceration.

Clinical Features:

1. Burning.
2. Foreign body sensation.
3. Mild photophobia.
4. Lid crusting.

On Examination: Hard brittle scales which leave behind bleeding ulcers when removed.

Complications:

1. Trichiasis, i.e., misdirection of eyelashes.
2. Madarosis.
3. **Poliosis,** i.e., graying of the eyelashes and **Tylosis,** i.e., thickening of the eyelid margin.
4. Scarred, notched and hypertrophic anterior lid margin.
5. External and internal hordeolum.
6. Recurrent attacks of acute bacterial conjunctivitis.

7. Secondary changes due to hypersensitivity to staphylococcal exotoxins are:
   a. Mild papillary conjunctivitis.
   b. Toxic punctate epitheliopathy.
   c. Marginal keratitis.
   d. Phlyctenulosis.
   e. Tear film instability.

Treatment:

1. Lid hygiene.
2. Antibiotic ointment.
3. Weak topical steroids for secondary changes in conjunctivitis.
4. Artificial tears.

Seborrhoeic Anterior Blepharitis

It is a disorder of glands of Zeis and Moll and is frequently associated with seborrhoeic dermatitis.

Two main forms are:

1. **The oily type:** Scaly eruptions are greesy.
2. **The dry type:** It is due to pityriasis capitis or dandruff.

C/F: Similar to staphylococcal blepharitis but less severe.

O/E: Soft scales, which **do not** leave a small ulcer when removed.

Complications are less frequent compared to staphylococcal blepharitis.

Treatment:

1. Antibiotic-steroid combination ointment.
2. Antibiotic-steroid combination drops for secondary changes in the conjunctiva.
3. Artificial tears.

Posterior Blepharitis

It is caused by dysfunction of the Meibomian glands.

Three main types are:

a. Meibomian seborrhoea.
b. Primary meibomitis.
c. Meibomitis with secondary blepharitis.

Clinical Features:

1. Copious secretions at the opening of the meibomian glands leading to very oily tear film.
2. In primary meibomitis there is diffuse inflammation at the orifice. These patients have associated acne rosacea and seborrhoeic dermatitis.
3. It is associated with papillary conjunctivitis and inferior punctate epitheliopathy.

Treatment:

Oral antibiotics are the mainstay of the therapy. It acts by inhibiting the production of bacterial lipase and free fatty acids. Tetracycline, Doxycycline and rarely erythromycin are given.

Other Measures:

1. Warm compresses to soften the solid secretions.
2. Lid hygiene.
3. Topical steroids.
4. Topical lubricating eye drops.

Ankyloblepharon

It denotes adhesions between the margins of upper and lower lid.

Etiology:

1. Chemical burns.
2. Thermal burns.
3. Ulcers.
4. Trauma.

Treatment:

Lids are separated by excision of adhesions between the lid margin and keeping them apart during the healing process.

Symblepharon

It denotes adhesions between the lids and palpebral conjunctiva, hence the lids become adherent with the eyeball.

Etiology:

1. Chemical burns.
2. Thermal burns.
3. Membranous conjunctivitis.
4. Injuries.
5. Ocular pemphigoid.
6. Stevens-Johnson syndrome.

Types: It is of three types:

1. *Anterior symblepharon:* When adhesions are present only in the anterior part.
2. *Posterior symblepharon:* When the adhesions are present in the fornix.
3. *Total symblepharon:* When the whole lid is involved.

Clinical Features:

1. Difficulty in lid movement.
2. Diplopia due to restricted ocular motility.
3. Lagophthalmos, i.e., inability to close the lids.
4. Cosmetic disfigurement.

Complications:

1. Dryness and thickening of the conjunctiva.
2. Corneal ulcerations.

Treatment:

Symblepharectomy with buccal mucosal graft.

Malignant Eyelid Tumors

a. **Basal cell carcinoma–Most common.**
b. Squamous cell carcinoma.
c. Sebaceous cell carcinoma.
d. Malignant melanoma.
e. Kaposis sarcoma.

Basal Cell Carcinoma: BCC is most common malignant eyelid tumour accounting for 90% of all cases. It most frequently arises from lower eyelid, followed in relative frequency by medial canthus, upper eyelid and lateral canthus. It is locally invasive.

Clinical Types:

1. Nodular.
2. Ulcerative.
3. Sclerosing.

Treatment:

a. **Small BCC**–*Local excision* of tumour together with 3 mm margin.
b. **Large BCC**–*Radical surgical excision.*
c. **Role of radiotherapy:**
   1. For small noduloulcerative BCC.
   2. BCCs which do not involve the medial canthal area.
   3. In patients who are either unsuitable for/or refuse surgery.
d. **Role of cryotherapy:** It is effective for small and superficial BCCs.
e. **Chemotherapy:** I/V cisplatin may be useful.
   i. In reducing the size of very large and advanced BCC before local excision.
   ii. For patients refusing exenteration.

Sebaceous Cell Carcinoma:

- Mostly affects elderly.
- Usually arises from meibomian glands. May arise from gland of Zeis; or sebaceous gland in the caruncle and the eyebrows.
- **May be misdiagnosed as recurrent chalazion or recurrent chronic blepharitis.**
- Metastasis occurs in: Regional lymph nodes, lungs, liver and brain.
- Two main types are:
  a. Nodular.
  b. Spreading.

NEET DRILL

1. Stye is an inflammation of hair follicle, sebaceous gland (gland of Zeis) and gland of moll (sweat gland).
2. Chalazion is a lipogranulomatous inflammation of the meibomian gland.
3. Recurrent chalazion should be checked for sebaceous cell carcinoma.
4. Most common malignant tumour of the lid is basal cell carcinoma.
5. Tylosis is thickening of the lid margin.
6. Poliosis is graying of the eyelashes.
7. Madarosis is loss of eyelashes or loss of eyebrows.
8. Vertical fissure height: It is the distance between upper and lower lid margins:

   Males: 7–10 mm.

   Females: 8–12 mm.
9. ULE, i.e., Upper Lid Excursion reflects levator function. It is graded as:

   Good: 12 mm or more.

   Fair: 6–11 mm; and

   Poor: 5 mm or less.
10. Frequency of blinking is 12–20 times per min.
11. Upper Lid Crease: It is the vertical distance between the lid margin and the lid crease in downgaze,

    In males: 8 mm.

    In females: 10 mm.
12. Most common site of sebaceous cell carcinoma is upper lid.
13. Wheelers operation is done for entropion.
14. Most common type of Ptosis is Aponeurotic.
15. Telecanthus is far apart medial canthus due to long canthal ligament, hence IPD (inter pupillary distance) is normal.
16. Hyperteleorism is far apart medial canthus due to bony defect, hence IPD is more.
17. The ideal material to do sling operation is fascia lata.
18. Hordeolum internum is acute inflammation of meibomian glands whereas Hordeolum externum is acute inflammation of hair follicle, gland of Zeis and gland of Moll.

MULTIPLE CHOICE QUESTIONS

1. Fasanella-Servat operation is specifically indicated in:

A. Congenital ptosis
B. Steroid-induced ptosis
C. Myasthenia gravis
D. Horner's syndrome

2. The operation of plication of inferior lid retractors is indicated in:

A. Senile ectropion
B. Senile entropion
C. Cicatrical entropion
D. Paralytic entropion

3. Ptosis with weakness of orbicularis – oculi is seen in:

A. Polymyositis
B. Myasthenia gravis
C. Eaton-Lambert syndrome
D. Thyrotoxicosis

4. A recurrent chalazion should be subjected to histopathological examination to exclude possibility of:

A. Squamous cell carcinoma

B. Sebaceous cell carcinoma

C. Malignant melanoma

D. Basal cell carcinoma

5. Ptosis occurs due to:

A. Facial nerve palsy

B. Oculomotor palsy

C. Trigeminal palsy

D. Trochlear palsy

6. Which of the following muscles is involved in ptosis?

A. Lateral rectus

B. Levator palpebrae superioris

C. Muller's muscle

D. Orbicularis oculi

7. Treatment of chalazion is:

A. Hot fomentation

B. Incision and curettage

C. Antibiotics

D. Diathermy

E. Injection of steroids

8. Chalazion is/are:

A. True meibomian cyst

B. Mucus cyst

C. Sebaceous cyst

D. Cyst of hair follicle

E. Obstruction of meibomian gland

9. Lid lag on ptotic side is caused by:

A. Neurogenic ptosis

B. Myogenic ptosis

C. Metabolic ptosis

D. Traumatic ptosis

10. Madarosis is seen in:

A. T.B.

B. Diabetes mellitus

C. Leprosy

D. Waardenburg syndrome

11. Most common malignant tumour of eyelid is:

A. Squamous cell carcinoma

B. Basal cell carcinoma

C. Malignant melanoma

D. Sebaceous cell carcinoma

12. Hordeolum internum is:

A. Acute on chronic suppuration of Meibomian glands

B. Acute suppuration of Molls gland

C. Chronic granulation of tarsal glands

D. Chronic granulation of Zeis' glands

13. Tylosis is:

A. Thickening of eyelid with ptosis

B. Thickening of eyelid margin

C. Ptosis

D. Enophthalmos

14. von-Graefe's sign:

A. Lid retraction

B. Lid lag

C. Staring look

D. Absence of convergence

15. Modified sweat glands:

A. Henle's glands

B. Zeis' glands

C. Meibomian glands

D. Moll glands

16. Painful lid margin is seen in:

A. Stye

B. Hordeolum internum

C. Eczema

D. Basal cell carcinoma

17. The most common fungal lesion of the eyelid is:
A. Candida
B. Aspergillosis
C. Sporothrix
D. Fusarium

18. Blaskovics operation is done for:
A. Proptosis
B. Ptosis
C. Lagophthalmos
D. Entropion

19. Wheelers operation is done in:
A. Ectropion B. Entropion
C. Ptosis D. None of the above

20. Sling operation should be avoided in cases of ptosis with:
A. Very poor levator function
B. Poor Bells phenomenon
C. Weak Muller's muscle
D. Multiple failed surgeries

21. All are complications of chronic staphylococcal blepharoconjunctivitis except:
A. Chalazion
B. Marginal conjunctivitis
C. Follicular conjunctivitis
D. Phlyctenular conjunctivitis

22. Which of the following is false?
A. External hordeolum is an acute inflammation of the Zeis' gland
B. Internal hordeolum is an acute inflammation of the Zeis' gland
C. Internal hordeolum is an acute suppurative inflammation of meibomian gland
D. Chalazion is a chronic granulomatous inflammation of the meibomian gland

23. A 2-year-old child is found to have ptosis of one eye with defective elevation of the eye. Opening the mouth causes elevation of the ptotic lid. The most likely clinical condition is:
A. Partial 3 nerve palsy
B. Congenital ptosis
C. Ocular myasthenia
D. Congenital ptosis with Marcus-Gunn phenomenon

24. Lid separation of fetus in intrauterine life occurs at which month?
A. 2 weeks B. 2 months
C. 6 months D. 7 months

25. Coloboma of the lid is most common in:
A. Lateral half of lower lid
B. Medial half of lower lid
C. Lateral half of upper lid
D. Medial half of upper lid

26. Adhesion of margins of two eyelid is called:
A. Symblepharon
B. Ankyloblepharon
C. Blepharophimosis
D. Blepharophimosis

27. Burrows operation is done for:
A. Ectropion
B. Entropion
C. Megalocornea
D. Nystagmus
E. Epibulbar dermoids

28. Muscle in the lid attached to posterior tarsal margin is:
A. Levator palpebrae
B. Superior oblique

C. Muller's muscle

D. Orbicularis oculi

29. Most common malignant tumor of eyelid:

A. Squamous cell carcinoma

B. Basal cell carcinoma

C. Malignant melanoma

D. Sebaceous cell carcinoma

30. A malignant tumour of eyelid is:

A. Cavernous hemangioma

B. Kaposi's sarcoma

C. Plexiform neuroma

D. Xanthoma

31. A 35-year-old female presents with recurrent chalazion of the upper eyelid. The curettage should be subjected to histopathological examination to rule out which of the following?

A. Sebaceous cell carcinoma

B. Squamous cell carcinoma

C. Basal cell carcinoma

D. Malignant melanoma

32. An elderly female presents with recurrent swelling of the upper eyelid. Further examination revealed it to be a chalazion. What would be the most likely histopathological finding?

A. Lipogranuloma

B. Suppurative granuloma

C. Foreign body granuloma

D. Xanthogranuloma

33. Lipogranulomatous inflammation is seen in:

A. Fungal infection

B. Tuberculosis

C. Chalazion

D. Viral infection

34. The operation for plication of lower lid retractors is done for:

A. Senile ectropion

B. Senile entropion

C. Cicatrial entropion

D. Paralytic entropion

35. Chalazion all are true except:

A. Vertical incision given to squeeze out contents

B. Horizontal incision to be made to squeeze out content

C. Incision and curettage done

D. It's a granulomatous condition

ANSWER AND EXPLANATION

1.	d	In Fasanella Servat operation, Muller's muscle is excised along with small part of conjunctiva and tarsal plate.
2.	b	Entropion is inward turning of the lid margin.
3.	b	Myasthenia gravis is a myopathy and involves both LPS and Orbicularis oculi.
4.	b	Meibomian gland is a sebaceous gland.
5.	b	LPS is supplied by the third nerve.
6.	b,c	Both LPS and Muller's muscles are the elevators of the upper eyelid.
7.	b,e	Chalazion is treated by intralesional injection of triamcilone acetate, or by incision and curettage.
8.	a,c,e	Chalazion is a chronic lipogranulomatous inflammation of the meibomian gland.

9. b It is a characteristic of congenital ptosis where LPS is not formed properly and hence there is both defective contraction and relaxation of the LPS.
10. c Madarosis term is used for both loss of eyebrows and eyelashes.
11. b Most common site of BCC is lower lid and then inner canthus.
12. a Hordeolum internum is an acute inflammation of the meibomian gland.
13. b Tylosis is a complication of chronic blepharitis.
14. b It is a feature of thyroid ophthalmopathy and occurs due to overaction of LPS.
15. d Gland of Moll is inflamed in patients of stye.
16. a Hordeolum externum, i.e., stye is a painful swelling on the anterior lid margin whereas Hordeolum internum is a painful swelling of the lid.
17. a Most common fungal infection of the lid is by candida albicans and dermatophytes.
18. b It is a method of LPS resection through conjunctival route.
19. b It is a treatment of involutional entropion.
20. b Poor Bell's phenomenon can cause exposure keratopathy, if ptosis is treated.
21. a Chalazion is not a staphylococcal infection.
22. b Acute inflammation of the Zeis' gland is Hordeolum externum.
23. d It occurs due to abnormal connection between the lateral Pterygoid muscle and LPS.
24. d Lids are formed by reduplication of the surface ectoderm during second month of gestation, these folds enlarge and their margins fuse. The final separation of the lids occurs by seventh month.
25. d Coloboma is absence of the part due to failure of formation in embryonic development.
26. b Symblepharon is adhesion of the palpebral conjunctiva with bulbar conjunctiva.
27. b Burrows operation is done for treatment of cicatrical entropion. In this procedure, a linear incision is made passing through conjunctiva, tarsal plate but not the skin along the sulcus subtarsalis.
28. c Muller's muscle is responsible for 2 mm elevation of the lower lid.
29. b Most common site of BCC is lower lid and that of sebaceous cell carcinoma is upper lid.
30. b Kaposi's sarcoma is a rare malignant tumour of the eyelid. Most common is BCC.
31. a Chalazion is a chronic lipogranulomatous inflammation of the meibomian gland which is a sebaceous gland, hence a recurrent lesion should be checked for sebaceous cell carcinoma.
32. a Chalazion is a chronic lipogranulomatous inflammation of the meibomian gland.
33. c Chalazion is a lipogranulomatous inflammation of meibomian glands and presents as a painless swelling on the lid.
34. b It is called Lester Jones operation.
35. b We avoid horizontal incision as it will damage the fibres of LPS.

RECENTLY ADDED QUESTIONS

1. **Identify the below finding:**

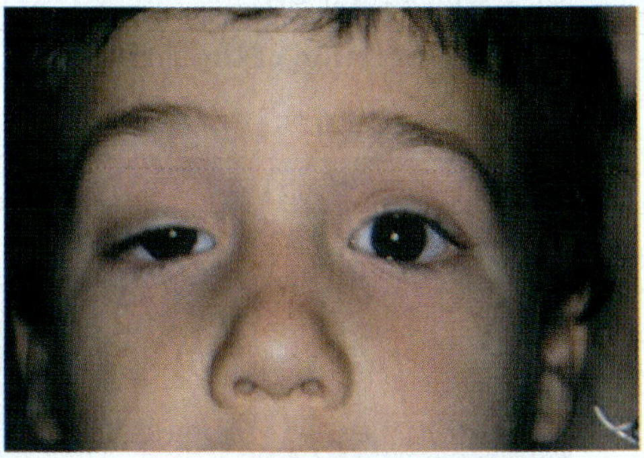

A. Ptosis of right eye
B. Entropion of right eye
C. Lagophthalmos right eye
D. Ectropion left eye

2. **True regarding tarsal plate is/are? (PGI)**

A. Acts a skeleton for eyelids
B. Wider in upper eyelids
C. Have meibomian glands
D. Attached to lateral palpebral superioris ligaments
E. Inferior plate is semilunar in shape

3. **Composition of upper eyelid includes? (PGI)**

A. Skin
B. Fat
C. Levator palpebrae superioris
D. Mueller's muscle
E. Orbicularis oris muscle

ANSWERS OF RECENTLY ADDED QUESTIONS

1.	a	Ptosis of right eye
2.	a,b,c,d	Tarsal plates are responsible for forming skeleton of the eyelids and are rich in meibomian glands. The superior tarsal plate is larger, wider and semilunar, while the inferior tarsal plate is smaller, thinner and elliptical in shape. LPS tendon is attached to the upper tarsal plate.
3.	a,b,c,d	Orbicularis oculi is present around the eyelid, not orbicularis oris.

IMAGE-BASED QUESTIONS

1. **The diagnosis is:**

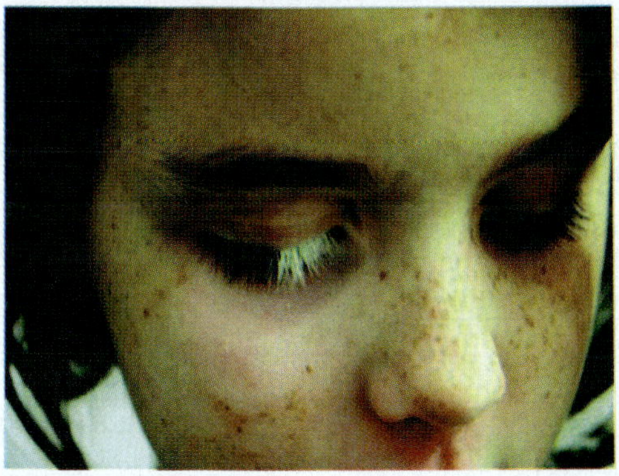

A. Tylosis
B. Poliosis
C. Trichiasis
D. Distichiasis

2. **The diagnosis is:**

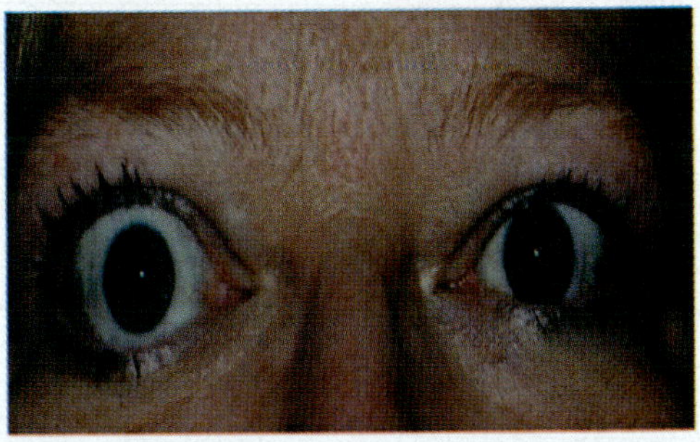

A. Stellwag sign B. Kochers sign
C. Von Graefe sign D. Dalrymple sign

3. The diagnosis is:

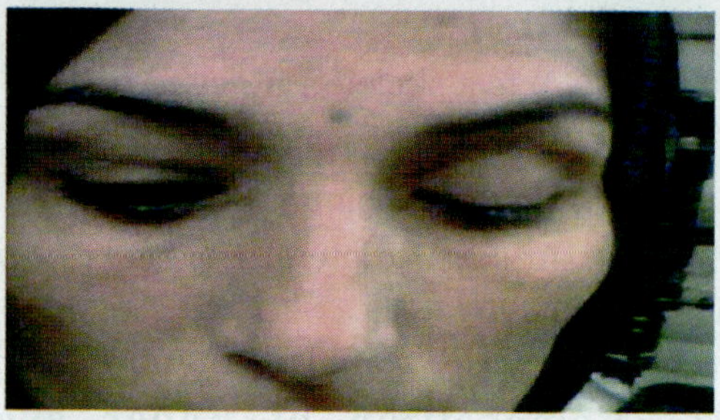

A. Lid lag B. Lid retraction
C. Ptosis D. Blepharospasm

4. The diagnosis is:

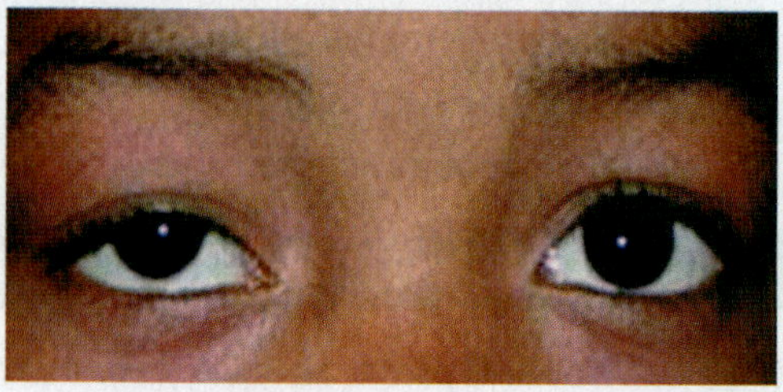

A. Ptosis of right eye
B. Lid retraction in the left eye
C. Ptosis of left eye
D. Lid retraction of the right eye

5. The diagnosis is:

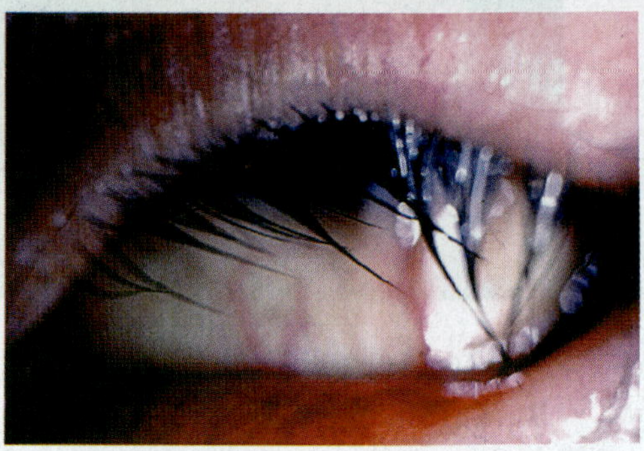

A. Trichiasis
B. Tylosis
C. Madarosis
D. Poliosis

ANSWERS OF IMAGE-BASED QUESTIONS

1. b The above slide is poliosis which is greying of eye lashes.
2. b The above slide shows staring look that is called kochers sign and occurs due to extreme lid retraction where upper sclera is also visible.
3. a The above slide shows lid lag of thyroid ophthalmopathy.
4. a The above slide shows normal lid position in left eye and ptosis in the right eye.
5. a The above slide shows trichiasis which is misdirection of eyelashes.

GUIDANCE

There is no need for you to be impatient. If you can achieve something very easily right from the start, you will find no sense of fulfilment or joy. It is in making tenacious all out efforts for construction, that profound happiness lies.

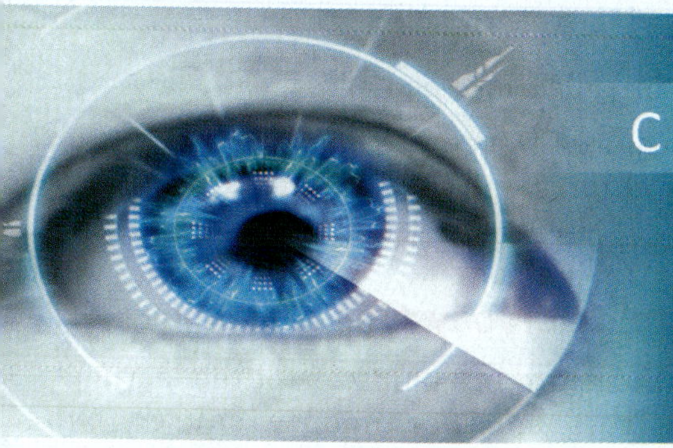

CHAPTER 9

Lacrimal Drainage System

ANATOMY

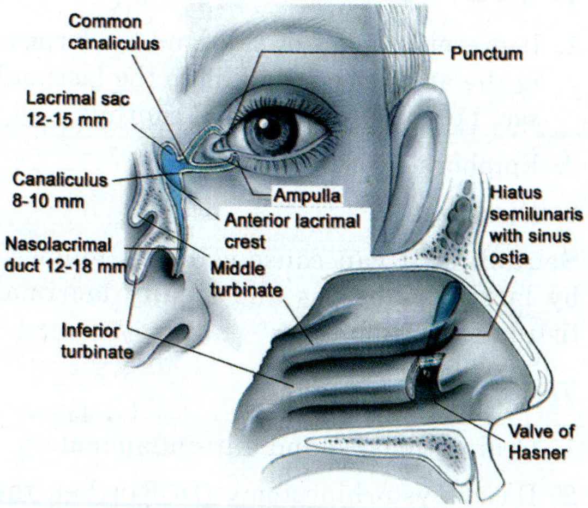

Fig. 9.1

Tearing or watering can be of two types:

1. Lacrimation.
2. Epiphora.

Epiphora: Abnormal overflow of tears due to obstruction of lacrimal drainage system is known as epiphora.

CAUSES OF EPIPHORA

1. **Anatomical**
   a. Strictures.
   b. Obstruction.
   c. F.B.
   d. Tumor.
2. **Physiological:**
   Lacrimal pump failure.

Obstruction may be at:

1. Lacrimal puncta.
2. Canaliculi.
3. Common canaliculi.
4. Lacrimal sac.
5. Nasolacrimal duct.

INVESTIGATIONS

1. **Syringing:** *Pressure syringing* is therapeutic in partial obstruction.
2. **Jones dye test:** It is indicated in patients with suspected partial obstruction of the drainage system. It has no value in total obstruction. It is divided into two parts: Primary and Secondary.

   Primary: It differentiates the partial obstruction from primary hypersecretion of tears. Fluorescein dye is instilled in the conjunctival sac and its presence checked in the inferior turbinate of nose with a cotton after 5 minutes. If positive the cause of watering is hypersecretion whereas if no dye seen then it indicates either partial obstruction or lacrimal pump failure.

Secondary: It is done when primary test is negative. In this test the drainage system is now irrigated using clear saline. If fluorescein stained saline is recovered then it indicates partial obstruction of the NLD and if unstained saline is recovered then, it is either a partial obstruction of upper drainage system (punctum, canaliculi or common canaliculi) or lacrimal pump failure.

3. **DCG-Dacryocystography:** It is a test in which contrast medium is injected into one of the canaliculi and posteroanterior and lateral radiographs are taken. This method demonstrates the exact location of the obstruction and helpful in the diagnosis of diverticula, fistulae and filling defects caused by stones or tumours. The dye used are Ethiodol and Pantopaque.
4. **Dacryoscintillography:** This involves the labeling of tears with a Gamma-emitting substance such as technetium-99M and monitoring their progress through drainage system by Gamma-camera. It helps to diagnose the functional defect in the lacrimal pathway.

INFECTIONS OF LACRIMAL PATHWAY

Chronic Canaliculitis

- By Actinomyces israeli (Streptothrix).
- Pouting punctum and concretions in canaliculi.

Treatment:

Removal of concretions by either simple curettage or by canaliculotomy followed by irrigation with penicillin solution. Topical and systemic tetracycline or erythromycin can also be given.

Dacryocystitis

It is the inflammation of the lacrimal sac.

Classification:

It is broadly classified as:

1. Acquired Dacryocystitis: It may be acute or chronic.
2. Congenital Dacryocystitis.

Acute Dacryocystitis

It is the acute inflammation of the lacrimal sac. It is most commonly caused by: Staphylococcus aureus.

Other organisms are: Streptococcus and Pneumococcus.

Clinical Features:

1. It presents as lot of pain and tenderness in the area corresponding to the lacrimal sac, i.e., below the medial canthus.
2. Epiphora.
3. Discharge.

Sequelae: It can cause cellulitis followed by lacrimal abscess and finally lacrimal fistula formation.

Treatment:

1. Oral antibiotics and anti-inflammatory.
2. Dacryocystorhinostomy (DCR) when the acute stage subsides. In DCR, an opening is made between lacrimal sac and **middle meatus** of the nose.

Chronic Dacryocystitis

- It is common in females (80%) between age 40 and 60 years.
- The causative organisms are: Staphylococci, Streptococci, Pneumococci, Pseudomonas pyocyanea. Rarely it is caused by T.B. Syphilis, Leprosy.

Clinical Features:

1. Epiphora with discharge.

2. **Encysted Mucocele:** It is a chronic condition due to tear collected into lacrimal sac causing permanent distension of lacrimal sac filled with mucous, called mucocele.

Sequelae: Chronic dacryocystitis can lead to mucocele formation which can further lead to pyocele formation (i.e., pus in the lacrimal sac) and finally there is fibrosis.

Treatment:

1. DCR, i.e., dacryocystorhinostomy if the obstruction is at the level of the NLD.
2. Canaliculocystorhinostomy if the obstruction is at the common canalicular level.
3. Conjunctivocystorhinostomy if the obstruction is more proximal.

Congenital Dacryocystitis

It is due to non-canalization of Nasolacrimal duct (NLD). Commonly this occlusion is membranous.

- In children, there can be *congenital dacryocele* where there is collection of amniotic fluid or mucus due to imperforate "valve of Hasner" (which is present at the end of the nasolacrimal duct). This condition presents as perinatal bluish cystic swelling below the medial canthus.

Clinical Features:

Epiphora and discharge, more commonly unilateral.

Treatment:

- Till 9 months–Antibiotics with massage (CRIGLERS MASSAGE).

  It increases the hydrostatic pressure of the nasolacrimal duct.
- 9 months to 4 years–Probing.
- 4 years onwards–DCR.

Crocodile Tears

It is a complication of VII nerve palsy, i.e., facial palsy. It is characterized by unilateral lacrimation with mastication and is due to faulty regeneration of parasympathetic fibres which now supply lacrimal gland instead of salivary glands.

Treatment:

Section of greater superficial pestrosal nerve or tympanic neurectomy.

NEET DRILL

1. NLD opens in inferior meatus of NOSE ANTERIORLY.
2. In DCR we make the opening in the middle meatus.
3. NLD is 18 mm in length.
4. The direction of NLD is downwards, backwards and laterally.
5. Most common cause of canaliculitis is actinomyces Israeli.
6. pH of tear is 7.4.
7. Average volume of the tear film is 7 microlitres.
8. Thickness of tear film after a blink is 9 microns and after 30 secs becomes 4 microns.
9. Average rate of tear secretion is 1.2 microlitres/minute.
10. Tear film has three layers:
    (a) Mucin layer: 0.02–0.05 microns.
    (b) Aqueous layer: 6.5–7.5 microns.
    (c) Lipid layer: 0.1 microns.
11. Most common feature of Rheumatoid Arthritis is KCS, i.e., Keratoconjunctivitis Sicca.
12. Most common etiological agent for both acute and chronic dacryocystitis is staphylococcus aureus.
13. Upper punctum is medial to lower punctum.
14. Tear production starts at 6 weeks.
15. Treatment of congenital dacryocystitis within 9 months is Criglers massage.
16. Chronic dacryocystitis is more common in females.

MULTIPLE CHOICE QUESTIONS

1. **A two months old child presents with epiphora and regurgitation. The most probable diagnosis is:**
   A. Mucopurulent conjunctivitis
   B. Buphthalmos
   C. Congenital dacryocystitis
   D. Encysted mucocele
2. **Epiphora is:**
   A. Cerebrospinal fluid running from the nose after fracture of anterior cranial fossa
   B. An epiphenomenons of a cerebral tumor
   C. An abnormal overflow of tears due to obstruction of lacrimal duct
   D. Eversion of lower eyelid following injury
3. **A 60-year-old man presented with watering from his left eye since one year. Syringing revealed a patent drainage system. Rest of ocular examination was normal. A provisional diagnosis of lacrimal pump failure was made. Confirmation of the diagnosis would be by:**
   A. Dacryoscintigraphy
   B. Dacryocystography
   C. Pressure syringing
   D. Canaliculus irrigation test
4. **Mucin layer deficiency occurs in:**
   A. Keratoconjunctivitis
   B. Lacrimal gland removal
   C. Canalicular block
   D. Herpetic keratitis
5. **Most common ocular finding in mumps is:**
   A. Chorioretinitis
   B. Anterior uveitis
   C. Haemorrhagic conjunctivitis
   D. Dacryocrystoadenitis
6. **Initial treatment of congenital dacryocystitis:**
   A. Massaging
   B. Probing
   C. Ointment
   D. DCR
   E. No treatment required
7. **Treatment of chronic dacryocystitis:**
   A. Dacryocystorhinostomy
   B. Antibiotics
   C. Probing
   D. Massage
8. **Crocodile tears are seen in:**
   A. Frey's syndrome
   B. Conjunctivitis
   C. Lacrimal tumour
   D. Abnormal VII nerve regeneration
9. **Most common cause of eye discharge in a 2 months old child is:**
   A. Ectropion
   B. Congenital nasolacrimal duct blockage
   C. Ophthalmia neonatorum
   D. Vernal catarrh
10. **Tears are produced in the newborn after:**
    A. 1 week B. 2 weeks
    C. 6 weeks D. 4 weeks
11. **In DCR the drainage is in:**
    A. Superior meatus
    B. Inferior meatus
    C. Middle meatus
    D. Superior fontanelle

12. Lacrimation is mediated by:

A. Greater petrosal nerve

B. Lesser petrosal nerve

C. Anterior ethmoidal nerve

D. Nasocilliary nerve

ANSWER AND EXPLANATION

1.	c	Epiphora is overflowing of the tears. Epiphora and regurgitation, both indicate that the child has dacryocystitis.
2.	c	Watering in the eyes is of two types: Lacrimation (increased production of the tears) and Epiphora (Overflowing of the tears).
3.	a	In dacryoscintillography, a radioactive dye is instilled in the tear and the path is followed by the gamma counter.
4.	d	KCS is deficiency of the aqueous layer of the tear film. Mucin layer deficiency occurs due to damage of the goblet cells which can occur in chronic infections.
5.	d	Most common ocular finding of measles is xerophthalmia.
6.	a	Treatment of dacryocystitis in a patient of less than 9 months: Massaging with antibiotic eye drops. Massaging increases the hydrostatic pressure of the NLD.
7.	a,b	Dacryocystorhinostomy is a procedure in which we make a fistula between the lacrimal sac and the middle meatus of nose.
8.	d	Crocodile tears are a complication of VII nerve palsy. It occurs due to faulty regeneration of parasympathetic fibres which now supply the lacrimal glands instead of salivary glands.
9.	b	Tear formation occurs at six weeks of age. Ophthalmia neonatorum will manifest within 1 week of birth.
10.	c	Tear production starts at 6 weeks.
11.	c	NLD opens in the inferior meatus of nose whereas in DCR we make the opening in the middle meatus.
12.	a	Lacrimation is mediated by: S – sup salivatory ganglion G – geniculate ganglion G – greater petrosal nerve P – pterygopalatine ganglion Z – zygomatic nerve

RECENTLY ADDED QUESTIONS

1. Phenol red thread test is used for dry eye. This test:

A. Requires topical anesthetic agent

B. Volume of tears is measured as it changes color on contact with tears

C. If the color changes to blue it depicts surface mucin deficiency

D. Requires pH meter for reading the result

2. NLD opens in the inferior meatus:

A. Anteriorly B. Posteriorly

C. Laterally D. Medially

3. Most common type of ptosis:

A. Aponeurotic

B. Mechanical

C. Neurogenic

D. Myogenic

ANSWERS OF RECENTLY ADDED QUESTIONS

1. b A cotton thread impregnated with phenol red dye is used. It is pH sensitive and changes from yellow to red when wetted by tears. The thread is placed on the lower conjunctival fornix for 15 seconds. Wetting of less than 9 mm is dry eye.
2. a NLD opens in inferior meatus anteriorly.
3. a Aponeurotic Ptosis occurs due to dehiscence of aponeurosis, which can be postoperative or involutional.

IMAGE-BASED QUESTIONS

1. The diagnosis is:

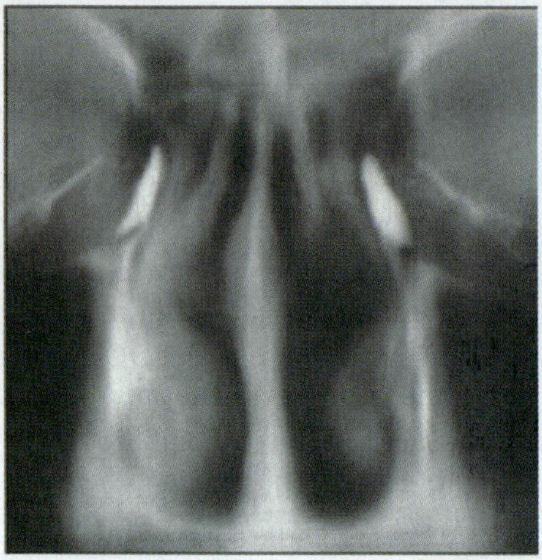

A. Chronic dacryocystitis
B. Lacrimal stone
C. Lacrimal tumour
D. Normal drainage system

2. The following slide indicates:

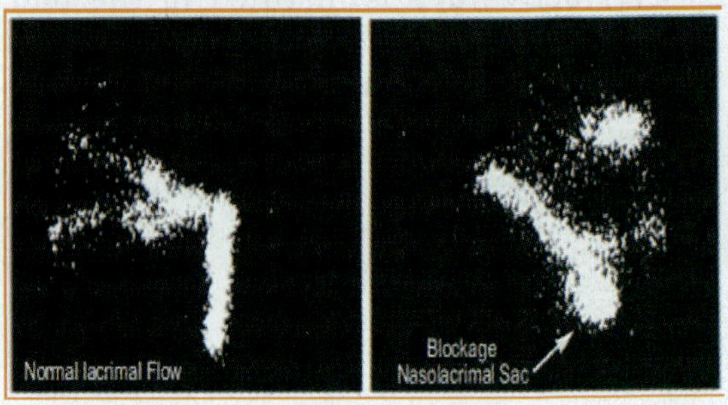

A. Dacryoscintillography
B. Dacryocystography
C. Syringing
D. Probing

ANSWERS OF IMAGE-BASED QUESTIONS

1. d The above slide shows normal lacrimal drainage system.
2. b It's a slide of dacryoscintillography where we use radioactive dye to study the lacrimal passage.

GUIDANCE

In all things, patience is the key to victory. Those who cannot endure cannot hope to win. Ultimate triumph belongs to those who can forbear.

CHAPTER 10

Neurophthalmology

ANATOMY

- The optic nerve is 3.5 cm to 5.5 cm long from optic disc to chiasma.
- It is divided into intraocular (1 mm), intraorbital (30 mm), intracanalicular (10 mm) and intracranial (6 mm) portions.
- **The longest part of the optic nerve is the intraorbital part and is 25 mm to 30 mm long.**

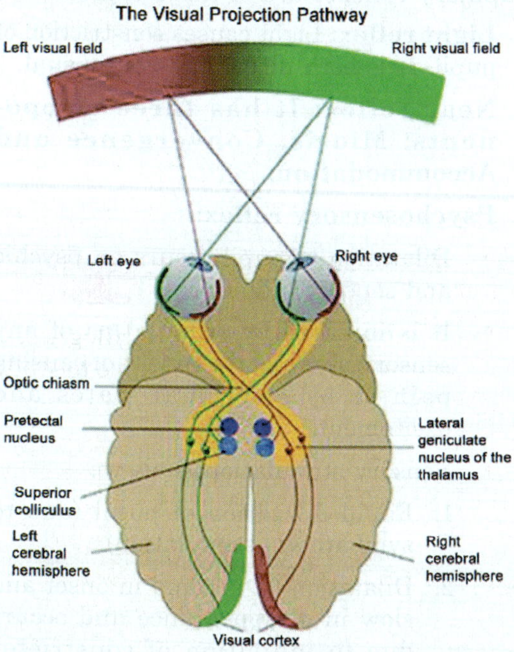

Fig. 10.1

Visual Field

The visual field has been defined as the island of vision in the sea of darkness.

Extent of Visual Field

In either eye, the field of vision is as follows:

Temporally—90°

Inferiorly—70°

Nasally—60°

Superiorly—50°

Maximum extent of peripheral visual field is temporally.

Perimetry: Visual field charting is known as perimetry.

The physiological scotoma of eye is the blind spot and is between 10° to 20° isopter. It is outlined by **Campimetry** [Central visual field assessment (on Bjerrums screen) is known as Campimetry].

Visual Pathway: It constitutes of optic nerve→optic chiasma→optic tract→lateral geniculate body→optic radiations→visual cortex.

Lateral Geniculate Body (LGB)

- LGB contains 6 well-defined layers. 1, 4, 6 receive input from contralateral eye whereas layers 2, 3 and 5 receive input from ipsilateral eye.

- In each layer of LGB there is point to point representation of the retina.
- Layers 1 and 2 of the LGB have large cells and are called. "*Magnocellular*" whereas 3–6 have small cells and are called "*Parvocellular*".
- **Magnocellular layer:**
  a. It receives input almost entirely from large gamma-Ganglion cells of the retina.
  b. It carries signals for detection of movement and flicker.
  c. It is colour blind and transmits only black and white information.
  d. Its point to point transmission is poor.
- **Parvocellular layer:**
  a. It receives input almost entirely from X-ganglion cells.
  b. It transmits colour vision. It also conveys very accurate point to point spatial information.
- **Functions of LGB:** It has two principal functions:
  1. *Relay station:* It relays visual information from the optic tract to the visual cortex by way of geniculocalcarine tract. The signals from the two eyes are kept apart in lateral geniculate body.
  2. *To gate the transmission of signals:* It gates the transmission of signals to the visual cortex, i.e., to control how much of the signals be allowed to pass to the cortex. It receives gating control signals from two major sources:
     i. Corticofugal fibres from the primary visual cortex.
     ii. The reticular area of mesencephalon.

Visual Cortex

The visual cortex is broadly divided into Primary visual cortex and Secondary visual cortex.

Primary Visual Cortex

1. It corresponds to Brodmann's area 17.
2. It is divided into six layers namely: 1 to 6. The fourth layer is the thickest and is further divided into a, b, c alpha, c beta. Maximum number of fibres from the optic radiations terminate into layer 4 of the visual cortex.

Secondary Visual Cortex

1. It corresponds to Brodmann's area 18 and 19.
2. It is also called Visual Association Areas.

Pathway for Colour Vision: Cones → Bipolar cells→Amacrine cells→Ganglion cell-**X cells**→Parvocellular layer of the Lateral geniculate body→Layer 4 c of the primary visual cortex→Secondary visual cortex→Fusiform and Lingual gyri.

NORMAL PUPILLARY REFLEXES

Pupillary reflexes are of three types:

1. **Light reflex:** Light causes constriction of pupil. It is both direct and consensual.
2. **Near reflex: It has three components: Miosis, Convergence and Accommodation.**
3. **Psychosensory reflex:**
   - Dilatation of pupil occurs on psychic and sensory stimuli.
   - It is initiated by stimulation of any sensory nerve to the extent of causing pain or by emotional states and excitement.
   - Sensory stimulation leads to:
     1. Rapid dilatation of pupil (due to sympathetic stimulation).
     2. Dilatation (It is rapid in onset and slow in disappearance and occurs due to inhibition of constrictor tone).

Light Reflex Pathway

It consists of 4 neurons:

From optic nerve
↓
Optic chiasma
↓
Optic tract
↓
Pretectal nucleus
↓
Edinger westphal nucleus of both sides (This bilateral supply is responsible for consensual reflex)
↓
Through inferior division of third nerve via, **the nerve to inferior oblique muscle**
↓
Ciliary ganglion
↓
Short ciliary nerves
↓
Sphincter pupillae

Hence as the fibres do not follow the optic tract till LGB but before that join the pretectal nucleus hence in lesions distal to this, light reflex will not be affected.

In unilateral afferent pupillary defect, when light is moved from normal to affected eye there will be dilatation of both pupils.

Near reflex pathway: It is almost the same as light reflex pathway, except that the impulse travels through the optic tract to some other nuclei ventral to the pretectal nucleus.

Third Nerve

The nuclear complex of the third (oculomotor) nerve is situated in the midbrain at the level of superior colliculus.

It is composed of:

1. Levator subnucleus—unpaired.
2. The superior rectus subnuclei—Paired and innervate **contralateral** subnucleus.

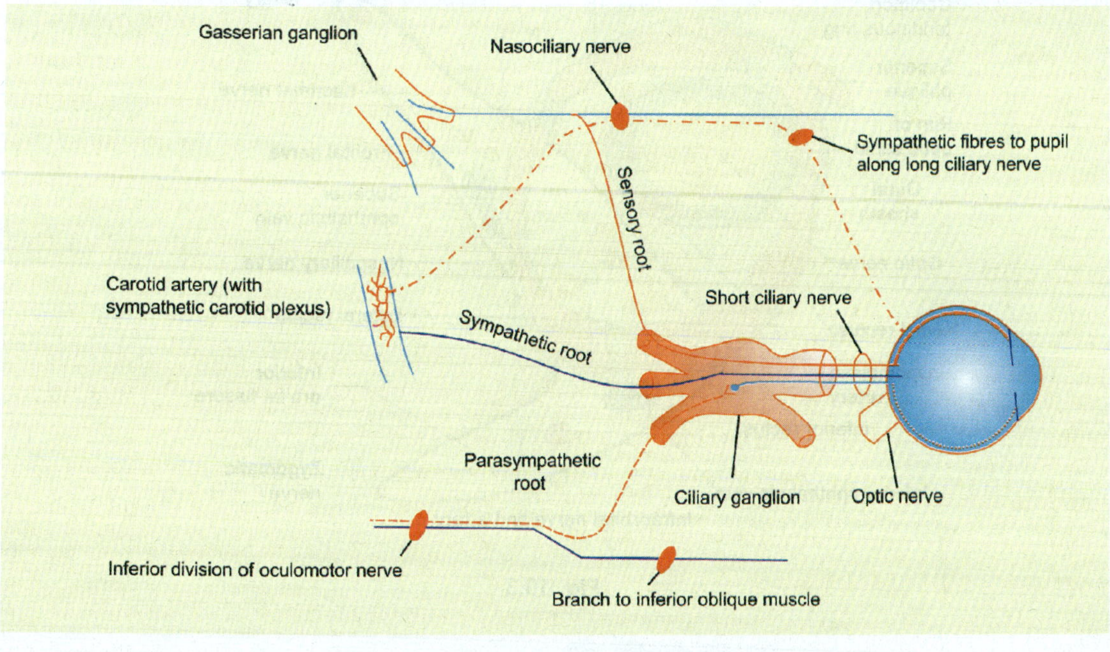

Fig. 10.2: Ciliary ganglion with its roots and branches

3. The medial rectus, inferior rectus and inferior oblique nuclei—These are paired and innervate their corresponding ipsilateral muscles.

Fourth Nerve

It is the only cranial nerve to emerge from the dorsal aspect of the brain and is the only crossed cranial nerve. Hence, it innervates the contralateral superior oblique muscle. It is the longest and most slender of all cranial nerves. Its nucleus is located at the level of the inferior colliculus.

Sixth Nerve

The nucleus of the sixth nerve lies in the midpoint of the pons closely related to the seventh nerve and horizontal gaze centre. Hence, an isolated sixth nerve palsy is never nuclear in origin.

OPTIC NEURITIS

Involvement of the optic nerve by disease process that impairs nerve conductivity.

Clinical Features:

1. Diminished visual acuity.
2. Visual field defects.
3. Afferent pupillary defect.
4. Impairment of color vision.
5. Diminished light brightness sensitivity.

CLASSIFICATION OF OPTIC NEURITIS

Anatomical

1. Papillitis.
2. Retrobulbar neuritis.
3. Neuroretinitis.

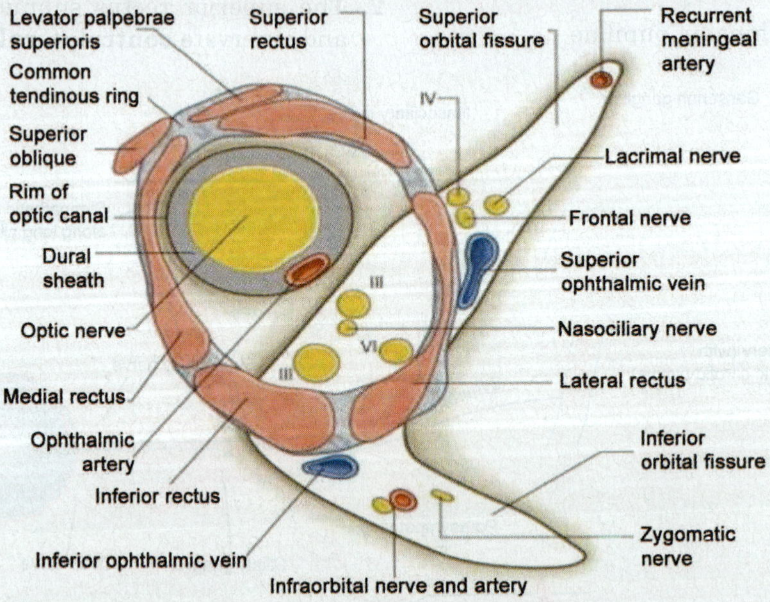

Fig. 10.3

Etiological

1. Inflammatory.
2. Degenerative.
3. Autoimmune.
4. Ischemic.
5. Toxic Amblyopia.
6. Hereditary.

Etiology of Optic Neuritis

a. **Idiopathic.**

b. **Hereditary:** Hereditary optic neuritis (Leber's disease).

c. **Demyelinating disorders (Degenerative):**

i. Multiple sclerosis.
ii. Neuromyelitis optica (Devic's disease).
iii. Diffuse periaxial encephalitis of schilder.
iv. Poliomyelitis.
v. Epidemic encephalitis.
vi. Acute disseminated encephalomyelitis: It occurs due to endogenous infections like measles, mumps, chickenpox, whooping cough, glandular fever.

d. **Due to metabolic dyscrasias:**

i. Diabetes mellitus.
ii. Anaemia.
iii. Pregnancy.
iv. Avitaminosis.
v. Starvation.

e. **Local causes (Inflammatory):**

i. Uveitis (specially sympathetic ophthalmitis).
ii. Retinitis.
iii. Meningitis (Syphilis and tuberculosis).
iv. Sinus disease (sphenoid and ethmoid infections).
v. Orbital cellulitis.

f. **Exogenous toxins (Toxic Amblyopia):** It is a degenerative optic neuritis:

i. Methanol.
ii. Ethyl alcohol.
iii. Oral contraceptives.
iv. Ethambutol.
v. Tobacco.
vi. Quinine.

g. **Ischemic**

Anterior Ischemic Optic Neuropathy

i. Arteritic.
ii. Non-arteritic.

Papillitis

Optic neuritis with involvement of optic disc is known as papillitis.

Ophthalmoscopic Features:

1. Swollen optic disc–upto 2 D.
2. Hyperaemic disc.
3. Disc margins blurred.

Signs and Symptoms:

It includes all the features of optic nerve disease.

1. Usually unilateral involvement.
2. Associated with ocular pain.
3. Sudden loss of vision.
4. Abnormal pupillary reaction.
5. Central scotomas.
6. Impairment of dark adaptation.
7. Impairment of color vision.

Retrobulbar Neuritis

Involvement of retrolaminar part of optic nerve with normal optic disc.

1. **Ophthalmoscopic feature**–Normal optic nerve head and retinal nerve fibre layer.

2. **S/S**–Similar to papillitis.

Neuroretinitis

Papillitis alongwith the involvement of the retina is known as neuroretinitis. Retinal involvement occurs in form of macular star, which are hard exudates deposited in the macular area due to increased capillary permeability, secondary to inflammation of retina.

Inflammatory Optic Neuritis

It includes all the causes of posterior uveitis that lead to papillitis and optic neuritis.

Degenerative Optic Neuritis

It includes optic neuritis occurring due to demyelinating disease such as multiple sclerosis.

Multiple sclerosis: It is a common idiopathic demyelination disorder of the central nervous system characterized by intermittent disturbance of neurological function. It does not affect the central nervous system.

Ocular Features:

1. Sudden monocular visual loss associated with periocular discomfort made worse on moving the eye, frontal headache and tenderness of the globe. Dimunition of visual acuity becomes maximum after 1–2 weeks and recovers after 4–8 weeks. Visual prognosis is good but there can be loss of other visual function like contrast sensitivity and colour vision.
2. *Fundus:* Normal in most cases or papillitis.
3. Impairment of colour vision is worse than would be expected at that level of visual impairment.
4. *Ocular motolity defects:*
   a. Internuclear ophthalmoplegia.
   b. Conjugate gaze paralysis.
   c. Isolated ocular nerve palsy.
   d. *Nystagmus:* It may be vertical or rotatory. Ocillopsia is the term used when the patient is aware of his nystagmus.

Treatment:

Treatment enhances recovery if the visual acuity is less than 6/12 in the first week. I/V methylprednisolone six hourly for 3 days followed by oral prednisolone for 11 days. Only oral dose does not work.

Toxic Amblyopia

It is a degenerative optic neuritis (commonly retrobulbar neuritis) occurring due to ingestion of drugs (exogenous poisons).

Causes of Toxic Amblyopia:

1. **Digoxin.**
2. **Chloroquine:** It is an antimalarial drug, also used in the treatment of rheumatological (e.g., rheumatoid arthritis, juvenile chronic arthritis, systemic lupus erythematosis) and dermatological diseases (e.g., discoid lupus).

   Ocular Side Effects:

   1. Optic neuritis.
   2. Retinotoxicity–Bull's eye maculopathy.
   3. Corneal deposits–Innocuous **(Vortex Keratopathy).**
3. **Ethambutol:** It is used in combination with Isoniazid and Rifampicin in the treatment of tuberculosis.

   Ocular Side Effects:

   1. Optic neuropathy.
   2. Risk of optic neuropathy is more if dose is greater than 15 mg/kg.

   Clinical Feature:

   Severe and dramatic visual loss with impairment of red green perception.

On Examination:

1. Either normal disc (Retrobulbar neuritis) or disc edema with superficial haemorrhage.
2. Visual field—Temporal defect.

Treatment:

If drug is stopped, prognosis is good. In minority of cases, there is permanent visual impairment due to optic atrophy.

Screening: At 4 weekly if dose > 15 mg/kg.

Other ATT drugs which may cause toxic optic neuropathy include:

a. Chloramphenicol.
b. Isoniazid.
c. Streptomycin.
d. Rifampicin.

4. **Ethyl alcohol:** Ethyl alcohol amblyopia generally occurs in association with tobacco amblyopia.

Clinical Features:

- Bilateral gradually progressive impairment in central vision.
- Patient complains of fogginess and difficulty in doing near vision.
- Bilateral centrocaecal scotomas.
- Fundus—normal or slight temporal pallor of disc.
- Optic neuritis occurs along with peripheral neuritis of chronic and debilitated alcoholics.

Treatment:

1. Complete cessation of tobacco and alcohol.
2. 1000 mg I/M injections of hydroxycobalamin weekly for 10 weeks. Prognosis—Poor.

5. **Methyl alcohol:**

- Unlike ethyl alcohol, poisoning by methyl alcohol is typically acute usually resulting in optic atrophy and permanent blindness.This is because it directly damages the ganglion cells.
- It occurs due to intake of wood alcohol or methylated spirit in cheap adulterated beverages.
- Methyl alcohol leads to formaldehyde formation which causes odema of ganglion cells and optic atrophy (primary optic atrophy).

6. **Tobacco:** It causes centrocaecal scotoma.
7. **Quinine:** It leads to degenerative optic neuritis and also causes **tubular vision.**

Note: After trauma, sudden loss of vision with defective *afferent pupillary* response indicates optic nerve compression, hence definitive treatment is optic canal decompression.

ANTERIOR ISCHEMIC OPTIC NEUROPATHY

It is a segmental or generalized infarction within the prelaminar or laminar portion of the optic nerve caused by **occlusion of short posterior ciliary arteries.**

Classification:

1. **Arteritic AION.**
2. **Non-Arteritic AION.**

Arteritic AION

Etiology:

It occurs due to Giant-Cell-Arteritis (GCA).

Clinical Features:

1. Transient visual obscuration (i.e., Amaurosis fugax) followed by uniocular, sudden and profound loss of vision.
2. Periocular pain.
3. Pale, swollen optic nerve head surrounded by small splinter-shaped haemorrhages.

Treatment:

I/V Hydrocortisone with oral prednisolone.

Amaurosis Fugax

It is the transient loss of vision in a curtain-like manner, which is totally regained after few seconds.

Causes of Amaurosis Fugax:

1. Arteritic AION.
2. Central retinal artery occlusion.
3. Transient ischemic attacks (TIA).
4. Carotid artery disease.
5. Uraemia.

Non-Arteritic AION

Etiology:

The exact etiology is not documented but the major risk factor is hypertension. Hypertensive patients suffer from nocturnal hypotension which is responsible for the ischemia of the optic nerve. Other causes include blood viscosity syndromes.

Clinical Features:

1. Monocular, sudden and painless visual loss.
2. No premonitory visual symptoms.
3. Diffuse or sectoral edema with hyperaemic optic nerve head surrounded by splinter-shaped haemorrhages, later the involved portion of the disc becomes pale.
4. Visual acuity in 1/3rd patients is either normal or slightly reduced. Remaining 2/3rd suffer from moderate to severe visual loss.
5. *Visual field defects:*
   i. **Altitudinal hemianopia:** Most commonly involves the inferior field.
   ii. **Central scotoma:** If there is infarction of papillomacular bundle.
6. *Colour vision:* It is diminished in **proportion** to the level of visual acuity **unlike degenerative optic neuritis.**

Investigations:

1. Serological studies, serum lipids, blood glucose, and factors affecting viscosity.
2. To exclude occult GCA and other auto-immune diseases.

Treatment:

- Treatment of underlying disease.
- To quit smoking and alcohol.
- Optic nerve sheath decompression if progressive visual loss.

Autoimmune Optic Neuropathy

- It denotes, optic nerve lesions which develop in patients with Systemic Lupus Erythematosis (SLE) and other systemic collagen vascular disorders.
- Pathogenesis is similar to AION and clinical features include all the features of optic neuritis.

Hereditary optic neuropathy: It is divided into two types:

A. *Lebers hereditary optic neuropathy.*

B. *Hereditary optic atrophies:* These may be autosomal dominant or autosomal recessive.

Lebers Hereditary Optic Neuropathy

- It is a rare disease which is the result of a **maternal mitochondrial DNA** mutation at **point 11778.**

Clinical Features:

- Commonly in adolescent males, atypically may involve females.
- Unilateral, acute, severe, painless optic neuritis followed by involvement of other eye.

On Examination:

a. Mild optic disc hyperaemia.
b. *Telangiectatic microangiopathy:* It is seen in the carriers of this disease.
c. Severe optic atrophy.

Treatment:

Prognosis is relatively poor with generally severe, bilateral and permanent visual loss.

1. High-dose systemic steroids are used in some cases.
2. Stop smoking and excessive drinking.

Papilloedema

Any edema around the optic disc is known as papilloedema.

Pathogenesis:

Due to disturbance of pressure gradient across the lamina cribosa
↓
Stasis of axoplasm in prelaminar area
↓
Axonal swelling
↓
Venous congestion
↓
Extracellular edema

Etiology:

A. Intracranial (Bilateral symmetric):

1. Haemorrhage.
2. Encephalitis, Meningitis.
3. Neoplasms—Glioma, Meningioma, Neurofibroma etc.
4. Brain abscess.
5. Pseudotumor cerebri (Benign intracranial hypertension).

B. Systemic:

1. Malignant HT.
2. Blood dyscrasias.
3. Endocrasias—Hyperthyroidism, Toxaemia of pregnancy.
4. Drugs: Intensive steroid therapy, OCPs, Salicyclate intoxication.

C. Orbital:

1. Orbital tumor.
2. Orbital cellulitis.
3. Orbital hemangioma.
4. Tumors of optic nerve.

D. Ocular (Secondary to hypotony):

1. Ocular trauma—Accidental/Surgical.
2. Sudden lowering of intraocular pressure–In cataract surgery, RD surgery.

Clinical Features:

Ophthalmoscopic Features:

1. Swelling of optic disc (6–8 D) which spills into periphery producing concentric folds in retina.
2. Hyperaemia of disc.
3. Blurring of disc margins.
4. Tortous and dilated veins.
5. Retinal haemorrhages.

Signs and Symptoms:

1. Transient obscuration of vision.
2. Mild decrease in VA (if markedly decreased, it is due to CME).
3. Normal color vision.
4. Normal pupillary reaction.
5. Visual field defect–**Enlargement of blind spot and later it leads to constriction of visual field.**
6. Associated symptoms (due to increased ICT)–Headache, Nausea, Vomiting, Diplopia.

Differential Diagnosis (*It includes all the causes of blurred disc margin*):

1. Optic neuritis.
2. Hyperopic discs.
3. Medullated nerve fibres.
4. Disc drusen.
5. Pseudotumor cerebri.
6. Skull malformations.
7. **Pseudopapilloedema/Pseudopapillitis:** *Pseudopapilloedema* can present in hypermetropic eyes where the size of disc area is small and the nerve fibres are crowded giving the appearance of blurred disc margin, hence termed as pseudopapilloedema.
   - Other causes are:
     1. Drusen.
     2. Medullated nerve fibres.
     3. Skull malformations.

Sequelae: Secondary optic atrophy.

Treatment: According to the cause.

Benign Intracranial Hypertension

Also called **"Pseudotumour cerebri"**.

Most common in women.

Pathophysiology: It occurs due to imbalance in the formation and absorption of the CSF, i.e., either the CSF is formed more in the choroid plexus or absorbed less from the arachnoid villi.

Etiology:

1. Obesity.
2. OCPs.
3. Tetracycline.
4. Hypervitaminosis A.

Signs and Symptoms:

- 5–10% patients are asymptomatic and papilloedema is detected on routine eye examination.
- Headache.
- Transient visual obscuration.
- Diplopia due to involvement of the sixth nerve.
- Painful neck stiffness.
- Tinnitus.

On Examination:

Papilloedema–Acute, chronic.

- *Visual field loss:*
  a. Enlargement of blind spot.
  b. Constriction of visual field.

Dandy's Diagnostic Criteria (For Pseudotumor Cerebri)

1. Patient is awake and alert.
2. S/S of increased intracranial pressure.
3. Absence of localized neurological signs except 6th nerve palsy (hence diplopia).
4. Opening pressure of CSF is > 200 mm of H_2O and is of normal composition.
5. Normal CT scan head and MRI head.

Associated Features:

1. Obesity.
2. Hypervitaminosis A.

Treatment:

1. Control of weight.
2. Carbonic anhydrase inhibitors–Furosemide, Digoxin.

Malignant Hypertension

It presents with features of hypertensive retinopathy; papilloedema being a common finding.

Optic Atrophy: It is the end result of any pathological process that damages the axons coursing between retinal ganglion cells and LGB.

CLASSIFICATION OF OPTIC ATROPHY

Ophthalmoscopically classified as:

A. Primary Optic Atrophy:

1. Chalky white disc.
2. Disc margins clear.
3. No sheathing of vessels.
4. Cup not full.

Etiology: Syphilis, Hereditary, Trauma.

B. Secondary Optic Atrophy:

1. Pale and dirty white in colour.
2. Disc margins blurred.
3. Sheathing of vessels.
4. Cup is full due to glial proliferation.

Etiology: Generally after papilloedema or papillitis.

C. Consecutive Optic Atrophy: A pale waxy disc.

Etiology:

1. Retinitis pigmentosa.
2. Diffuse chorioretinitis.

D. Glaucomatous Optic Atrophy OR Cavernous Optic Atrophy

- It is also known as **"Schnables' atrophy"**.

Features:

1. Atrophy of nerve fibres.
2. No glial cell proliferation.
3. Mucoid degeneration of glial cells leading to formation of lacunae or clear pools.

Occurs in:

1. Glaucoma.
2. Methyl alcohol poisoning.
3. High myopia.

E. Partial Optic Atrophy:

It is characterized by temporal pallor.

Pathologically classified as:

1. Ascending optic atrophy.
2. Descending optic atrophy.
3. Cavernous optic atrophy–Occurs in *Chronic simple glaucoma.*

Foster-Kennedy Syndrome:

- Ipsilateral optic atrophy with contralateral papilloedema.
- Occurs due to tumor in orbital surface of frontal lobe, olfactory groove or pituitary body on the ipsilateral side.

ABNORMAL PUPILLARY REACTIONS

a. Marcus Gunn Pupil or Relative Afferent Pupillary Defect (RAPD)

- It is caused by incomplete optic nerve lesion or severe retinal disease.
- **Features are: They are depicted by "Swinging flash light test"**, which denotes that when abnormal pupil is stimulated by direct light, it dilates instead of constricting.

b. Total Afferent Pupillary Defect (TAPD):

- Due to complete optic nerve lesion.
- **Features are:**

1. Involved eye is completely blind.
2. Both pupils are equal.
3. When affected eye is stimulated neither pupil reacts but when the normal eye is stimulated both pupil react normally.
4. Near reflex is normal in both eyes.

c. Argyll-Robertson Pupil: The lesion is mainly in the pretectal and Edinger-westphal nucleus.

- It is caused by Neurosyphilis.
- **Features are:**

1. Usually bilateral but asymmetrical.

2. Pupil are small and irregular.
3. Light reflex absent or very sluggish.
4. Near reflex is normal.
5. Pupils are very difficult to dilate.

Note:

Other causes of Light–Near dissociation

- Pineal lesions.
- Parinaud's syndrome (Dorsal mid-brain syndrome).

d. Holmes-Adie Pupil:

- It is due to denervation of postganglionic supply to sphincter pupillae and ciliary muscle which may follow a viral illness.
- **Features are:**

1. It is unilateral in 80% of cases.
2. Diminished tendon reflexes.
3. Affected pupil is large and regular.
4. Light reflex is very slow.
5. Constriction to near is very slow and tonic and associated with **vermiform movement of the iris.**
6. Accommodation is slow.
7. *Pharmacological testing:* Constriction of pupil with as small dose of pilocarpine–0.125% which occurs due to denervation hypersensitivity.

e. Horner's Syndrome (Oculosympathetic palsy): Horner's syndrome occurs due to disruption of sympathetic pathway.

Sympathetic Supply: It consists of three neurons:

1. The first starts in *posterior hypothalamus* and descends uncrossed down the brainstem to terminate in **"Ciliospinal centre of Budge"** located between C8 and T2.
2. The second passes from ciliospinal centre to *superior cervical ganglion* in the neck, being closely related to apical pleura during its course.
3. The third ascends along the internal carotid artery into the skull to join the *ophthalmic division of trigeminal nerve.* Sympathetic fibres from here reach the ciliary body via *nasociliary nerve* and then reach dilator pupillae through *long ciliary nerves.*

Causes of Horner's Syndrome:

1. Pancoast's tumour of lung.
2. Carotid and aortic aneurysms.
3. Lesions in neck like trauma, tumour, surgery.
4. Brainstem—Vascular or demyelinating disease.
5. Congenital.
6. Idiopathic.

Features of Horner's Syndrome:

1. Lesion is usually unilateral.
2. Mild ptosis due to weakness of Muller's muscle.
3. Slight elevation of inferior eyelid as a result of weakness of inferior tarsal muscle.
4. Miosis due to unopposed action of sphincter pupillae.
5. Normal pupillary reactions (both light and near).
6. Reduced ipsilateral sweating if *lesion is below superior cervical ganglion.*
7. Apparent enophthalmos.
8. Heterochromia iridis, if the cause of Horner's syndrome is congenital.

Third Nerve Palsy

1. *Ptosis:* LPS involved, neurogenic ptosis.

2. *Eye is—Down and Out.* Third nerve supplies all extraocular muscles except SO and LR, hence, when paralysed the eye is down and out due to uninhibited action of the above two muscles. These two muscles are supplied by 6th nerve and 4th nerve **remembered as LR6 SO4.**
3. Defective adduction, elevation and depression.
4. Dilated pupil with defective accommodation.
5. **Webino (Wall-Eyed Bilateral Internuclear Ophthalmoplegia):** Due to lesions involving paired medial rectus subnuclei. It leads to defective convergence and adduction.
6. **Benedikt's Syndrome:** Ipsilateral third nerve palsy and contralateral hemitremor.
7. **Weber's Syndrome:** Ipsilateral third nerve palsy and a contralateral hemiparesis.
8. Intorsion of eye on attempted downgaze due to superior oblique muscle action.
9. Crossed diplopia.
10. Head posture may change if pupillary area remains uncovered.

A patient presented with normal eyesight and absence of direct and consensual light reflexes indicates involvement of third nerve.

Internal Ophthalmoplegia

The term refers to III nerve palsy confined to internal eye muscles, i.e., iris sphincter and ciliary muscles. When this condition is accompanied by paralysis of external ocular muscles **(External ophthalmoplegia)** we call it as **Total ophthalmoplegia.**

- Internal ophthalmoplegia is also termed as tonic pupil.
- Internal ophthalmoplegia occurs when the efferent pathway of pupillary fibres (III nerve) are affected, i.e.:
  a. Lesions of ciliary ganglion, e.g., in orbital tumors, orbital infection, orbital pseudotumour, orbital trauma.
  b. Lesions of short ciliary nerves, e.g., trauma orbital floor.

Hence, causes of internal ophthalmoplegia can be documented as:

A. *Inflammatory*—HZO, chickenpox, measles, sarcoidosis.
B. *Trauma*—Orbital floor fracture, penetrating orbital trauma.
C. *Orbital tumor.*
D. *Generalized peripheral neuropathy*—Alcoholism, diabetes mellitus, Guillain Barré syndrome, Sky Drager syndrome, Amyloidosis, Charcot-Marie tooth disease, trichlor ethylene intoxication.
E. *Idiopathic*—Adie's tonic pupillary syndrome.

Clinical Features:

1. Segmental palsy of iris sphincter.
2. Tonic response to both light and near.
3. Light–near dissociation.
4. Denervation hypersensitivity to diluted cholinergic agents.

Fourth Nerve Palsy

1. Hyperdeviation.
2. *Excyclotorsion:* Compensated by head tilt to opposite shoulder.
3. Limited depression in adduction.
4. *Diplopia:* **Vertical** Worse on looking down.
5. *Bielchowsky's sign:* This is a test to confirm SO palsy. On tilting the head on the same side, if hypertropia increases, its SO palsy.

Sixth Nerve Palsy

1. Defective abduction.

2. Convergent strabismus.
3. Horizontal diplopia.
4. Face turn into field of action of paralysed eye.
5. **Millard Gubler Syndrome:** Ipsilateral sixth nerve palsy with contralateral hemiplegia.

SUPRANUCLEAR CONTROL OF EYE

- The eye movements are controlled by the frontal and occipital lobe which in turn control the gaze centres both horizontal and vertical.
- Horizontal gaze centre is present at pons known as PPRF (Pontine parareticular formation).
- In any horizontal gaze, PPRF manages the sixth nerve nucleus (which causes abduction) whereas the adduction of the contralateral eye is managed by the MLF (which gets the information from PPRF).
- **Vertical Gaze Centre:** It is situated in the Rostral Interstitial Nucleus of MLF and Nucleus of Cajal. It lies in the midbrain just dorsal to the red nucleus. From vertical gaze centre impulses pass through subnuclei of each eye muscle controlling vertical gaze in each eye.

Supranuclear disorders of the eye: Progressive supranuclear palsy is a severe degenerative disease presenting in old age.

Features are:

1. **Gaze palsies:** It initially affects downgaze, then upgaze, then horizontal gaze and finally global palsy.
2. Normal vestibulo-ocular reflexes.
3. Absence of diplopia.

Internuclear Ophthalmoplegia (INO): It occurs due to lesion of medial longitudinal fasciculus.

Clinical Features:

1. Defective adduction of ipsilateral eye.
2. Ataxic nystagmus of the contralateral abducting eye.

PERINAUD'S DORSAL MIDBRAIN SYNDROME

Clinical Features:

1. Supranuclear upgaze palsy.
2. Straight eyes in primary positions.
3. Normal downgaze.
4. Large pupils with light-near dissociation.
5. Lid retraction (Collier sign).
6. Paralysis of convergence.
7. Convergence–Retraction nystagmus.

Etiology:

1. Tumour.
2. Trauma.
3. Inflammatory.
4. Demyelinating diseases.

LESIONS OF VISUAL PATHWAY

A. **Optic nerve lesions: Ipsilateral blindness.**

B. **Lesions through proximal part of optic nerve:** Ipsilateral blindness with contralateral hemianopia.

C. **Chiasma:** Bitemporal hemianopia or Junctional Scotoma of Traquair (Any lesion at the junction of chiasma and the optic nerve will lead to ipsilateral central scotoma and contralateral superotemporal quadrantopias. It occurs specifically in pituitary tumours). **Chiasmal lesions are always heteronymous. Hence chiasmal lesions can cause bitemporal hemianopia, superior quandrantopia**

or inferior quadrantopia depending upon the exact site of lesion.

D. Optic tract

1. *Incongruous homonymous hemianopia:* Left optic tract lesion denotes lesion of temporal fibres of left eye and of nasal fibres of right eye, which will lead to left eye nasal field defect and right eye temporal field defect, hence causing right homonymous hemianopia.
2. *Wernicke's hemianopic pupil:* The optic tracts contain both visual and pupillomotor fibres. The visual fibres terminate in the lateral geniculate body but pupillary fibres leave the optic tract anterior to lateral geniculate body and terminate in pretectal nucleus. An optic tract lesion may give rise to afferent pupillary conduction defect. This pupillary light reflex will be normal when unaffected hemiretina is stimulated and absent when involved hemiretina is stimulated. This is **Wernicke's hemianopic pupillary reaction.** It is difficult to elicit due to scatter of light and a fine beam of light is needed.
3. **Optic atrophy.**
4. **Contralateral pyramidal signs.**

E. Lesions of Optic Radiations:

1. Incongruous or congruous homonymous hemianopia.

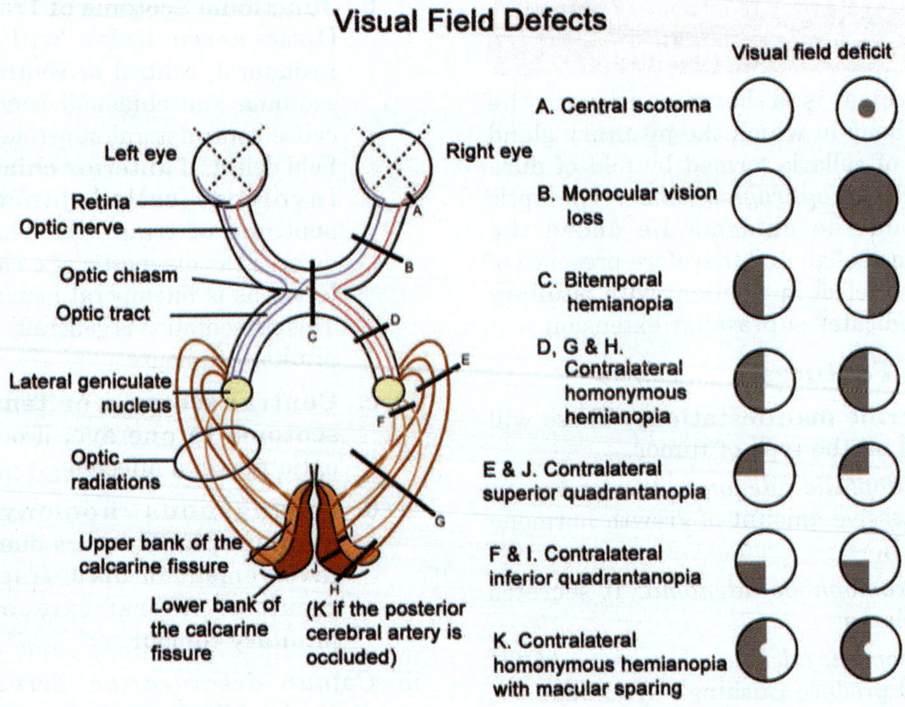

Fig. 10.4: Lesions of visual pathway

2. No optic atrophy.
3. *Temporal lobe lesions lead to* – Contralateral superior quadrantopia **("Pie in sky")**.
4. *Parietal lobe lesions lead to* – Contralateral inferior quadrantopia **("Pie on floor")**.

F. Striate Calcarine Cortex:

1. **Pupillary reactions are normal.**
2. **Macula-sparing congruous homonymous hemianopia**–Due to occlusion of posterior cerebral artery.
3. **Congruous homonymous macular defects**–Due to damage to tip of occipital cortex, due to involvement of middle cerebral artery.

PITUITARY ADENOMA (AFFECTS CHIASMA)

Sella turcica is a bony cavity in the sphenoid bone in which the pituitary gland lies. Roof of sella is formed by fold of dura mater called *diaphragma sellae*. The optic nerves and the chiasma lie above the diaphragma sellae and therefore presence of visual field defect in a patient with pituitary tumour indicates suprasellar extension.

Clinical Features:

A. Endocrine manifestations: These will depend on the type of tumor.

i. *Acidophilic adenoma*: It secretes an excessive amount of growth hormone (GH).
ii. *Chromophobe adenoma:* It secretes prolactin.
iii. *Basophilic adenoma:* It secretes ACTH and produce Cushing's syndrome.

B. Neurologic manifestations:

- *Headache:*
  a. Severe, bursting headache located in frontal, bitemporal or retro-orbital region.
  b. Frequently associated with nausea and vomiting due to increased ICT.
- *Seizures:* Due to lateral extension of tumor in temporal lobe.
- *Hydrocephalus:* Due to:
  a. Compression of foramen of monro; or
  b. Compression of aqueduct of sylvius.

C. Ocular manifestations:

i. *Gradual loss of vision*, which may be preceded by attacks of amaurosis.

ii. *Visual field defects:*

a. **Bitemporal Hemianopia:** When chiasma lies just above the pituitary gland.

b. **Junctional Scotoma of Traquair:** Optic nerve lesion will cause ipsilateral, central or centrocaecal scotoma and chiasmal lesion will cause contralateral superotemporal field defect, **if anterior chiasma is involved (called junctional scotoma of traquair)**. This field defect is as diagnostic of a chiasmal lesion as is bitemporal hemianopia. This presentation is generally seen in pituitary tumours.

c. **Central scotoma or temporal scotoma in one eye,** if only one optic nerve is affected.

d. **Incongruous homonymous hemianopia:** It occurs due to the involvement of optic tract as a result of lateral extension of pituitary tumour.

iii. *Colour desaturation across the vertical midline.*

iv. *Optic atrophy:* It is bilateral but not symmetrical.

v. *Ocular motor palsy:*

- Rare.

- Occurs when lateral expansion leads to involvement of cavernous sinus.

vi. *Proptosis:* Due to pressure on cavernous sinus leading to stasis of orbital venous return.

vii. *See-saw nystagmus:* Dissociated vertical rotatory nystagmus may occur.

Treatment:

A. Surgery.

B. *Bromocriptine:* It shrinks a prolactin secreting tumor.

C. *Radiotherapy:* It is effective in selected cases.

NYSTAGMUS

It is the repetitive, involuntary to and fro oscillation of the eyes.

Nystagmus can be caused by lesions in midbrain, pons, cerebrum, cerebellum and lesions of craniocervical junction. It is most commonly associated with cerebellar lesions.

Classification:

According to Clinical Types:

a. Pendular:

Velocity of movement is equal in each direction.

b. Jerk:

Movement of eye has a slow drift and a fast phase.

c. Mixed:

Pendular in primary position and jerk in lateral gaze.

According to the Etiology:

A. Physiological

i. **End-point nystagmus:** Some people have nystagmus in extremes of gaze.

ii. **Optokinetic nystagmus:** It constitutes the pursuit and saccadic movements. Pursuit and saccadic movements are binocular movements in which the two eyes move symmetrically in the same direction.

Saccadic Movements

- Its function is to place the object of interest on the fovea rapidly or to move the eyes from one object to another.
- These movements are abrupt.
- It can be a voluntary movement or can occur as a reflex triggered by presence of an object in the peripheral visual field.
- Its pathway originates in the premotor cortex of the frontal motor area, and pass to the **contralateral** horizontal gaze centre (PPRF—Pontine, Para-Reticular Formation).

Pursuit Movements

- Its function is to maintain fixation on the target once it has been located by the saccadic system.
- These movements are slow and smooth.
- Its pathway originates in peristriate cortex of the occipital motor area and **ipsilateral** horizontal gaze centre in the PPRF.

iii. **Vestibular nystagmus (COWS):** Cold water in the ear leads to nystagmus in opposite direction and hot water leads to nystagmus on the same side.

B. Motor Imbalance

i. **Congenital Nystagmus:**

- Present at birth.
- Persists throughout life.

- Dampened by convergence.
- Absent during sleep.

ii. Spasmus Nutans:

- Present between 4th and 12th month and ceases by age of 3 years.
- Pendular and asymmetrical. It may be associated with neurological lesion.
- Associated with abnormal head posture and head nodding.

iii. Latent Nystagmus:

Presents in early childhood in patients of **infantile esotropia.**

iv. Ataxic Nystagmus:

It occurs in abducting eye of patients of **Internuclear Ophthalmoplegia.**

v. Downbeat Nystagmus:

- Jerk nystagmus with fast phase beating downwards.
- It occurs in patients with lesions of craniocervical junction at the foramen magnum such as *Arnold Chiari malformation*, brainstem and cerebellar stroke, alcoholism and multiple sclerosis.

vi. Upbeat Nystagmus:

- Jerky nystagmus with fast phase beating upwards.
- It is caused by:
  a. Drugs, e.g., phenytoin.
  b. Lesions of posterior fossa.

vii. Convergence Retraction Nystagmus:

- It is stimulated by attempted upward gaze in which the fast phase brings the two eyes towards each other in a convergence movement. This is associated with retraction of globe.
- **Causes are:**
  1. Lesions of pretectal area such as pinealomas and vascular accidents.
  2. Perinaud's dorsal mid-brain syndrome.

viii. See-Saw Nystagmus of Maddox:

- It is seen in patients with bitemporal hemianopia due to chiasmal lesions.
- There is alternating movement of eye; one eye rises and intorts and other falls and extorts.

ix. Periodic Alternating Nystagmus:

- There is rhythmic changes in amplitude and direction usually every 2 minutes.
- **Causes**—Vascular or Demyelinating brainstem lesions.

C. Ocular Nystagmus or Nystagmus due to Sensory Deprivation

- Pendular nystagmus.
- It is due to sensory deprivation to the macula, e.g., congenital cataract, macular hypoplasia, Rubella keratitis etc.

D. Nystagmoid Movements

These are the movements which mimic nystagmus.

a. Ocular Flutter

- Horizontal oscillation and inability to fixate after change of gaze.
- Due to interruption of cerebellar connection to brainstem.

b. Opsoclonus

- Combined horizontal, vertical and/or torsional oscillations.
- Associated with myoclonic movement of face, arms and legs.

- **Cause:** Encephalitis.

c. **Superior Oblique Myokymia**

- Monocular, rapid, intermittent, torsional vertical movements.
- Best seen on slit-lamp.

d. **Ocular Bobbing**

- Rapid downward deviation of the eyes with slow updrift.
- Due to pontine dysfunctions.

Miners Nystagmus: It is rotatory. It occurs in persons working in coal mines for a long duration.

Oculogyric Crisis

In this condition there is spasmodic conjugate deviation of the eyes (usually upwards) accompanied by synergic movements of the head and neck.

Etiology:

1. Encephalitis lethargica.
2. Phenothiazines idiosyncrasy.

Treatment:

Benzedrine upto 30 mg/day.

COLOUR BLINDNESS

In this, faculty to appreciate one or more primary colours is either defective (anomalous) or absent (anopia). It may be congenital or acquired.

Congenital

Males are affected more.

It is of the following types:

A. *Anomalous trichromatic colour vision:* Colour perception is present but defective.

It is of following types:

1. *Protanomalous:* Defective red colour appreciation.
2. *Deuteranomalous:* Defective green colour perception.
3. *Tritanomalous:* Defective blue colour perception.

B. *Dichromatic colour vision:* Faculty to perceive one of the three primary colors is completely absent.

1. *Protanopia:* Complete red colour defect.
2. *Deuteranopia:* Complete green colour defect.
3. *Tritanopia:* Complete blue colour defect.

C. *Monochromatic colour vision:* Only one primary colour can be appreciated.

D. *Achromatic colour vision:*

- Extremely rare condition.
- Due to congenital absence of cones.
- Day blindness and Nystagmus.
- Also called **Total colour blindness.**

Acquired

Causes:

1. Damage to macula or optic nerve (red-green discrimination affected). It is usually associated with central scotoma or decreased visual acuity.
2. Acquired blue colour defect (blue blindness) may occur in old age due to increased sclerosis of the crystalline lens. It is due to increased absorption of blue rays by the amber coloured pigment in the nucleus.

Distribution of Colour Vision in the Retina

- The very center of fovea (1/8th degree) is blue blind.
- Trichromatic colour vision mechanism extends 20° to 30° from point of fixation.

- Peripheral to this (30°), red and green become indistinguishable.
- In far periphery, all colour sense is lost, although cones are still found in this region of retina.
- Hence, when a red object is brought from periphery in the field of vision the individual first becomes aware of a colourless object in the periphery. Then as the object is advanced, it is seen successively as salmon pink or yellow and eventually as red.

CONGENITAL OPTIC DISC ANOMALIES

1. Tilted disc.
2. *Optic disc drusen:* These are depositions in the substance of optic nerve head. Drusens are composed of hyaline like calcific material. It is commonly seen in patients of Angiod streaks and Retinitis pigmentosa. It presents as pseudopapillitis.
3. *Optic disc pit:* It presents as a round oval pit on the disc. More than 50% cases are associated with serous detachment of the macula and is confused with CSR.
4. *Optic disc coloboma:* Coloboma indicates absence of part of the tissue. It presents as very large excavation which is usually situated inferiorly. It occurs due to incomplete closure of fetal fissure.
5. *Morning-Glory Anomaly:* Dysplastic coloboma of the optic disc. Ophthalmoscopy shows an enlarged and excavated optic nerve head with a central core of whitish glial tissue of persistent hyaloid remnants within its base. The blood vessels emerge in radial pattern like the spokes of the wheel. Visual acuity is very poor. Majority of the cases are unilateral.
6. *Optic nerve hypoplasia.*
7. *Myelinated nerve fibres:* Normally myelination occurs behind the eyeball, i.e., retrolaminar. If it occurs prelaminar and visible on the optic disc. It is called myelinated nerve fibres. It presents as pseudopapillitis.
8. *Aicardi's Syndrome:*
   a. Large colobomatous discs.
   b. Chorioretinal atrophy.
   c. Retinal pigmented epithelial changes.

NEET DRILL

1. Length of the optic nerve: 5 cm.
2. Pie-in-sky is a feature of temporal lobe lesion.
3. Ophthalmoplegic migraine is migraine with 3rd nerve palsy.
4. Central nystagmus is due to lesion at the midbrain and cerebellum whereas peripheral nystagmus is due to problem in the vestibular system.
5. Length of the longest part of the optic nerve: 25 mm–30 mm.
6. Length of the smallest part (intraocular) of the optic nerve is: 1 mm.
7. Structures passing through the optic foramen: optic nerve and ophthalmic artery.
8. Nerves passing through the superior orbital fissure outside the annulus of Zinn are learnt by LFT, i.e., lacrimal nerve, frontal and trochlear nerve.

MNEMONIC

LFT **(Lacrimal, Frontal and Trochlear)**

9. First sign of optic nerve disease is APD, i.e., afferent pupillary defect.
10. RAPD is a feature of RBN, diagnosed by Swinging Flashlight Test.

11. Primary optic atrophy is chalky white in color with a clear disc margin.
12. Field defect in papilloedema is Enlargement of Blind Spot.
13. ARP, i.e., Argyll Robertson Pupil: Light reflex is absent and near reflex is present.
14. Wernicke's hemianopic pupil is a feature of optic tract lesion.
15. Position of eye in third nerve palsy is down and out.
16. Shortest part of nerve is intraocular, it is 1 mm.
17. Altitudinal field defect is a feature of NON-Arteritic AION.
18. Pseudo Foster Kennedy syndrome is a feature of NON-Arteritic AION.
19. INO, Internuclear ophthalmoplegia is a lesion of MLF, i.e., medial longitudinal fasciculus.
20. Bielchowsky sign: Increase of hypertropia on same side tilt is superior oblique palsy.
21. Horizontal gaze centre is located in PONS called PPRF, i.e., paramedian pontine reticular formation.
22. One-and-a-half syndrome: It is due to lesion of PPRF and MLF of the same side. It is characterised by defective adduction and abduction of the ipsilateral side and defective adduction of the contralateral side.
23. Vertical gaze centre is: riMLF (rostral interestitial nucleus of MLF) and nucleus of Cajal.

MULTIPLE CHOICE QUESTIONS

1. All statements are true about papilloedema except:

A. Extracellular edema
B. Disruption of neurofilament
C. Stasis of axoplasmic flow
D. Axonal swelling

2. Lamina Cribosa is absent in:

A. Morning-Glory syndrome
B. Nanophthalmos
C. Coloboma of retina
D. Optic nerve agenesis

3. Paralysis of 3rd, 4th and 6th nerves with involvement of ophthalmic division of 5th nerve, localizes the lesion to:

A. Cavernous sinus B. Apex of orbit
C. Brainstem D. Base of skull

4. Oculogyric crisis is known to be produced by all of the following drugs except:

A. Trifluoperazine B. Atropine
C. Perchlorperazine D. Perphenazine

5. The parvocellular pathway from lateral geniculate nucleus to visual cortex is most sensitive for the stimulus of:

A. Colour contrast
B. Luminance contrast
C. Temporal frequency
D. Saccadic eye movements

6. The fibers from the contralateral nasal hemiretina project to the following layers of the lateral geniculate nucleus:

A. Layers 2, 3 and 5
B. Layers 1, 2 and 6
C. Layers 1, 4 and 6
D. Layers 4, 5 and 6

7. Horner's syndrome is characterized by all of the following except:

A. Miosis B. Enophthalmos
C. Ptosis D. Cycloplegia

8. The most common condition of inherited blindness due to mitochondrial chromosomal anomaly is:

A. Retinopathy of prematurity
B. Leber's hereditary optic neuropathy
C. Retinitis pigmentosa
D. Retinal detachment

9. In the normal human right eye, the peripheral field of vision is usually least:

A. On the left side (nasally)
B. In the downward direction
C. In the upward direction
D. On the right side (temporally)

10. Any spectral colour can be matched by mixture of three monochromatic lights (red, green, blue) in different proportions. If a person needs more of one of the colour for matching than a normal person, then he has a colour anomaly. More red colour is needed in the case of:

A. Deuteranomaly
B. Tritanomaly
C. Protanomaly
D. Tritanopes

11. The colour best appreciated by the central cones of our foveomacular area are:

A. Red and blue
B. Blue and green
C. Red and green
D. Blue and yellow

12. Oculomotor nerve palsy affects all of the following muscles, except:

A. Medial rectus
B. Inferior oblique
C. Lateral rectus
D. Levator palpebrae superioris

13. Wernicke's hemianopic pupillary response is seen in lesions at:

A. Optic tract
B. Optic chiasma
C. Optic radiation
D. Lateral geniculate body

14. Chalky white optic disc on fundus examination is seen in all, except:

A. Syphilis
B. Lebers hereditary optic neuropathy
C. Post papilloedema optic neuritis
D. Traumatic injury to optic nerve

15. All of the following can cause optic neuritis except:

A. Rifampicin
B. Digoxin
C. Chloroquine
D. Ethambutol

16. A 40-year-old lady presents with bilateral papilloedema. CT scan shows normal ventricles. Diagnosis is:

A. Benign intracranial hypertension
B. Malignant hypertension
C. Papillitis
D. Raised intraocular pressure

17. Which of the following is not seen in increased intracranial tension?

A. Disc edema
B. Macular edema
C. Normal vision
D. Afferent pupillary defect

18. All the following are caused by third nerve palsy except:

A. Ptosis
B. Mydriasis
C. Medial deviation of eyeball
D. Pupillary reflex lost

19. In unilateral afferent pupillary defect, when light is moved from normal to affected eye there is:

A. Dilatation in affected eye and constriction in normal eye

B. Dilatation in normal eye and constriction in affected eye

C. Dilatation in both eyes

D. Constriction in both pupils

20. Right eye superotemporal quadrantopia, left eye centrocaecal scotoma with headache. Site of lesion is:

A. Left optic nerve + chiasma

B. Left optic tract + chiasma

C. Right optic nerve + chiasma

D. Right optic tract + chiasma

21. Functional defect of optic nerve can be diagnosed by:

A. Direct ophthalmoscopy

B. Indirect ophthalmoscopy

C. Perimetry and field charting

D. Retinoscopy

22. All of the following constitute Horner's syndrome except:

A. Ptosis

B. Exophthalmos

C. Anhydrosis

D. Loss of ciliospinal reflex

23. All are true about papilloedema except:

A. It is purely non-inflammatory phenomenon

B. Transient loss of vision

C. 1st sign is blurring of nasal side of optic disc

D. Sudden painful eye movement

24. The afferent pathway for light pupillary reflex is:

A. Trigeminal nerve

B. Optic nerve

C. Abducent nerve

D. Ciliary nerve

25. Bitemporal hemianopic field defect is characteristic of:

A. Glaucoma

B. Optic neuritis

C. Pituitary tumour

D. Retinal detachment

26. A female presented with loss of vision in both eyes and on examination has normal pupillary responses and normal fundus. Her visually evoked response (VER) examination shows extinguished responses. The most likely diagnosis is:

A. Hysteria

B. Cortical blindness

C. Optic neuritis

D. Retinal detachment

27. Idiopathic nyctalopia is due to a hereditary:

A. Absence of rod function

B. Absence of cone function

C. Absence of both rod and cone function

D. Decrease of cone function

28. A patient has a right homonymous hemianopia with saccadic pursuit movements and defective optokinetic nystagmus. The lesion is most likely to be in the:

A. Frontal lobe

B. Parietal lobe

C. Occipital lobe

D. Temporal lobe

29. Which of the following best defines the "Saccade"?

A. Voluntary slow eye movements
B. Involuntary slow eye movements
C. Abrupt, involuntary slow eye movements
D. Abrupt, involuntary rapid eye movements

30. Which one of the following extra-ocular muscles is served by a contra-lateral brainstem subnucleus?

A. Superior rectus
B. Medial rectus
C. Inferior oblique
D. Inferior rectus

31. A patient presented with normal eyesight and absence of direct and consensual light reflexes. Which of the following cranial nerves is suspected to be lesioned?

A. Oculomotor B. Trochlear
C. Optic D. Abducent

32. A case of injury to right brow due to a fall from scooter presents with sudden loss of vision in the right eye. The pupil shows absent direct reflex but a normal consensual pupillary reflex is present. The fundus is normal. The treatment of choice is:

A. Intensive intravenous corticosteroids as prescribed for spinal injuries to be instituted within six hours
B. Pulse methylprednisolone 250 mg four times daily for three days
C. Oral prednisolone 1.5 mg/kg body weight
D. Emergency optic canal decompression

33. An optic nerve injury may result in all of the following except:

A. Loss of vision in that eye
B. Dilatation of pupil
C. Ptosis
D. Loss of light reflex

34. Ophthalmoplegic migraine means:

A. When headache is followed by complete paralysis of the III and VI nerve on the same side as the hemicrania
B. When the headache is followed by partial paralysis of the III nerve on the same side as the hemicrania without any scotoma
C. Headache associated with III, IV and VI nerve paralysis
D. Headache associated with optic neuritis

35. Horner's syndrome is best described by:

A. Miosis + ptosis
B. Miosis + anhydrosis
C. Anhydrosis + enophthalmos
D. Miosis + enophthalmos

36. Lesion in Meyers' loop of optic radiation causes:

A. Upper homonymous quadrantanopia
B. Lower homonymous quadrantanopia
C. Unilateral anopia
D. Contralateral hemianopia

37. Protanopia is inability to see which colour?

A. Yellow B. Green
C. Blue D. Red

38. Internuclear ophthalmoplegia results due to involvement of:

A. Medial longitudinal bundle
B. Pontine reticular formation
C. Cerebellum
D. Motor nuclear sparing Edinger-Westphal nucleus

39. Which of these is not useful in arriving at a diagnosis of moderate papilloedema in a patient of head injury?

A. Impaired pupillary reflex

B. Hyperaemia

C. Filling of the physiological cup

D. Blurring of the margins

40. Basanti, a 20-year-old female, presents with complaints of difficulty in reading near print. On examination there is ptosis and diplopia in looking in all directions. What is the most probable diagnosis?

A. Lateral rectus palsy

B. Oculomotor palsy

C. Presbyopia

D. Myasthenia gravis

41. A patient with suprasellar extension of pituitary tumor presents with:

A. Bitemporal hemianopia

B. Binasal hemianopia

C. Pie in the sky

D. Right homonymous hemianopia

42. Homonymous (superior) quadrantanopia is seen in lesion of:

A. Temporal lobe

B. Frontal lobe

C. Occipital lobe

D. Parietal lobe

43. Abducent nerve palsy cause:

A. Convergent squint

B. Limitation in upward movement

C. Limitation in downward movement

D. Divergent squint

44. Which is not a clinical feature of right sided VI nerve palsy?

A. Medial convergent squint

B. Face turn to left

C. Inability to abduct right eye

D. Diplopia

45. All are features of optic nerve disease, except:

A. Afferent pupillary defect

B. Sudden loss of vision

C. Headache and vomiting

D. Pain on movement of eyeball

46. Optic chiasma lesions will cause:

A. Bitemporal hemianopia

B. Superior quadrantanopia

C. Unilateral blindness

D. Inferior quadrantanopia

E. Nasal blindness

47. Homonymous hemianopia is seen in lesion of:

A. Optic tract

B. Optic chiasma

C. Optic radiation

D. Optic nerve

E. Occipital cortex

48. The visual pathway consists of all of these except:

A. Optic tract

B. Geniculocalcarine tract

C. Inferior colliculus

D. Lateral geniculate body

E. Pretectal region

49. Components of pupillary light reflex are:

A. Retina

B. Pretectal nucleus

C. Lateral geniculate body

D. Edinger-Westphal nucleus

E. Calcarine sulcus

50. Field defect seen in pituitary adenoma:

A. Bitemporal hemianopia

B. Binasal hemianopia

C. Quadrantanopia

D. "Pie in sky" defect

E. Amaurosis in one eye and temporal hemianopia in other eye

51. Optic neuritis is seen in all except:

A. DM

B. Methanol poisoning

C. Multiple sclerosis

D. SLE

52. Loss of convergence with slight light reflex is seen in:

A. ARP

B. Holmes Adie pupil

C. Marcus Gunn pupil

D. Wernicke's pupil

53. Pupil that responds to convergence but light reflex is absent:

A. Adie's pupil

B. Argyll Robertson pupil

C. Hutchison pupil

D. Myotonic pupil

54. Down beat nystagmus could be due to:

A. Cerebellar lesion

B. Arnold-Chiari malformation

C. Optic neuritis

D. Pontine lesion

55. In pupillary reflex nerve tested is:

A. 2nd

B. 3rd

C. Both 2nd and 3rd

D. 4th

56. Homonymous hemianopia is seen in:

A. Pituitary adenoma

B. Optic nerve damage

C. Post chiasmic damage

D. Cortical lesion

57. Bitemporal hemianopia can be due to:

A. Third ventricle tumour

B. Meningioma of sella turcica

C. Calcarine cortex infarction

D. Aneurysm circle of Willis

58. Pseudopapilloedema is characterized by all except:

A. Field defect

B. Myopia

C. Drusen

D. Spontaneous venous pulsations

59. Pupillomotor fibres of third cranial nerve travel alongwith:

A. Nerve to medial rectus

B. Nerve to superior rectus

C. Nerve to inferior rectus

D. Nerve to inferior oblique

60. Bilateral internal ophthalmoplegia is seen in:

A. Diabetes mellitus

B. Myasthenia gravis

C. Multiple sclerosis

D. Thyrotoxicosis

61. Lesion in Argyll Robertson pupil is in:

A. Edinger-Westphal nucleus and optic radiation

B. Edinger-Westphal nucleus and ciliary ganglion

C. Pretectal nucleus and Edinger-Westphal nucleus

D. Ciliary muscle

62. Arterial blood supply of visual cortex is by:

A. Posteromedial branch of posterior cerebral artery

B. Posterolateral branch of posterior cerebral artery

C. Posterior inferior cerebellar artery

D. Vertebral artery

63. Dilator pupillae is supplied by:

A. Cholinergic fibres of oculomotor nerve

B. Ophthalmic division of trigeminal nerve

C. Facial nerve

D. Adrenergic fibres of oculomotor nerve

64. Optic tract lesion of left side manifests:

A. Left Homonymous hemianopia

B. Right homonymous hemianopia

C. Bitemporal hemianopia

D. Total left eye blindness

65. Lesion at optic chiasma causes:

A. Homonymous hemianopia

B. Heteronymous hemianopia

C. Quadrantanopia

D. Unilateral blindness

66. Which is a feature of Foster-Kennedy syndrome?

A. Ipsilateral atrophy

B. Ipsilateral papilloedema

C. Contralateral papilloedema

D. Glioma of optic nerve

67. Optic neuritis is a complication of heavy dose of:

A. Methyl alcohol

B. Ethyl alcohol

C. Disulfiram

D. Piracetam

68. All are true about Adie's pupil except:

A. Miosis

B. Slow dilatation

C. Slow contraction

D. Absent knee jerk

69. Nystagmus is caused by lesion of:

A. Pons

B. Medulla

C. Cerebrum

D. Cerebellum

70. The graph of the movement of the eye is called:

A. Electroretinogram

B. Electroencephalogram

C. Electronystagmogram

D. Electrocardiogram

71. Hutchinson's pupil is:

A. Seen in syphilis

B. Unilateral miosis followed by mydriasis

C. Irregular pupil

D. Argyl Robertson pupil

72. Angry sun appearance is a feature of:

A. Primary optic atrophy

B. Papilloedema

C. Papillitis

D. Drusen's rings

73. Miners nystagmus is of which type?

A. Lateral B. Vertical

C. Rotatory D. Jerky

74. The field defect in tobacco amblyopia is:

A. Central

B. Centrocaecal

C. Altitudinal

D. Enlargement of blind spot

75. Second order neurons in optical pathway are present in:

A. Retina

B. Lateral geniculate body

C. Medial geniculate body

D. Superior colliculus

76. Pupillary reaction will be altered in injury to the following pathway:

A. Optic nerve

B. Optic tract

C. Optic chiasma

D. Optic radiations

77. Macular sparing is seen in the affection of:

A. Optic nerve

B. Optic chiasma

C. Optic tract

D. Occipital lobe

78. Marcus Gunn pupil is due to:

A. Defect anterior to optic chiasma

B. Defect at optic chiasma

C. Defect posterior to optic chiasma

D. Defect in ciliary muscles

79. Which is not a feature of tobacco amblyopia?

A. Bilateral involvement

B. Normal fundus

C. Ganglion cell degeneration

D. Peripheral scotoma

80. Sudden loss of vision occurs in all of the following except:

A. Retrobulbar neuritis

B. Central retinal artery occlusion

C. Papilloedema

D. Retinal detachment

81. Ipsilateral loss of all movements of eyeball except lateral rotation with contralateral hemiplegia is due to lesion in the:

A. Pons B. Medulla

C. Midbrain D. Motor cortex

82. Most common type of color blindness is:

A. Protanopes

B. Tritanopes

C. Deutaranopes

D. Both A and C

83. Blind spot enlargement indicates:

A. Retinal detachment

B. Avulsion of the optic nerve

C. Papilloedema

D. Papillitis

84. Twilight vision is due to:

A. Rods B. Cones

C. Both D. None

85. In Weber's syndrome there is:

A. 3rd nerve palsy

B. 4th nerve palsy

C. 6th nerve palsy

D. 7th nerve palsy

86. In uraemic amaurosis the pupils are:

A. Constricted

B. Dilated and do not react to light

C. Dilated and react to light

D. Normal sized pupil

87. Scintillating scotoma is seen in:

A. Migraine

B. Hypertension

C. Transient ischemic attacks

D. Myasthenia gravis

88. The most common cranial nerve involved in ophthalmoplegic migraine:

A. 2nd nerve

B. 3rd nerve

C. 6th nerve

D. 4th nerve

89. Most common adverse effect on eye in using oral contraceptive is:

A. Colour blindness

B. Ring scotoma

C. Optic neuritis

D. Nystagmus

90. Diplopia with limitation of adduction of right eye with abduction saccades of left eye and normal convergence is due to:

A. Duane's retraction syndrome

B. Partial 3rd nerve palsy

C. Internuclear ophthalmoplegia

D. Absence of medial rectus

91. Young man with blurring of vision in right eye, followed by left eye after 3 months, showing disc hyperemia, edema, circumpapillary telangiectasia with normal pupillary response with centrocaecal scotoma on perimetry, the cause can be:

A. Typical optic neuritis

B. Lebers hereditary optic neuropathy

C. Papilloedema

D. Toxic optic neuritis

92. All are seen in Argyl Robertson pupil except:

A. Near reflex normal

B. Direct reflex absent

C. Consensual reflex normal

D. Vision normal

93. A patient presents with headache with bitemporal hemianopia with 6/6 vision this condition is seen with:

A. Trauma

B. Chiasmal lesion

C. Bilateral cavernous sinus thrombosis

D. Optic neuritis

94. Pupillary sparing 3rd nerve palsy is seen with:

A. Diabetes

B. Tumor

C. Raised ICT

D. Saccular aneurysm

95. Not associated with Horner's syndrome:

A. Miosis

B. Apparent exophthalmos

C. Anhydrosis of local area

D. Heterochromia

96. Pseudopapillitis is seen in:

A. Myopia B. Squint

C. Presbyopia D. Hypermetropia

97. Pupil that respond to convergence but light reflex is absent:

A. Adie's pupil

B. Argyll Robertson pupil

C. Hutchinson's pupil

D. Myotonic pupil

98. Field defect in pituitary adenoma is:

A. Bitemporal hemianopia

B. Binasal hemianopia

C. Quandrantopia

D. Pie-in sky

99. Blind spot enlargement indicates:

A. Retinal detachment

B. Optic nerve injury

C. Papilloedema

D. Papillitis

100. Topical administration of 1% pilocarpine failed to produce pupillary constriction in a patient who had a large dilated pupil. What could be most probable reason?

A. Diabetic III cranial nerve palsy

B. Adie's tonic pupil

C. Pharmacological blockade

D. Uncal herniation

101. Dilator pupillae is supplied by:

A. Post ganglionic parasympathetic fibers from Edinger-Westphal nucleus

B. Post ganglionic sympathetic fibers from cervical sympathetic chain

C. III nerve

D. Sympathetic fibers from fronto orbital branch of V nerve

102. All are seen in 3rd nerve palsy except:

A. Ptosis

B. Diplopia

C. Miosis

D. Outwards eye deviation

103. A 25-year-old lady presents with sudden, severe bilateral loss of vision more so on right side with no perception of light. Rest of the examination including Pupillary reflex, fundus and optokinetic nystagmus are normal. She was able to touch tips of her finger with right eye closed but not with left eye closed. Most likely diagnosis:

A. Optic neuritis

B. Anterior ischaemic optic neuropathy

C. CMV retinitis

D. Funtional visual loss

104. Fundoscopy of a patient shows chalky white optic disc, rest of the retina is absolutely normal, probable diagnosis is:

A. Primary optic atrophy

B. Post neuritic optic atrophy

C. Glaucomatous atrophy

D. Consecutive optic atrophy

105. Optic atrophy is not seen in:

A. Retinitis pigmentosa

B. CRAO

C. Choroidal vasculopathy

D. Methanol poisoning

106. Painless loss of vision is seen in all except:

A. Papilloedema

B. Papillitis

C. Angle closure glaucoma

D. CRAO

107. Methyl alcohol causes blindness by acting on:

A. Ganglion cells

B. Nerve fibers

C. Rods amd Cones

D. Rods only

108. Keyhole shaped visual field defect is a feature of:

A. LGB

B. Occipital lobe lesion

C. Optic tract

D. Optic radiations

ANSWER AND EXPLANATION

1. b Axons are not damaged in papilloedema. There is only axonal swelling due to stasis of axoplasmic flow.
2. a It is a dysplastic coloboma of the optic disc. Lamina Cribosa is a part of sclera at the optic disc.
3. a All the nerves, i.e., 3, 4, 5 and 6 pass through the cavernous sinus. Sixth passes through the body of the sinus alongwith internal carotid artery whereas the rest of the nerves pass along the wall.
4. b It is a spasmodic conjugate movement of eyes along with the synergic movement of head and neck. It occurs due to phenothiazine idiosyncrasy.
5. a Pathway of color vision passes from the X ganglion cells through the parvocellular layer of the LGB to the layer IV c of the visual cortex.
6. c LGB: 1, 4, 6 has contralateral supply, whereas 2, 3, 5 has ipsilateral supply.
7. d Horner's syndrome is caused by the lesion of the sympathetic chain.
8. b Leber's hereditary optic neuropathy occurs due to mutation in the maternal mitochondrial DNA.
9. c Visual field in the normal eye is least superiorly and maximum temporally.
10. c Defective red color appreciation protanomalous, defective for green color is deuteranomalous and defective blue color is tritanomalous.
11. c The very centre of the fovea is blue blind.
12. c LR-6/SO-4, i.e., lateral rectus is supplied by sixth nerve whereas Superior oblique is supplied by fourth nerve.
13. a Wernicke's hemianopic pupil is when the pupil reacts to light thrown into the eye from one direction whereas in the same eye, it does not react when the light is shown from the opposite direction.
14. c Chalky white optic disc is a characteristic of primary optic atrophy. Post papilloedema there is secondary optic atrophy.
15. a The degenerative optic atrophy caused by these drugs is called toxic amblyopia.
16. a It is also called Pseudotumour cerebri and is characterized by increased intracranial tension with normal intracranial findings and normal composition of the CSF.
17. d Increased ICT causes papilloedema and the pupillary reactions are normal. APD is seen in optic neuritis and not in papilloedema.
18. c The position of the eye in third nerve palsy is down and out.
19. c This is due to absence of both direct and consensual light reflex in the diseased eye.
20. a This type of field defect is seen in meningiomas where the lesion is at the junction of optic nerve and the chiasma. This is called "junctional scotoma of Traquair".
21. c Non-seeing area in the visual field is called scotoma and is diagnosed by perimetry, i.e., field charting.
22. b In Horner's there is enophthalmos and not exophthalmos. This enoph-

thalmos is apparent enophthalmos due to unilateral ptosis.

23. d Papilloedema is a painless condition and not painful.

24. b Afferent pathway of the pupillary light reflex travels from the optic nerve to the chiasma, optic tract, pretectal nucleus and Edinger-Westphal nucleus.

25. c Pituitary adenoma causes chiasmal lesion leading to Bitemporal hemianopia.

26. b In cortical blindness the pupillary reactions are normal. VEP shows the activity from the ganglion cells to the cortex.

27. a Rods are responsible for the night vision whereas cones are responsible for day vision and color vision.

28. b Optokinetic nystagmus is a physiological nystagmus. If defective, the first diagnosis is parietal lobe lesion.

29. d Saccadic movement refixes the object on the fovea whereas pursuit is a following movement.

30. a Innervation of superior rectus is contralateral, rest all recti have ipsilateral innervation.

31. a Efferent pathway for the pupillary light reflex is through third nerve.

32. d Absent direct light reflex with normal consensual reflex indicates optic nerve injury and hence the best course of management is to decompress the orbital cavity immediately to save the nerve.

33. c LPS is supplied by third nerve and hence ptosis is a feature of the oculomotor palsy.

34. b Ophthalmoplegic migraine involves the paralysis of the third nerve.

35. a Anhydrosis, i.e., loss of sweating, does not occur in all cases of Horner's syndrome. Enophthalmos in Horner's is apparent enophthalmos due to ipsilateral ptosis.

36. a Meyer's loop constitutes inferior fibres of the optic radiations looping around the temporal horn.

37. d Protanopia-red/deteuranopia-green/tritanopia-blue.

38. a INO occurs due to lesion of the MLF. It can occur due to both vascular and degenerative cause.

39. a Pupillary reactions are normal in papilloedema.

40. d Diplopia in all directions indicates involvement of all muscles which can occur in a myopathy.

41. a Pituitary adenoma in suprasellar extension will involve the chiasma.

42. a Superior quadrantanopia is a feature of temporal lobe lesion also called Pie-in-sky.

43. a Abducent supplies lateral rectus and hence its palsy will cause convergent squint.

44. b In right-sided sixth nerve palsy the face will turn to the right.

45. c Headache and vomiting are signs of increased intracranial tension.

46. a,b,d Chiasmal lesions will manifest according to the location of the lesion. If few fibres of the chiasma are involved, as in junctional scotoma of Traquair then it will lead to quadrantanopia.

47. a,c,e The only lesions which are heteronymous are chiasmal lesions.

48. c,e Pretectal nucleus is a part of pupillary light reflex pathway.

49. a,b,d Light reflex pathway does not reach the lateral geniculate body but deviates from the optic tract.
50. a,c It is due to involvement of the chiasma.
51. a Diabetes mellitus commonly causes ophthalmoplegia (III nerve) with pupillary sparing.
52. b Holme's Adie pupil occurs due to lesion of the ciliary ganglion and short ciliary nerves. It affects the accommodation and convergence with mild reaction to the light.
53. b It is called Light-Near dissociation. Light reflex is absent but accommodation reflex and convergence are present.
54. b Downbeat nystagmus is a jerky nystagmus with fast phase downwards.
55. c Afferent is through the optic nerve whereas efferent is through third nerve.
56. c,d Any damage below the chiasma is homonymous.
57. b,d Cortical lesions are always homonymous. Both aneurysm of Circle of Willis and meningioma can affect the chiasma.
58. b Blurred disc margins with neither papilloedema nor papillitis are called Pseudopapillitis or pseudopapilloedema.
59. d Pupillomotor fibres travel through the inferior division of the third nerve, then through the nerve to inferior oblique, it reaches the ciliary ganglion.
60. a Internal ophthalmoplegia is third nerve palsy involving only the internal muscles, i.e., iris sphincter and ciliary muscles.
61. c ARP is light reflex absent and near reflex present.
62. b Visual cortex has dual blood supply, i.e., posterior cerebral artery and middle cerebral artery.
63. b Dilator pupillae has sympathetic supply whereas iris sphincter has parasympathetic supply.
64. b Field defect is always opposite to the side of the lesion because projection is always in opposite direction.
65. b Chiasma constitutes of the nasal fibres of both eyes and hence the lesion is heteronymous.
66. c FK syndrome is ipsilateral optic atrophy and contralateral papilloedema.
67. b Ethyl alcohol, when taken for a long time causes optic neuritis due to deficiency of vitamin B.
68. a In Adie's pupil, the pupil is mid-dilated.
69. d Cerebellar lesions cause past-pointing nystagmus.
70. c Nystagmus is involuntary to and fro movement of the eyeball.
71. b In Hutchinson's pupil, initially there is constriction followed by the dilatation of the pupil.
72. b Papilloedema is characterized by blurred disc margin and tortuous veins.
73. c Miner's nystagmus occurs in people who work in mines.
74. b Tobacco causes degenerative optic neuritis.
75. a Second order neurons are the ganglion cells whereas first order neurons are the bipolar cells.

76. a Pupillary reaction will be altered in the lesion of all three pathways, i.e., optic nerve, optic chiasma and optic tract.

77. d Macula sparing homonymous hemianopia occurs if posterior cerebral artery is blocked.

78. a Marcus Gunn pupil is also called relative afferent pupillary defect and occurs in retrobulbar neuritis.

79. d It causes central or centrocaecal scotoma. Fundus in later stages may show the picture of optic neuritis but we mark the best possible option.

80. c Visual acuity is normal in papilloedema.

81. c This condition is termed as Webers syndrome and is characterized by third nerve palsy with contralateral hemiplegia due to involvement of the cerebral peduncle.

82. c Most common is defective perception of green colour.

83. c Field defect in papilloedema is enlargement of the blind spot.

84. a Rods are responsible for night vision.

85. a See 81.

86. c Amaurosis is total loss of vision.

87. a Migraine can be preceded by visual aura, seen as scintillating scotoma.

88. b Migraine with III nerve palsy is ophthalmoplegic migraine.

89. c OCPs can cause optic neuritis.

90. c INO is lesion of the MLF with defective ipsilateral adduction, and contralateral abducting eye shows ataxic nystagmus.

91. b Lebers hereditary optic neuropathy presents as optic neuritis but it is atypical as the pupillary reactions are normal.

92. c ARP, i.e., Accommodation Reflex Present.

93. b Bitemporal hemianopia is a feature of chiasmal lesion.

94. a In diabetes it is the vasa nervorum (at the core of the third nerve) which is involved first and hence there is pupillary sparing (pupillary fibres are at the surface of the nerve).

95. b In Horner's syndrome there is enophthalmos and not exophthalmos. (It is not a true enophthalmos but an apparent enophthalmos).

96. d Pseudopapillitis in hypermetropia is due to small size of lamina cribosa which leads to a picture of blurred disc margin.

97. b ARP is light-near dissociation, i.e., light reflex absent and accommodation reflex present.

98. a Pituitary adenoma involves the chiasma.

99. c Papilloedema is edema around the optic disc and since optic disc is blind spot in the field chart therefore in papilloedema there is enlargement of blind spot.

100. c In Adie pupil there is denervation hypersensitivity and hence the pupil reacts even with very low dose of pilocarpine. In diabetic 3rd nerve palsy there will be pupillary sparing whereas in uncal herniation there will be surgical 3rd nerve palsy, hence pupillary fibres will be involved but it should react to pilocarpine.

Pharmacological blockade indicates that patient has used a mydriatic and hence there is no action of pilocarpine.

101. b Ophthalmic division of trigeminal, i.e., ophthalmic nerve arises from the

trigeminal ganglion, and in the cavernous sinus it divides into three branches, i.e., lacrimal, frontal and nasociliary. Nasociliary enters the orbit through SOF and one of its branches is long ciliary nerves. These long ciliary nerves carry the motor sympathetic nerve to dilator pupillae. They also carry sensory nerves to cornea, iris and ciliary body.

102. c 3rd nerve supplies iris sphincter, and hence its palsy will lead to mydriasis.

103. d Pupillary reactions will not be normal in optic neuritis and anterior ischemic optic neuropathy and fundus shows blurred disc margin. In CMV retinitis, fundus shows sauce and cheese retinopathy. The above symptoms are more in favour of functional visual loss.

104. a Chalky white optic disc is diagnostic of primary optic atrophy. In primary optic atrophy the cause is not in the eye but in the brain and hence both anterior and posterior segment is normal.

105. c This is the least common among all options.

106. c Angle closure glaucoma is painful due to high pressure. Though papilloedema visual acuity is normal but this is the best possible option.

107. a Methyl alcohol directly damages the ganglion cells.

108. a Keyhole shaped scotoma is a feature of LGB lesion, and keyhole vision is a feature of bilateral occipital lobe lesion, where there is macula sparing homonymous hemianopia of both sides causing tubular or keyhole vision.

RECENTLY ADDED QUESTIONS

1. **Which of the following is the nucleus for upwards gaze?**
   A. Paramedian pontine reticular formation
   B. Nucleus raphe magnus
   C. Cuneiform nucleus
   D. Nucleus of Cajal
2. **In diabetic 3rd nerve palsy all are seen except:**
   A. Normal pupillary reflex
   B. Ptosis
   C. Outward downward rolling of pupil
   D. Impaired pupillary reflex
3. **Visual pathway defect at the level of optic chiasma will result in:**
   A. Binasal hemianopia
   B. Bitemporal hemianopia
   C. Central scotoma
   D. Bilateral hemianopia
4. **A 50-year-old patient presented with a history of STD and came to OPD with neurological abnormality. Which of the following is true?**
   A. Normal light reflex, accommodation reflex lost
   B. Absent light reflex, accommodation reflex normal
   C. Both lost
   D. Both normal
5. **Unilateral enlarged pupil is seen in:**
   A. Horner syndrome
   B. Adie's tonic pupil
   C. Marcus-gunn pupil
   D. Argyll-Robertson pupil
6. **A person present with painful unilateral dimness of vision. He gives a history of persistence of after images. What is the likely diagnosis?**
   A. Retrobulbar neuritis
   B. Papilledema
   C. Ocular ischemic syndrome
   D. CRVO

ANSWERS OF RECENTLY ADDED QUESTIONS

1. d The centre for upward gaze is rostral interestitial nucleus of MLF and nucleus of Cajal.
2. d The pupillary fibres of third nerve are spared in medical cause of third nerve palsy like diabetes and hypertension.
3. b **Bitemporal hemianopia**

   Lesion at the optic chiasma most commonly causes bitemporal hemianopia.

   The most common lesions producing the chiasmal lesion include:
   - Pituitary adenoma.
   - Parasellar meningioma.
   - Craniopharyngioma; and
   - Parasellar internal carotid artery aneurysm.
4. b The history suggests that the patient is suffering from syphilis. We expect Argyll Robertson pupil (i.e., light reflex absent and accommodation reflex present).
5. b In Adie's tonic pupil, unilaterally enlarged pupil is seen. There is absent/very sluggish light reflex and also very sluggish accommodation reflex.
6. a Persistence of after image is called palinopsia and may be a feature of optic neuritis.

   Retrobulbar neuritis can be caused by a variety of conditions, including:
   - Infections such as meningitis, syphilis, and various viral illnesses.
   - Multiple sclerosis.
   - Tumors.
   - Exposure to certain chemicals or drugs.
   - Allergic reactions.

   However, in many cases, the cause is unknown.

   Optic neuritis affects women twice as often as men and usually affects adults between the ages of 20 and 40.

IMAGE-BASED QUESTIONS

1. **The diagnosis is:**

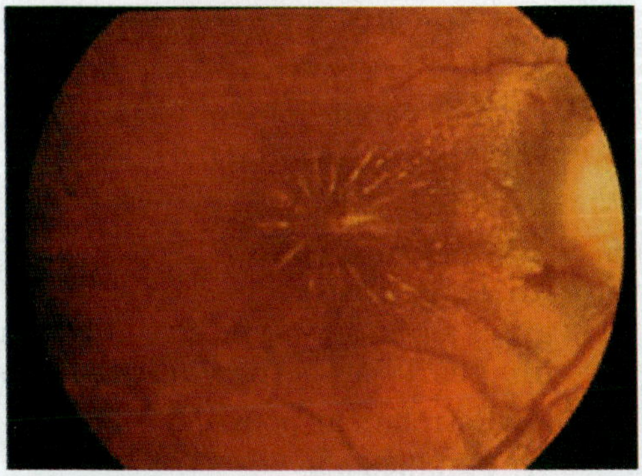

A. Papillitis
B. Neuroretinitis
C. Retrobulbar neuritis
D. Macular hole

2. **What is the visual field defect in the below given condition?**

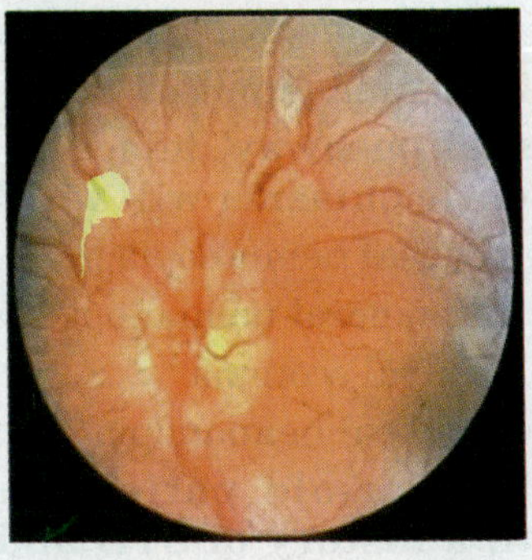

A. Central scotoma
B. Paracentral scotoma
C. Centrocaecal scotoma
D. Enlargement of blind spot

3. All are causes of the below given condition except:

Primary Optic Atrophy

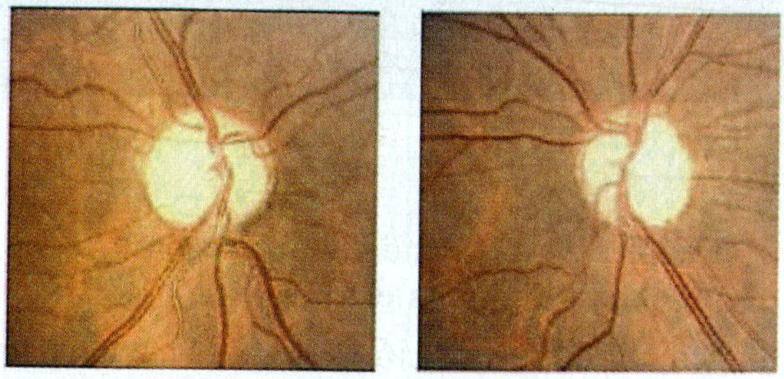

A. Multiple sclerosis
B. Neurosyphilis
C. Trauma
D. Papillitis

4. The diagnosis is:

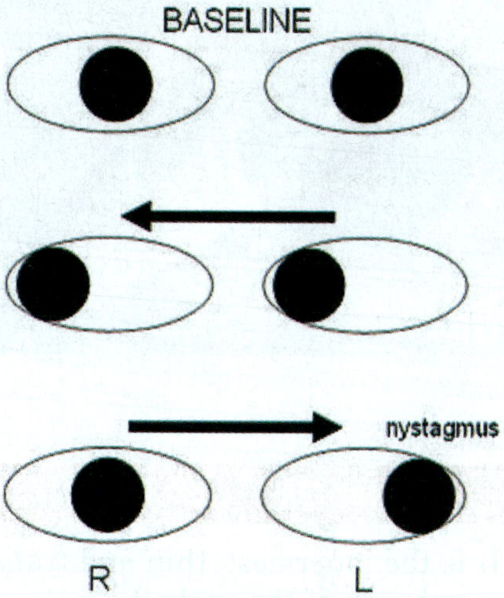

A. Right MLF lesion
B. Left MLF lesion
C. Right PPRF lesion
D. Left PPRF lesion

ANSWERS OF IMAGE-BASED QUESTIONS

1. b The slide shows macular star which is deposition of hard exudates at the macula and is a feature of neuro-retinitis.
2. d The above slide shows papilloedema, and hence the field defect is enlargement of blind spot in the early case and in late stage we get 'constriction of the visual field'.
3. d This is a slide of primary optic atrophy. Papillitis will lead to secondary optic atrophy.
4. a There is defective adduction on right side with nystagmus on the abducting eye, therefore the diagnosis is INO (internuclear ophthalmoplegia).

   Since there is defective adduction on the right side hence it's a right MLF lesion.

GUIDANCE

Strength is the source of happiness. We mustn't shy away from life's challenges. We mustn't be defeated. Refusing to be defeated equals victory.

CHAPTER 11

Fundus

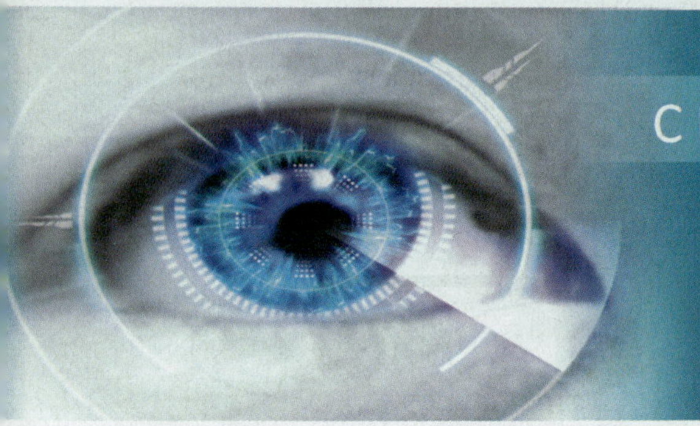

ANATOMY OF RETINA

- It is the innermost, thin and transparent membrane of the eyeball.
- Retina extends from optic disc to ora serrata and is ophthalmoscopically divided into 3 regions, i.e., optic disc, macula lutea, rest of peripheral retina.
- **Optic disc:** It is the area of exit of nerve fibres**. It is 1.5 mm in diameter**.
- **Macula:** It is an area of 5.5 mm situated at the posterior pole of the eyeball. It corresponds to 15° of the visual field. Photopic vision and colour vision are the primary functions of this area.
- Macula contains *Macula Lutea* which is 3 mm area of yellow coloration.
- **Fovea centralis:**
  - It is responsible for maximum visual acuity of the eye.
  - **It is the most sensitive part of the retina.**
  - It has the lowest threshold for light.
  - It is the central depressed part of macula.

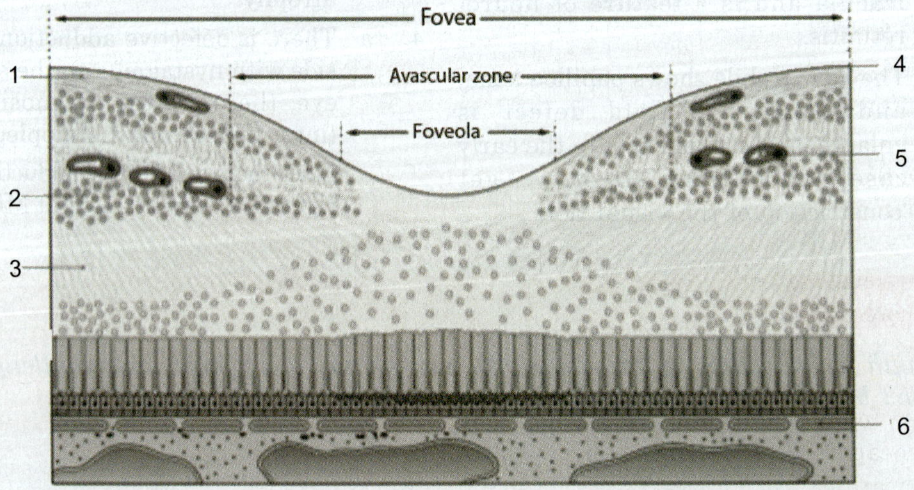

Fig. 11.1: 1. Nerve fibre layer, 2. Inner nuclear layer, 3. Outer plexiform (Henle's) layer, 4. Inner limiting membrane, 5. Retinal capillaries, 6. Choriocapillaries

- It is 1.85 mm in diameter.
- It accounts for 5° of visual field.
- It contains central area of 0.35 mm called *foveola*.
- **FAZ** (Foveal Avascular Zone): It constitutes the area inside the fovea but outside foveola.

- **Foveola:**
  1. It is 0.35 mm in diameter.
  2. It is 2 DD away from temporal margin of optic disc.
  3. It constitutes only of cones.
  4. **Umbo:** It is a tiny depression at the centre of foveola. This is what is seen as a foveal reflex.
- **Peripheral retina:** It is divided into four regions: (a) Near periphery (b) Mid periphery (c) Far periphery (d) Ora Serrata (serrated peripheral margin of retina).
- **Thickness of retina:**

Posterior pole	: 0.5 mm
Equator	: 0.2 mm
Ora serrata	: 0.1 mm.

- **Normal A : V (Artery : Vein) ratio is 2 : 3.**

  The above ratio is increased in certain situations like:

  a. **Hypertensive retinopathy:** Here due to the attenuation of arterioles, the ratio becomes 1:3.

  b. **Papilloedema:** Here due to dilatation of veins the ratio may become 2:4 or more.

Blood Supply of the Retina

1. Outer four layers are supplied by the choriocapillaris, i.e., the short posterior ciliary arteries.
2. Inner six layers are supplied by the central retinal artery.
3. The retina around the optic disc is supplied by the Circle of Haller and Zinn which is an anastomosis between short posterior ciliary arteries.

MICROSCOPIC STRUCTURE OF RETINA (OUT TO IN)

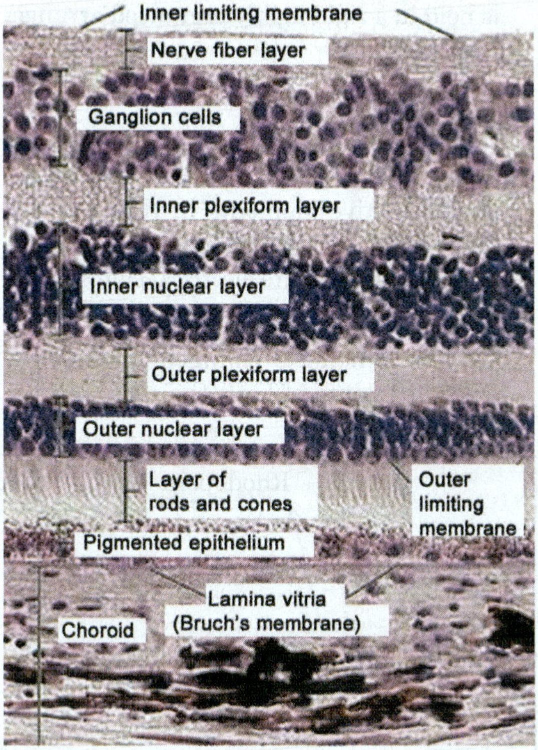

Fig. 11.2

1. **RPE.**
2. **Rods and cones.**
3. **External limiting membrane.**
4. **Outer nuclear layer.**
5. **Outer plexiform layer.**
6. **Inner nuclear layer.**
7. **Inner plexiform layer.**
8. **Ganglion cell layer.**
9. **Nerve fibre layer.**
10. **Internal limiting membrane.**

Rhodopsin (Visual purple)

- It is the photosensitive visual pigment present in the discs of the rod outer segments.
- It consists of a protein opsin (i.e., scotopsin) and a carotenoid called retinal. Rhodopsin is thus a membrane bound glycolipid which is held in a rigid highly organized arrangement.
- Human rhodopsin has a molecular weight of 40,000.
- Light falling on retina is absorbed by the photosensitive pigments in the rods and cones and initiates photochemical changes which in turn initiate electrical changes and in this way the process of vision sets in.
- The photochemical changes occur in the outer segments of both the rods and the cones.

Dietary vitamin A (Carotenes in plant food and retinol in animal food)

↓

Digestion and absorption of vitamin A from the food.

Transport in intestinal lymphatics

↓

1. Storage of vit. A in liver cells as retinol
2. Production of retinol – binding protein (the carrier protein)

↓

Transport of retinol bound to retinol binding protein

↓

1. Formation of rhodopsin used in night vision.
2. Maintenance of healthy corneal and conjunctival epithelial cells.

- In rods following changes occur: (i) rhodopsin bleaching (ii) rhodopsin regeneration (iii) visual cycle.

Visual Cycle (See Figure 11.3)

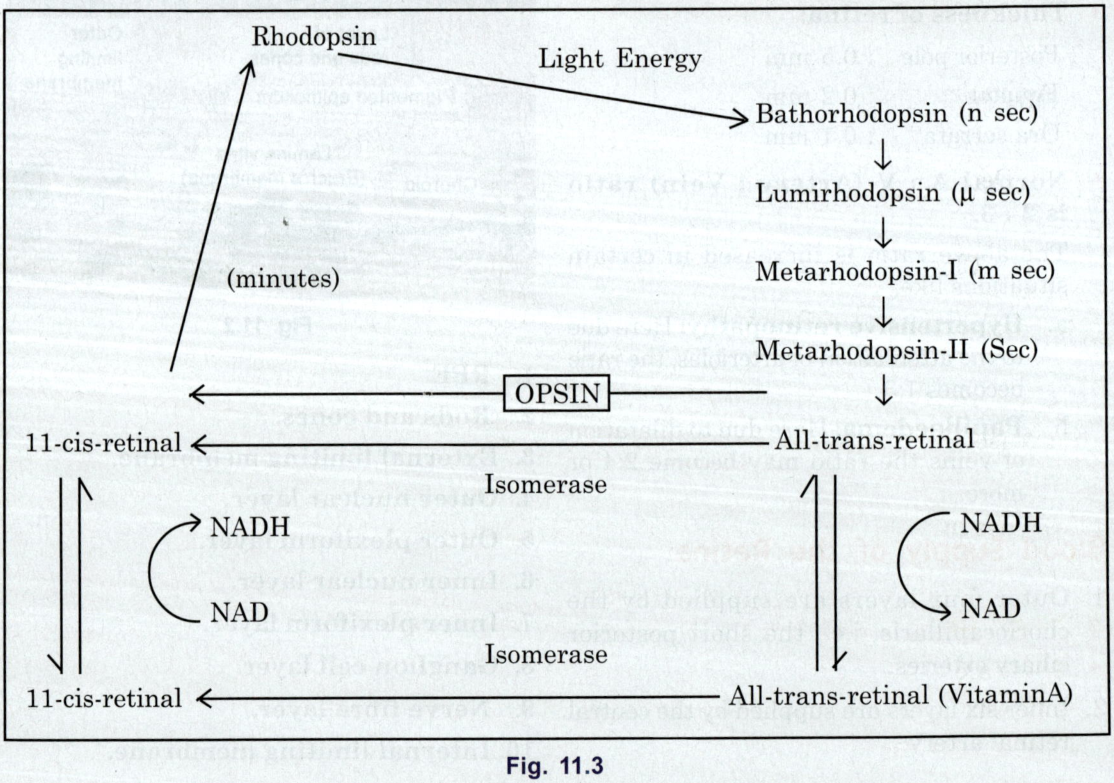

Fig. 11.3

Cone pigments: Like rhodopsin, cone pigments also consist of protein opsin (called photopsin) and the retinene (11 cis-retinal). Photopsin differs slightly from scotopsin (rhodopsin). There are three classes of cone pigments: red sensitive (Erythrolabe), green sensitive (Chlorolabe) and blue sensitive (Cyanolabe).

Photoreceptor Cells

Sequence of events involved in phototransduction process in the photoreceptors are:

Rhodopsin

↓ Incident light

All trans Retinal + Opsin ← Metarhodopsin II

↓

Activation of transduction

↓

Activation of phosphodiesterase

↓

Decreased intracellular cGMP

↓

Closure of Na+ channels

↓

Hyperpolarization

↓

Decreased release of synaptic transmitter

↓

Response in bipolar cells and other neural elements

Bipolar Cells

- These are the neurons of first order of visual pathway.
- Their dendrites are stimulated by the light induced hyperpolarization of the photoreceptors.
- Some bipolar cells depolarize and some hyperpolarize when the photoreceptors are excited. This may be because some receive direct excitation from photoreceptors and others indirectly through horizontal cells. This reciprocal relationship between bipolar cells provide a mechanism for lateral inhibition **(Spatial information processing).**

Muller Cells

These are supportive cells.

Retinal Astrocytes

- Astrocytes are a type of neuroglial cell (i.e., all non-neuronal cells of central nervous system).
- Astrocytes are highly branched cells whose footplates rest on capillary in the nervous tissue. They play both nutritive and structural role.

Amacrine Cells

Amacrine cells receive information at the synapse of the bipolar cell axon with ganglion cell dendrites, and use this information for temporal processing at the other end of the bipolar cell. Amacrine cell adjusts the bipolar cell in a negative feedback arrangement as to the subsequent response that will be projected onto the ganglion cell.

Horizontal Cells

Horizontal cells transmit signals horizontally in the outer plexiform layer from rods and cones to the bipolar cells. Their main function is to enhance the visual contrast by causing lateral inhibitions. Hence when a minute spot of light strikes the retina, the central most area is excited but the area around is inhibited by the horizontal cells. This allows high visual accuracy in transmitting contrast borders in the visual image.

Ganglion Cells

The electrical response of bipolar cells after modification by the amacrine cells is transmitted to the ganglion cells which in turn transmit their signals by means of action potential to the brain.

Types:

A. On center cell (increased discharge on illumination) and Off center cell (decrease their discharge on illumination).

B. W, X, Y cell.

W-ganglion

- Small sized.
- Widespread dendrites.
- Responsible for rod vision.
- Sensitive to directional movement.

X-ganglion

- Medium sized.
- Very small field as dendrites do not spread.
- **Responsible for color vision.**

Y-ganglion

- Largest.
- Very broad dendritic field.
- Respond to rapid changes in visual image either rapid movement or rapid change in light intensity.

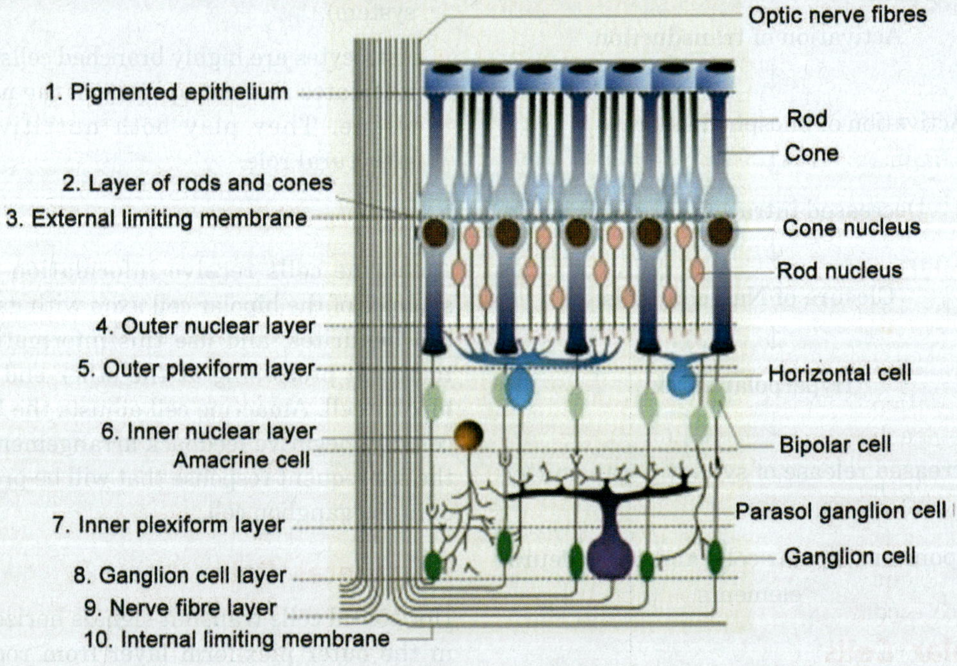

Fig. 11.4

METHODS OF EVALUATING MACULAR DISEASE

A. Clinical

1. Distortion of image, wavy lines, blurred areas or blank spots.
2. Positive scotoma.
3. Metamorphopsia.
4. Micropsia.
5. Visual acuity: Diminished.
6. Pupillary light reaction: Normal in eyes with macular disorders.
7. Colour vision: Not significantly impaired.

B. Amsler Grid Test

It evaluates 10° of visual field surrounding fixation. The Amsler grid chart consists of a 10 cm square divided into smaller 5 mm squares. When viewed at one third of a meter, each small square subtends an angle of 1°.

Uses:

a. For screening of macular disease.
b. Diagnosis of subtle optic nerve lesions.

C. Ophthalmoscopy

Specially with red-free light (Green light).

D. Photostress Test

This test is a gross version of dark adaptation test in which the visual pigments are bleached by light.

Procedure:

- Take the best corrected visual acuity.
- Patient fixes at a pen torch 3 cm away for 10 seconds.
- Record the time taken to read any three letters of the pre test acuity line (Photostress recovery time) – (PSRT).
- Results are compared in other eye.

PSRT is raised in macular lesion like (CME/CSR) but not in optic nerve lesions.

Methods of Evaluating Macular Disease in Opaque Media

1. *Two-point discrimination test:* It gives rough estimate of macular function.
2. *Pin hole test:* The pin hole aperture increases the depth of focus and limits the scattering effect of corneal scars and lenticular opacities.
3. *Maddox rod test:* The continuity of the rod produced by placing the Maddox rod in front of eye is assessed in all quadrants. Appearance of a break or distortion implies retinal pathology.
4. *Amsler–Grid:* To exclude the presence of metamorphopsia or scotoma.
5. *Purkinje vessel shadows:* It is based on entoptic phenomenon. Entoptic phenomenon refers to visualization of reproducible visual perceptions arising from within the eyes. It may be sensations arising from the normal intraocular structures or from opacities in the ocular media. Shadow of retinal vasculature should be visible if no retinal pathology.
6. *Blue-field Entoptoscope:* If no retinal pathology, flying dots (WBCs) should be visualized to be moving in a sinous manner in series of acceleration and deceleration in all four quadrants. This method is again based on entoptic phenomenon.
7. *Interferometers:* It is useful in eyes with immature cataract. The test provides a measure of the resolving power of the macula by using two coherent light beams to create a three dimensional fringe pattern on retina (in form of black and white bands). The patient is asked to indicate the orientation of the bands.

Initially larger gratings are used and then they are gradually diminished.

8. *PAM–Potential Acuity Meter:* It projects a standard snellen chart through a small clear area of an immature cataract. It is most accurate in eyes with visual acuities of 6/60 or better.
9. *Electrophysiological tests:*
   a. ERG–Electroretinogram.
   b. VEP–Visual Evolved Potential.

OPHTHALMIC ELECTRODIAGNOSTIC TESTS

1. ERG (Electroretinogram)

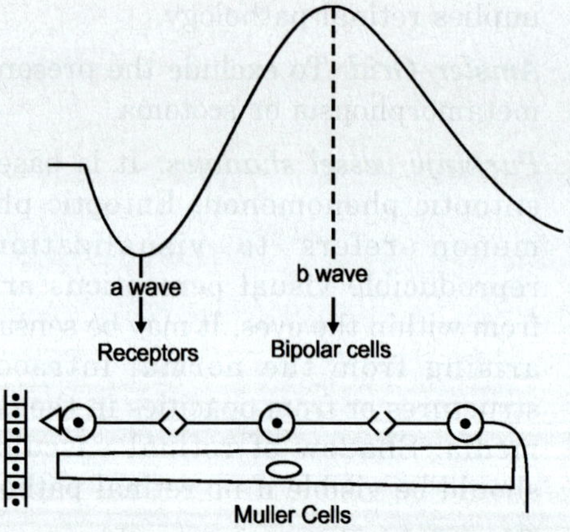

Fig. 11.5: Origins of electroretinogram

- Electroretinogram is the record of an action potential produced by the retina when it is stimulated by light of adequate intensity. It is elicited both in photopic and scotopic state.
- *Usual response is biphasic:*
  a. a wave (Due to Photoreceptor activity).
  b. b wave (Due to Bipolar cell activity).

  b wave has two components:
  b1 and b2.
  b1–both rod and cone activity.
  b2–only cone activity.
- Rod responses can be isolated by stimulating fully dark adapted eye with a flash of dim light.
- Cone responses can be isolated by fully light—adapted eye with bright flash of light, **OR** by using a flicker light stimulus of 30–40 Hz.
- **In RP:**
  i. ERG amplitudes are markedly subnormal.
  ii. Mainly scotopic ERG is affected whereas photopic response is unaffected.

2. VEP (Visual Evoked Potential)

When light falls on the retina there is series of nerve impulses generated and passed to the visual cortex. Hence it is EEG recorded in the visual cortex. It indicates the activity from ganglion cell layer to the visual cortex.

3. EOG (Electrooculogram)

Electrooculogram measures the standing action potential between the electrically negative cornea and electrically positive back of the eye. It reflects the activity of the RPE and the photoreceptors. **It is only affected by widespread diseases of the RPE.**

FLUORESCEIN ANGIOGRAPHY (FA)

FA is used in studying the normal physio-logy of the retinal and choroidal circulation and to detect any changes in vasculature produced by various fundus disorders.

Technique: Injection of 5 ml of 10% solution of sterile sodium fluorescein dye in **antecubital vein** and taking serial photographs of fundus. First photograph is taken **after 5 seconds,** then every second for next 20 seconds and every 3–5 seconds for next one minute. Last pictures are taken after 10 minutes.

The structures examined by the fluorescein angiography are the uveal tissue, i.e., iris, ciliary body and choroid and the retina. Avascular structures like lens and cornea cannot be seen.

Results: It may be normal, hypofluorescence or hyperfluorescence.

Hypofluorescence: It may be due to blocked fluorescence as a result of any haemorrhage or exudates or CNP, i.e., capillary nonperfusion.

Hyperfluorescence: It may be due to leakage or RPE defects. A leakage will increase in size, but size of RPE defects will remain normal.

D/D: Sudden painless loss of vision.

1. Central retinal artery occlusion.
2. Vitreous haemorrhage.
3. Retinal detachment.
4. Central retinal vein occlusion.
5. Central serous retinopathy.
6. Optic neuritis.
7. Methyl alcohol amblyopia.

D/D: Sudden painful loss of vision.

1. Acute congestive glaucoma.
2. Acute iridocyclitis.
3. Chemical injuries to eyeball.
4. Mechanical injuries to the eyeball.

DIABETIC RETINOPATHY (DR)

Definition

It's a microangiopathy affecting the retinal precapillary arterioles, capillaries and venules.

Pathogenesis of Diabetic Retinopathy

Following factors play role:

1. *Hypoxia:* This is due to:
   a. Decreased 2, 3 diphosphoglycerate leads to decreased oxygen release.
   b. Increased levels of glycosylated haemoglobin: These have greater oxygen binding capacity.
2. *Excessive glucose:* Polyol pathway intracellular accumulation of sorbitol and fructose increased osmotic pressure cellular edema.
3. *Impaired glucose metabolism:* Release of growth hormone increase in fibrinogen and alpha-2 globulin hyperaggregation of RBCs and platelets.

Hence retinal changes in diabetes are due to glycosylated end products, whereas cataract due to diabetes is due to sorbitol accumulation.

Pathophysiology

In diabetic retinopathy, loss of pericytes

↓

Mechanical weakening of capillary wall

↓

Focal dilatation (along with disruption of blood retinal barrier)

↓

Formation of Microaneurysms

Hence microaneurysms are commonly found around areas of capillary fallout. Microaneurysms are seen ophthalmoscopically as red dots and on fluorescein angiography as hyperfluorescent dots.

Risk Factors of DR

1. *Duration of diabetes:* Most important factor.
2. *Metabolic control:* Control of the blood glucose level delays the development of DR by few years.
3. *Misc factors:* Pregnancy, anaemia, hypertension, renal disease.

CLASSIFICATION

A. Simple background DR.

B. Pre-proliferative DR.

C. Proliferative DR.

A. Simple Background DR (BDR)

Clinical Features:

1. **Microaneurysms:** First clinically detectable lesion of DR.

In diabetic retinopathy–loss of pericytes

↓

Mechanical weakening of capillary wall

↓

Focal dilatation (along with disruption of blood retinal barrier)

↓

Formation of Microaneurysms

- Microaneurysms are commonly found around areas of capillary fall out.
- Microaneurysms are seen ophthalmoscopically as red dots and on fluorescein angiography as hyperfluorescent dots.

2. **Haemorrhages:** Dot and blot; flame-shaped.
3. Hard exudates and few soft exudates. Hard exudates are leaked lipids whereas soft exudates are axonal debris.
4. Retinal edema.
5. **Macular oedema:** Retinal thickness or hard exudates within 1DD of center of fovea (1500 um).

Involvement of fovea by edema or hard exudates is the most common cause of visual impairment in diabetic patients particularly with NIDDM.

CSMO (Clinically significant macular edema): It is defined as the presence of one or more of the following features:

1. Retinal edema within 500 um of center of fovea.
2. Hard exudates within 500 um of fovea, if associated with adjacent retinal thickening (which may be outside the 500 um limit).
3. Retinal edema that is one disc area (1500 um) or larger any part of which is within one disc diameter of the center of fovea (1 DD is 1.5 mm).

Treatment:

1. Medical treatment:
   - Strict glycemic control.
   - Anti-hypertensives if associated with high BP.
   - Anti-oxidants.
2. If CSMO present, do laser photocoagulation–focal or grid following fluorescein angiography.

B. Pre-Proliferative DR

Clinical Features:

1. Vascular changes:
   a. Venous looping, beading and sausage-like segmentation.
   b. Arterioles–Narrow and obliterated.
2. Dark blot haemorrhages which are haemorrhagic retinal infarcts.
3. Multiple cotton-wool spots.
4. IRMA (Intraretinal microvascular abnormalities)–These are A-V shunts due to capillary closure.

Treatment:

1. Strict follow-up to watch for changes of PDR.

2. If CSMO is present, then manage it accordingly.
3. The usual medical treatment including strict control of blood sugar.

C. Proliferative DR (PDR)

Clinical Features:

1. *Neovascularisation:* NVD (Neovascularisation at disc), NVE (Neovascularisation elsewhere).
2. Vitreous detachment, generally incomplete.
3. *Haemorrhage:* Intravitreal, pre-retinal (These are also called prehyaloid haemorrhages and are typically boat-shaped).

Complications of PDR:

1. Persistent intra-gel vitreous haemorrhage.
2. *Retinal detachment:* Both tractional and rhegmatogenous can occur.
3. Opaque membranes on posterior surface of detached hyaloid face of vitreous.
4. *Rubeosis iridis:* It can lead to neovascular glaucoma (NVG).
5. *Burnt-out stage:* It refers to increase in fibrous component.

Treatment:

1. **Medical treatment:**
   - Strict glycemic control.
   - Anti-hypertensives.
   - Antioxidants.
2. **Panretinal photocoagulation (PRP)** by either Argon laser, double frequency NdYAG, i.e., Yellow laser or Diode laser is preferred choice of treatment. The aim of PRP is to convert the hypoxic area to anoxic area, so that there is involution of new vessels and no further neovascularisation.

   (Pre-retinal haemorrhages hamper the visualization of the retina for PRP and laser treatment may increase the incidence of further retinal haemorrhage and vitreous haemorrhage. Hence PRP should be avoided in cases of preretinal haemorrhage).

   Method of PRP: In PRP, generally either **Goldmann or Panfundoscopic** lens is used.

   Initial burns are in a double arc, 2 disc diameters (3 mm) temporal to macula. This serves as visual barrier against an accidental burn to the fovea. It involves placement of about 2000–3000 burns in a scatter pattern.
3. **Surgical management:**

   In complicated cases of proliferative diabetic retinopathy:
   1. Pars plana vitrectomy.
   2. Retinal detachment surgery.
   3. Extraction of diabetic cataract.

   If thcre is recurrence of neovascularisation, following modalities can be used:
   1. Further Argon laser PRP to fill in the gaps.
   2. Xenon-arc photocoagulation applied over previous laser scars.
   3. Cryotherapy to anterior retina.
   4. **The latest mode of treatment is to give Anti-VEGF (Vascular endothelial growth factor) injections in the vitreous cavity for the resistant cases of DR.**
      - **Gradual progressive painless loss of vision in a diabetic**

patient is most commonly due to cataract.**

- **Most common cause of moderate vision loss in a diabetic patient is CME.**
- **Floaters in a diabetic patient, most commonly indicate vitreous haemorrhage.**

D/D of Soft Exudates/Cotton-wool Spots

1. Diabetic retinopathy.
2. Hypertensive retinopathy.
3. Toxaemia of pregnancy.
4. HIV.
5. Collagen disorders like: DLE, PAN, Scleroderma.
6. Putschers retinopathy.

Conditions which can cause rubeosis iridis are:

1. CRVO.
2. Diabetic retinopathy.
3. Eales disease.
4. Sickle cell retinopathy.
5. Carotid occlusive disease.
6. Ocular ischemic syndrome.
7. Fuch's heterochromic cyclitis.
8. Exfoliation syndrome.

Studies Done in DR

1. *DRS:* Diabetic retinopathy study.
2. *ETDRS:* Early treatment diabetic retinopathy study.
3. *DRVS:* Diabetic retinopathy vitrectomy study.
4. Wisconsin's epidemiological study of diabetic retinopathy.

Schedule of Examination

Age at onset of diabetes	Time of First Examination	Follow-up
0-30	5 years after onset	Every year
31 years and older	At time of diagnosis of DM	Every year
During pregnancy	In first trimester	3 monthly

CENTRAL RETINAL VEIN OCCLUSION

It is common next to diabetic retinopathy.

Predisposing Factors:

1. *Increasing age:* 6th and 7th decade.
2. *Systemic hypertension:* **It is the most significant risk factor.**
3. *Blood dyscrasias:* Hyperviscosity due to chronic leukemias and polycythaemia.
4. Raised intraocular pressure.
5. *Hypermetropia:* Increased risk of branched retinal vein occlusion.
6. Congenital anomaly of central retinal vein.
7. *Periphlebitis:* Due to Sarcoidosis, Behcet's disease etc.

Classification of CRVO

a. Non-ischemic.
b. Ischemic.
c. In young adults (papillophlebitis).

Clinical Features:

1. Decreased visual acuity, much more in ischemic type of CRVO.
2. RAPD (Relative afferent papillary defect), is a feature of ischemic CRVO.
3. Tortuosity and dilatation of retinal veins.

4. Dot and blot; flame-shaped haemorrhages specially around the disc.
5. Cotton-wool spots, more in number in case of ischemic CRVO.
6. Optic disc oedema and hyperaemia.
7. Macular edema; may show cystoid changes.

100 days glaucoma/90 days glaucoma: It refers to neovascular glaucoma occurring after ischemic CRVO. It is found to occur after 90 to 100 days.

Splashed sauce appearance: This is the typical feature of CRVO where the fundus picture is multiple flame-shaped haemorrhages around the disc.

Treatment:

Fluorescein angiography is done to know the type of occlusion. If ischemic then prompt panretinal photocoagulation is required to prevent neovascular glaucoma. In case of non-ischemic type, the haemorrhages resolve by their own or sometimes peribulbar or intravitreal (IVTA) injections of steroids are given to enhance its absorption.

CENTRAL RETINAL ARTERY OCCLUSION (CRAO)

Etiology:

1. Due to emboli from heart or carotid artery.
2. Vaso-obliteration by atheroma or arteritis.
3. Raised intraocular pressure, rarely when very severe.

Clinical Features:

1. Acute and profound painless loss of vision, it may be preceded by transient loss of vision called amaurosis fugax.

   Patients who have a dual blood supply of the macula, i.e., by central retinal artery and cilioretinal artery may have some preserved central vision even after CRAO.
2. Marcus-Gunn pupil also called relative afferent pupillary defect.
3. White cloudy retina due to intracellular edema.
4. **Cherry-red spot** at the centre of fovea.
5. Marked narrowing of retinal arterioles, which become thread-like.
6. Segmentation of blood column in venules and arterioles known as **"Cattle-track appearance"**.
7. Optic atrophy at a later stage.

Treatment:

It is an ocular emergency:

1. Patient should lie flat.
2. Firm ocular massage to decrease the intraocular pressure.
3. Intravenous acetazolamide (500 mg), helps in sudden lowering of pressure.
4. Inhalation of mixture of 5% CO_2 and 95% of O_2, to relax the patient.
5. Anterior chamber paracentesis: It also helps in sudden lowering of intraocular pressure.

Differential Diagnosis of Cherry-Red Spot

1. CRAO.
2. Tay-Sach's disease. It is a gangliosidosis.
3. Niemann-Pick disease. It is a sphingo-lipidosis.
4. Other gangliosidosis:
   - Type I—Generalised.
   - Type II—Sandoff's disease.
5. Sialidosis (Cherry-red spot myoclonus syndrome).

6. Gaucher's disease.
7. Metachromatic leucodystrophy.
8. *Blunt trauma:* Cherry red spot in blunt trauma occurs due to **Berlin's edema** at the macula (also known as **'commotio—retinae'**). It manifests as milky white cloudiness involving considerable area in the foveal region. It may disappear or lead to pigmen-tary changes. If long standing may lead to lamellar hole which in turn leads to full thickness macular hole.

HYPERTENSIVE RETINOPATHY

Pathogenesis

Fundus picture is characterised by:

1. Vasoconstriction.
2. Leakage.
3. Arteriosclerosis.

Hollen-Horst plaques are a type of retinal emboli containing **cholesterol**. These plaques may be responsible for BRAO and CRAO. In hypertensive retinopathy, these plaques may be mentioned in relation to the associated atherosclerotic changes.

Other types of retinal emboli include:

A. Platelet—fibrin.
B. Calcific.

Clinical Features:

1. Arteriolar attenuation.
2. A-V Crossing findings indicating atherosclerotic changes in the vessels.
3. *Haemorrhages:* They are generally flame shaped. Sometimes vitreous hemorrhages may be found.
4. *Exudates:* Both hard and soft exudates may be found. Hard exudates at the macular area are placed radially and known as **macular star. Soft exudates are seen in great number in cases of malignant hypertension.**
5. Retinal edema which may involve the macula.
6. Swelling of optic nerve head, i.e., papilloedema in severe cases.

Significant loss of vision in hypertensive retinopathy occurs due to:

1. Retinal haemorrhages involving macula.
2. Macular edema.

It will not occur due to papilloedema, as visual acuity is not affected in this condition.

Grading of Hypertensive Retinopathy

Grade I: Mild generalised arteriolar attenuation.

Grade II:

1. Severe generalised and focal arteriolar attenuation.
2. Salus sign: It is S-shaped deflection of veins at the A-V junction.

Grade III:

1. Haemorrhages.
2. Exudates.
3. Copper-wiring of arterioles.
4. Bonnet sign/Gunn's sign.

Grade IV: Papilloedema with features of Grade III and silver wiring of arterioles.

Other Ocular Manifestations of Hypertension

1. Central vein occlusion and branched vein occlusion.
2. Retinal artery occlusion.
3. Elschnig's spots–Ischemic choroidal infarcts seen in patients of malignant hypertension.
4. Macroaneurysms.
5. Non-arteritic anterior ischemic optic neuropathy.

6. Ocular motor nerve palsies.
7. Subconjunctival haemorrhages.
8. Occipital infarct.

TOXAEMIA OF PREGNANCY

Eclamptic retinopathy also known as toxaemia of pregnancy presents with characteristics of hypertensive retinopathy.

Clinical Features:

1. Initially there is narrowing of retinal arteries **usually nasal branches first.**
2. Edema may be so profuse and generalized so as to cause retinal detachment.
3. Severe persistent retinal vessel spasm causes severe retinal hypoxia leading to cotton-wool spots and superficial haemorrhages.
4. Macular star and flat macular detachment due to edema.

   Advent of hypoxic retinopathy (soft exudates, edema, haemorrhages) should be considered an indication for termination of pregnancy, otherwise permanent visual loss may occur.

RETINITIS PIGMENTOSA

It is a generic name for a group of hereditary disorders characterised by progressive loss of photoreceptors, hence it is a photoreceptor dystrophy. Damage to the rod system is predominant. It is most commonly sporadic.

Inheritance:

1. *AD:* Autosomal dominant. It has the best prognosis, next common to sporadic cases.
2. *X-linked recessive:* It has the worst prognosis and is least common.
3 *AR:* Autosomal recessive.

Clinical Features:

1. Nyctalopia.
2. Impaired dark adaptation.
3. Decreased visual acuity: It may occur due to associated cystoid macular edema.
4. **Fundus features:** Typical RP primarily involves the mid-periphery of the retina. It presents as a classical triad of:
   a. Arteriolar attenuation.
   b. Retinal bone-spicule pigmentation.
   c. Pale, waxy disc (Consecutive optic atrophy).

Other Ocular Features:

1. CME-Cystoid macular edema.
2. OAG-Open-angle glaucoma.
3. PSC-Posterior sub-capsular cataract.
4. PVD-Posterior vitreous detachment.
5. Keratoconus.
6. Myopia.
7. Disc drusen.

Investigations:

1. Subnormal amplitude of ERG mainly scotopic.
2. *Perimetry:* It shows **Ring scotoma** (due to mid-peripheral involvement).

   Double arcuate scotoma found in patients of open angle glaucoma is also termed as: "*ring scotoma*".

Atypical Retinitis Pigmentosa

1. **Retinitis punctata albescens:** In this variant, instead of bony spicules there are white dots.
2. **Sector RP:** The whole midperiphery is not involved but only a sector of retina.
3. **Pericentric RP:** In contrast to the mid-peripheral involvement, the disease starts from the central retina.

4. **RP with exudative vasculopathy.**
5. **Retinitis pigmentosa sine pigmento:** In this condition, bony spicules are not present, instead there is pigment dispersion in form of salt and pepper fundus.

Systemic Associations

1. **Bassen-Kornzweig syndrome:** It's a triad of Retinitis pigmentosa, abetalipoproteinemia and acanthocytosis.
2. **Refsum's syndrome:** It is a defect in phytanic acid metabolism which infiltrates many body tissues including the eye.
3. **Ushers syndrome:** It is Retinitis pigmentosa associated with deafness. **It is the most common systemic association of RP.**
4. **Cockaynes syndrome:** It is manifested as childhood dwarfism.
5. **Kearns-Sayre syndrome:** It's a triad of Retinitis pigmentosa, ocular myopathy and heart defects.
6. **Mucopolysaccharidosis.**
7. **Bardet-Biedl syndrome:** It is characterized by mental handicap, polydactyly and retinitis pigmentosa.
8. **Laurence-Moon syndrome:** It is characterized by features of Bardet-Biedl syndrome and spastic paraplegia.
9. **Friedreich's ataxia:** It is characterized with ataxia and nystagmus.

Differential Diagnosis of Night Blindness

1. Xerophthalmia.
2. Retinitis pigmentosa.
3. High myopia.
4. Advanced cases of open angle glaucoma.
5. Congenital stationary night blindness.
6. Fundus albipunctatus.
7. Oguchi's disease.
8. Choroideremia.

Treatment: There is no effective treatment, hence progression of disease is not altered.

RETINAL DEGENERATIONS

A. Benign Peripheral Retinal Degenerations:

1. Microcystoid degenerations.
2. Snowflake degenerations.
3. Paving-stone degenerations.
4. Honey-comb retinal degenerations.
5. Drusen.
6. Oral pigmentary degenerations.

B. Predisposing Vitreo-Retinal Degenerations: These degenerations can lead to Rhegmatogenous RD.

1. **Lattice Degenerations:**
   a. Common in high myopes.
   b. Circumferentially oriented, spindle shaped areas of retinal thinning.
   c. May be associated with holes or retinal tears leading to retinal detachment.
2. **Snail-track Denegerations:**
   a. Bands of tightly packed snowflakes.
   b. Has large round holes; hence retinal detachment is common.
3. **Others:**
   a. *Acquired retinoschisis:* Retinoschisis is splitting of the sensory retina into two layers, choroidal and vitreous layer.
   b. White with pressure.
   c. White without pressure.

RETINAL DETACHMENT

It is the separation of sensory retina from retinal pigment epithelium (RPE) by subretinal fluid.

Types:

a. **Rhegmatogenous:** It is due to formation of retinal tear or hole. This can occur due to PVD, i.e., posterior vitreous detachment in old age, high myopes, aphakia and trauma.

b. **Tractional:** It is due to traction bands formed secondary to neovascularisation. It occurs in diseases causing neovascularisation.

c. **Exudative:** It occurs secondary to any choroidal pathology, leading to the percolation of fluid into the subretinal space. It occurs due to accumulation of fluid under the retina due to inflammatory or vascular lesions. It occurs in all causes of posterior uveitis, vascular diseases like CSR and Coats' disease, tumours like choroidal melanoma, retinoblastoma etc. and due to sudden hypotony as seen in intraocular operations or perforation of the globe.

Clinical Features:

a. **Floaters:** Opacities in the vitreous is known as floaters. It occurs due to dispersion of pigments from the retinal pigment epithelial cells. It is present in rhegmatogenous RD and in very few cases of exudative RD (due to presence of vitreous cells), but not in tractional RD.

b. **Photopsia:** These are flashes of light seen by the patients due to irritation of photoreceptor cells. It is commonly a feature of rhegmatogenous RD, and sometimes also seen in tractional RD, but not in exudative RD.

c. **Visual field defects:** The defect corresponds to the area of the retina involved in the detachment.

d. **Diminished visual acuity:** It is seen when the central retina is involved.

On Examination:

1. **Grey reflex:** It occurs due to retinal detachment as a result of loss of background choroidal glow. The retinal detachment is generally convex shaped both in exudative and rhegmatogenous type, whereas in tractional type it is concave shaped.
2. **Fluid shift:** It generally occurs in exudative retinal detachment.
3. **Line:** Pigmented line at the inter-section of attached and detached retina occurs in old retinal detachment.
4. **Hole:** Occurs in rhegmatogenous RD but not necessarily in tractional RD and never in exudative RD.

Investigations:

Examination of retina can be done in the following ways:

A. **+90D lens/Hruby lens:** These primarily help to see the centre of the retina.

B. **3 mirror contact lens:** It helps to examine the whole retina.

C. **Direct ophthalmoscopy:** It is useful to see only the central fundus.

D. **Indirect ophthalmoscopy** (With or without scleral indentation): It particularly helps to see the periphery of the retina.

Other Investigations helpful are:

a. **ERG:** Subnormal.

b. **Ultrasonography:** It is specially helpful in hazy media.

   i. B scan depicts the detached retina.

   ii. A scan is also helpful, as in RD there will be effective shortening of the axial length.

Treatment:

Rhegmatogenous retinal detachment: Aim of treatment is closure of break:

DACE Procedure

a. **D**rainage of SRF.

b. **A**ir injection into vitreous: The substances used for injection into the vitreous are: air, saline, expanding gases, silicone oil and perflourocarbons. Perfluorocarbons are heavy liquids with specific gravity double of the water but viscosity is low and hence easily injected.

c. **C**ryotherapy: Laser photocoagulation is not the usual mode of treatment (usually cryotherapy is used) but it may be used for posteriorly located breaks where cryotherapy is not possible.

d. **E**xplant: These are used to buckle or encircle the area corresponding to the retinal holes so as to indent it. Indentation prevents any reopening of the sealed holes.

Exudative retinal detachment: Management is treatment of the cause of retinal detachment like choroidal tumours, age-related macular degeneration etc.

Tractional retinal detachment: PRP is done to manage the hypoxia, and the traction bands have to be surgically removed and retina is reposed back.

BULL'S EYE MACULOPATHY

It is so-called as there is central foveolar hyperpigmentation surrounded by depigmented zone and encircled by a hyperpigmented ring. There is moderate reduction in VA-6/18 to 6/24.

D/D of Bulls Eye Maculopathy

1. Chloroquine toxicity.
2. Batten's disease.
3. Benign concentric annular macular dystrophy.
4. Bardet-Biedl syndrome.
5. Cone dystrophy.
6. Occasionally Leber's Amaurosis.

Chloroquine Toxicity

The three main potential ocular side effects are:

A. **Retinotoxicity.**

B. **Corneal deposits:** It is also called **"Cornea Verticillata"or Vortex Keratopathy** and is characterized by bilateral golden corneal epithelial deposits which appear in vortex fashion from point below pupil and swirl outwards sparing the limbus.

C. **Optic neuritis.**

Retinotoxicity: The risk of retinotoxicity increases when the additive dose exceeds 300 g or duration of treatment is greater than 1 year.

Chloroquine Maculopathy: It can be divided into following stages:

1. **Premaculopathy:**
   a. Normal visual acuity.
   b. Scotoma to red target between 4° and 9° from fixation.
   c. Defect in Amsler grid test.
2. **Established maculopathy:**
   a. Visual acuity–6/9 to 6/12.
   b. Loss of foveolar reflex.
   c. Subtle parafoveal halo of RPE pallor.
   d. Mild central scotoma to a white target may be present.

   Till stage 2 the changes are reversible on stopping the drug.
3. **Bull's eye maculopathy:**
   a. Visual acuity–6/18 to 6/24.
   b. Central foveolar hyperpigmentation surrounded by a depigmented zone and encircled by hyperpigmented ring.
4. **Severe maculopathy:**
   a. Visual acuity–6/36 to 6/60.

b. Pseudohole at fovea with widespread surrounding RPE atrophy.

5. **End stage maculopathy:**
   a. Severe reduction of visual acuity.
   b. Marked atrophy of RPE with unmasking of larger choroidal blood vessels.
   c. Attenuated retinal arterioles with pigment clumping in the peripheral retina.

CME (CYSTOID MACULAR EDEMA)

It is the accumulation of fluid in the outer plexiform (Henle's) and inner nuclear layers of the retina, centred about the foveola. It is generally innocuous.

Etiology:

a. **With Retinal Vascular Leakage:** DR, BRVO, Intermediate uveitis, Aphakic or Pseudophakic CME.
b. **Without Retinal Vascular Leakage/ Degenerative:** RP.
c. **Postoperative:** CME may occur post-operatively after cataract surgery called as **"Irvine Gass syndrome"**. Its etiology is attributed to either vitreous traction or prostaglandins released during the inflammatory cascade.
d. **Inflammatory:** It may occur secondary to all causes of posterior uveitis.

Sequelae:

Long-standing cases→Large cystic space →Lamellar hole (Decrease in VA)→Full-thickness macular hole.

Types of Macular Edema:

1. **Cystoid:** It is due to disturbance of the blood retinal barrier, with no structural alteration of foveal tissue.
2. **Non-cystoid/or Amorphous:** There is distorted capillary architecture at the macula, e.g., in neovascularization or by traction forces.

Investigations:

Fluorescein Angiography: The pathognomic feature of CME is **Flower-Petal Pattern.**

Treatment:

1. Systemic carbonic anhydrase inhibitors.
2. Laser photocoagulation in some vascular cases.
3. Systemic steroids.

CENTRAL SEROUS RETINOPATHY

Idiopathic, self-limiting disease of young or middle-aged adult males.

Pathogenesis:

Dysfunction of RPE

↓

Accumulation of fluid in subretinal space

↓

Local detachment of sensory retina at macula

Clinical Features:

1. Sudden onset of blurred vision in one eye.
2. Relative scotoma.
3. Micropsia.
4. Metamorphopsia.
5. VA is 6/9 to 6/12 and correctable by addition of plus lens.

On Examination:

Elevation of sensory retina at posterior pole, borders of which are outlined by glistening reflex or ring reflex.

Fluorescein Angiography: It manifests two pictures:

1. Smoke-stack appearance.
2. Ink-blot appearance.

Classification:

A. Histological Classification (Spitnaz Classification)

Type I—Detachment of sensory retina.

Type II—RPE detachment.

Type III—Intermediate type, both sensory retina and RPE are elevated.

B. Clinical Classification

I. **Typical CSR**

i. Best corrected visual acuity (BCVA) 6/6 or better.

ii. Macular detachment <3 DD.

iii. Pinpoint inkblot or smoke—stack leakage on FFA.

iv. Spontaneous resolution.

II. **Atypical CSR**

i. Profound loss of vision, BCVA<6/60.

ii. Large area of macular detachment (>3 DD).

iii. Irregular, double or multiple leakage on FFA with large collection of serous fluid.

iv. No spontaneous resolution.

Treatment:

- Spontaneous resolution is common (by 6–12 months).
- *Laser photocoagulation:* It hastens symptomatic relief by speeder resolution of serous detachment.

MYOPIC MACULOPATHY

Fundus Changes in Pathological Myopia

1. Annular crescent around optic disc.
2. Islands of chorioretinal atrophy at posterior pole.
3. *Laquer cracks:* These are break in Bruch's membrane. They can lead to choroidal neovascularisation.
4. Posterior staphyloma.
5. *Foster-fuchs spot:* These are haemorrhage with secondary pigmentary proliferation at the macular area. They are also called Fuchs flecks.
6. Macular holes.
7. Lattice degenerations and peripheral retinal holes.
8. *Tigroid fundus:* Choroid tessellation.
9. *Degenerated vitreous:* The gel vitreous becomes fluid like due to degeneration.
10. *Retinal detachment:* Rhegmatogenous RD occurs due to hole formation in the peripheral degenerative areas.
11. Subretinal neovascularization.

FUNDUS FINDINGS IN HYPERMETROPIA

1. **Watered silk or shot silk retina:** Sharp foveal reflex at macula.
2. **Pseudopapillitis:** Decreased C:D ratio and blurring of margins of the disc.
3. **Vessels:** Undue tortuosity and abnormal branchings.
4. Macula is situated farther from disc than in emmetropic eye.

Other Findings

- Pseudodivergent squint, i.e., pseudo-exotropia due to large angle kappa or angle alpha.
- Small eye with shallow anterior chamber.

EALES' DISEASE (PERIPHLEBITIS RETINAE)

- Mainly affects young males. It causes sudden painless loss of vision with no trauma.
- **Etiology:**
  1. Idiopathic.
  2. Hypersensitivity to tubercular protein leads to peripheral retinal vasculitis.
- **Presentation:** Sudden blurring of vision as a result of vitreous haemorrhage. It is commonly recurrent.
- **On Examination:**
  1. Sheathing of small peripheral retinal veins.
  2. Massive proliferative retinopathy leads to extensive vitreous or retinal haemorrhage causing TRD, i.e., tractional retinal detachment.

Complications:

1. Rubeosis irdis which later leads to neovascular glaucoma (NVG).
2. Cataract.

Treatment:

1. PRP.
2. Pars plana vitrectomy.

ARMD (AGE RELATED MACULAR DEGENERATION)

Definition: Presence of some degree of visual loss in association with drusen and geographical atrophy of the RPE or changes associated with sub-retinal neovascularization in individual over 50 years old.

Two main types of ARMD are:

a. Non-exudative.

b. Exudative.

A. Non-Exudative ARMD: (Geographical atrophy)

Most common—90% of cases.

Clinical Features: Gradual, mild to moderate impairment of vision over several months or years.

On Examinations:

1. Initially Drusens.
2. Sharply circumscribed circular areas of RPE atrophy associated with varying degrees of loss of the choriocapillaries called Geographical atrophy.

Pathology: Slowly progressive atrophy of RPE and photoreceptors.

Treatment:

- No effective treatment.
- Low visual aids.

B. Exudative ARMD:

- Less common but effect on vision is more devastating.
- **Clinical features:** Visual impairment is within days and may lead to loss of all central vision.
- **On examination:**
  1. RPE detachment.
  2. Choroidal neovascularisation.

RPE detachment: Sharply circumscribed dome-shaped elevation at posterior pole of varying size, may lead to:

a. Spontaneous resolution.

b. Detachment of sensory retina.

c. Tear of RPE.

CHOROIDAL NEOVASCULARISATION

Proliferation of fibrovascular tissue from choriocapillaris through defects in Bruch's membrane into sub-RPE space and later into the subretinal space.

D/D of Sub-Retinal Neovascular Membrane

1. Wet ARMD.
2. POHS–Presumed ocular histoplasmosis syndrome.
3. Severe myopia.
4. Angiod streaks.
5. Choroidal naevus.
6. Choroidal rupture.
7. Inappropriate laser photocoagulation.
8. Optic disc drusen.

Treatment of Wet ARMD: It depends upon the location of the neovascular membrane.

Membranes can be:

a. **Extrafoveal**–More than 200 microns from centre of FAZ (foveal avascular zone).
b. **Subfoveal**–Involving centre of FAZ.
c. **Juxtafoveal**–Not involving centre but closer than 200 microns.
   - Laser photocoagulation is done for mainly extrafoveal membranes. Membrane is destroyed by blue-green laser. Can also be done in some cases of juxtafoveal membranes.
   - **For subfoveal and extremely juxtafoveal lesions:**
     A. PDT—Photodynamic therapy.
     B. TTT—Transpupillary Thermo-therapy.
     C. Anti-VEGF drugs (vascular endothelial growth factor): Intravitreal injections of these drugs are given to arrest neovascularisation.

PDT—It relies on photochemical injury to the vessel wall and selective damage to the target tissue while sparing the adjacent normal tissue.

PDT requires two components:

A. *Photosensitizer*—It accumulates in neovascular tissue. Commonly used are benzoporphyrin derivative—**Verteporfin.**
B. A specific laser light corresponding to the absorption peak of the dye (690 nm, i.e., diode laser).

TTT–It closes the choroidal neovascular lesions by means of hyperthermia.

- Helpful in subfoveal lesions.
- Use of low irradiance, long-pulse diode laser. Heat is delivered to the choroid and RPE through pupil using a modified diode (810 nm) laser.

Other Modalities of Treatment in ARMD

1. Submacular surgery.
2. Macular translocation surgery.
3. Trace metals and antioxidants.
4. Anti-angiogenic factors (Interferon alpha, Interleukin 12, Fumagillin derivatives, thalidomide).

RETINOPATHY OF PREMATURITY (ROP)

It is a proliferative retinopathy which affects preterm infants exposed to high ambient oxygen concentrations. Retina is unique among tissues in that it has no blood vessels until the fourth month of gestation at which time vascular complexes emanating from the hyaloid vessels at the optic disc, grow towards the periphery. These vessels reach the nasal periphery after 8 months of gestation and to the temporal periphery not before 1 month after delivery. This incompletely vascularized retina is particularly susceptible to oxygen damage. **Hence it is the prematurity which is the most important factor for development of ROP.**

Clinical Features:

It is divided into two types:

A. Active ROP.

B. Cicatricial ROP.

Active ROP

It is divided into five stages:

Stage I (Demarcation line): Development of a thin, tortous, grey-white line which runs roughly parallel with the ora serrata. It separates avascular immature peripheral retina from vascularised posterior retina.

Stage II (Ridge): Demarcation line develops into a ridge of tissue which extends out of plane of retina.

Stage III (Ridge with extra-retinal fibrovascular proliferation): Generally this stage occurs 35 weeks post-conception. Ridge becomes pink due to development of fibrovascular proliferation on surface of retina and into vitreous. It may be associated with retinal haemorrhage and vitreous haemorrhage.

Stage IV (Sub-total Retinal Detachment): Tractional RD which starts at periphery and progresses centrally.

Stage V: Total Retinal Detachment.

Treatment of ROP:

1. Ablation of avascular immature retina by either cryotherapy or laser photo-coagulation.
2. Vitamin–E therapy–Role is controversial and based on following pathogenesis:

Excessive free radicals

↓ → Vitamin E (Antioxidant)

Inhibit spindle cell migration

↓

Produces angiogenic factors

↓

ROP

3. If retinal detachment is present, we do Scleral Buckling.

Screening of ROP: Eyes of all infants < 36 weeks or weighing less than 1500 g who have received supplemental oxygen should be screened for ROP.

Ideal time of screening: Add 4 weeks to postnatal age or between 31 and 33 weeks.

- **Before 32 weeks** screening is of limited value because pupils are difficult to dilate and visualization of fundus is impaired by vitreous haze caused by **Tunica vasculosa lentis.**
- **After 36 weeks:** ROP rarely develops.

Toxic Maculopathy

It can be caused by following drugs:

1. Chloroquine.
2. Quinine.
3. Phenothiazines
   a. Chlorpromazine (Largactil).
   b. Thioridazine (Melleril).
4. Tamoxifen.
5. Canthaxanthin.

PURTSCHER'S RETINOPATHY

Etiology:

1. Head trauma, chest trauma.
2. **Systemic causes:**
   a. Acute pancreatitis.
   b. Systemic lupus erythematosus.
   c. Chronic renal failure.
   d. Thrombotic thrombocytopenia.

Pathogenesis:

Blockage of retinal capillaries by emboli (fat, air) leading to retinal atrophy and optic atrophy.

Clinical Feature: Multiple cotton-wool exudation and haemorrhages around optic disc.

Treatment:

- No known treatment.
- No significant recovery of vision.
- Medical or surgical therapy for the underlying condition prevents further damage.

COATS' DISEASE

- It is the most severe form of retinal telangiectasia.
- Invariably unilateral.
- More common in boys than in girls.

Clinical Features:

1. Leukocoria.
2. Strabismus.
3. Visual loss.

Ophthalmoscopy

Large areas of intra and sub-retinal yellowish exudates often associated with overlying dilated and tortuous retinal blood vessels at the posterior pole and periphery.

Complications:

1. Massive sub-retinal exudation.
2. Exudative retinal detachment.
3. Retrolental mass.
4. Secondary cataract.
5. Rubeosis iridis.
6. Uveitis.
7. Secondary glaucoma.
8. Pthisis bulbi.

PERSISTENT HYPERPLASTIC PRIMARY VITREOUS (PHPV)

PHPV is caused by failure of regression of the primary vitreous. It can be divided into anterior and posterior types:

A. Anterior PHPV.

B. Posterior PHPV.

Anterior PHPV

1. Most common.
2. Usually unilateral.
3. In microphthalmic eye.
4. Presents as retrolental mass into which elongated ciliary processes are inserted.

↓

If contract

↓

Ciliary processes are pulled forward

↓

Tear in posterior capsule of lens

↓

Cataract

↓

Swelling of lens

↓

Secondary angle-closure glaucoma

Posterior PHPV

1. Less common, usually unilateral and associated with microphthalmos.
2. White dense membrane extending from optic disc to peripheral retina or retrolental region.
3. May be associated with pale optic disc and retinal detachment.

Epidemic Dropsy

- It occurs due to contamination of mustard oil with argemone oil.
- Toxic alkaloid, **sanguinarine** in argemone oil is responsible for epidemic dropsy. This toxic substance interferes with the oxidation of pyruvic acid which accumulates in the blood.

Clinical Features:

A. Systemic Features

1. Sudden, non-inflammatory, bilateral swelling of legs.
2. Diarrhea.
3. Dyspnoea.
4. Cardiac failure and death.

B. Ocular Features

1. Hypersecretory glaucoma.
2. Fundus – There is increased capillary permeability and tortuosity of vessels leading to disc edema, retinal edema and deposition of hard exudates.

PHOTORECEPTOR DYSTROPHIES

A. Retinitis Pigmentosa (Mainly involves the Rods).

B. Cone Dystrophy

Clinical Features:

1. Day–Blindness.
2. Progressive loss of visual acuity.
3. Defective colour vision.

Ophthalmoscopy:

1. Bulls–eye maculopathy.
2. Attenuated arterioles, pale waxy disc and bony spicules may be present.
3. Subnormal or unrecordable photopic ERG.

C. Leber's Amaurosis

Clinical Features:

i. Blindness at birth or within first few years of life.
ii. Pupillary light reactions are absent or severely diminished.
iii. A characteristic feature is **oculodigital syndrome** in which constant rubbing of the eyes by the child causes enophthalmos as a result of resorption of fat.
iv. Unrecordable ERG.

Ophthalmoscopy:

a. Salt pepper fundus.
b. Bull's eye maculopathy.
c. Optic disc pallor (Waxy) and attenuation of arteries.

D. Congenital Stationary Night Blindness

i. Normal fundus.
ii. Non-progressive night blindness.
iii. Absence of dark adaptation.

E. Congenital Stationary Night Blindness with Fundus Changes:

1. ***Fundus Albipunctatus:***

   i. *Fundus*

   - Tiny yellow-white spots extending from posterior pole to periphery.
   - Macula is spared hence visual acuity is unaffected.
   - Unlike retinitis punctata albescens, retinal blood vessels, optic disc and peripheral visual field remain normal.

   ii. *Non-progressive night blindness.*

2. ***Oguchi's Disease:*** Oguchi disease, (also called congenital stationary night blindness), is an autosomal recessive form of congenital stationary night blindness associated with fundus discoloration and abnormally slow dark adaptation. It is characterised by **Mizou's phenomena**: If a patient of Oguchi's disease is made to sit for one hour in dark, then there is no night blindness and fundus is normal.

   It occurs due to overstimulation of rods.

DYSTROPHIES OF THE RETINAL PIGMENT EPITHELIUM

A. Best's Vitelliform Macular Dystrophy

Clinical Features:

Divided in to 5 stages:

Stage I (Pre-vitelliform):

- Abnormal EOG.
- Asymptomatic.
- Fundus normal.

Stage II (Vitelliform):

- Yellow spots (lipofuscin granules) at the level of RPE.
- "Egg-yolk lesion" or "Sunny side up".
- Yellow material accumulated in subretinal space at the macula.

Stage III (Pseudohypopyon):

When part of this "egg–yolk" lesion is absorbed.

Stage IV (Vitelliruptive):

- Egg-yolk breaks and assumes a "scrambled–egg" appearance.
- Visual impairment.

Stage V:

- *Macula:* Hypertrophic scar.
- Vascularised scar with choroidal neovascularisation.

B. Adult Foveomacular Vitelliform Dystrophy

- Benign condition with minimal visual symptoms.
- Compared to Best's disease, foveal lesions are smaller, present later and do not demonstrate evolutionary changes.
- EOG—Normal or slightly abnormal.

C. Stargardt's Macular Dystrophy—Fundus Flavimaculatus

- **It is a macular dystrophy mainly involving RPE.**
- Stargardt's macular dystrophy and Fundus flavimaculatus are regarded as variants of same disorder.
- Inheritance – Autosomal recessive (AR).
- Both sexes are equally effected.

Stargardt's Disease

- Stargardt's disease is characterized by:

a. Presents in 1st or 2nd decade of life.

b. Impaired visual acuity.

c. *Ophthalmoscopy:*

Nonspecific Mottling at Fovea

↓

Oval lesions at macula, 1.5 DD in size, having "**Snail-lime**" or "**beaten-bronze**" reflex

↓

Atrophic changes in RPE and choriocapillaris and secondary changes in photoreceptors

↓

Marked visual impairment

- Prognosis–Poor.

Fundus Flavimaculatus

Clinical Features:

1. Presentation in 4th and 5th decades of life.
2. Patients may remain asymptomatic for many years unless foveola is involved.
3. *Ophthalmoscopy:*

   a. Ill-defined yellow white spots or flecks at the level of RPE (either round, oval, linear, fish-tail like) scattered throughout the posterior pole and mid periphery of both eyes.

b. New lesions form peripherally and older reabsorb.

c. Fundus has vermilion colour in 50% cases.

d. ERG and EOG—Abnormal only in advanced cases.

e. Peripheral visual field and night vision is normal.

ANGIOD STREAKS

They are due to dehiscence in the collagenous and elastic portions of Bruchs membrane with secondary changes in the RPE and the Choriocapillaris. Its systemic associations are:

1. **Pseudoxanthoma elasticum.**
2. **Paget's disease.**
3. **Ehler Danlos syndrome.**

CHOROIDAL DYSTROPHIES

A. Choroideremia

i. Affect only males with female carriers.

ii. Night blindness.

iii. Diffuse mottled depigmentation of RPE which later progresses into large patches of RPE and choroidal atrophy in mid-retinal zone.

iv. In contrast to primary retinal dystrophies, retinal blood vessels are normal.

v. Scotopic ERG–Non-recordable.
Photopic ERG–Severely reduced.

B. Gyrate Atrophy

i. Very rare disease.

ii. Due to deficiency of mitochondrial matrix enzyme—*Ornithine Aminotransferase*. Hence there is increased ornithine in plasma, urine, CSF and aqueous humour.

iii. Night blindness.

iv. Development of axial myopia.

v. Scalloped circular patches of chorioretinal atrophy in retinal periphery with vitreous degeneration. Retinal vessel attenuation in late cases.

vi. *Other ocular features:*

a. Blunting of ciliary processes.

b. Iris atrophy.

c. Posterior cataract.

d. Macular edema.

vii. *ERG and EOG*—Non-recordable.

viii. **Treatment:**

1. Pyridoxine (Vitamin B_6).
2. A diet low in proteins and arginine.

C. Central Areolar Choroidal Dystrophy

1. Primarily involves macula, hence there is impairment of visual acuity (atrophic lesion).
2. Localised disease, hence ERG and EOG normal.

D. Generalised Choroidal Atrophy

i. Diffuse atrophy of RPE and choriocapillaris.

ii. Night blindness and decreased visual acuity.

NEET DRILL

1. Thinnest part of the retina is ora serrata with a thickness of 0.1 mm.
2. Distance between temporal margin of disc and foveola is 2 DD.
3. Ratio of rods: Ganglion cells is 3:1.
4. Ratio of cones: Ganglion cells is 1:1.
5. EOG is depicted as Arden ratio, i.e., ratio of light peak/dark trough. The normal ratio is 1.85.
6. In Best disease EOG is abnormal with Arden ratio of less than 1.5.
7. Rods: Cones at the periphery is 20:1.

8. Most common type of CRVO (75%) is non-ischemic.
9. Most common gas used in RD surgery is: perfluorocarbon, i.e., C3F8.
10. 90% of infants with ROP are in milder category and do not require treatment.
11. Most sensitive part of the retina is fovea centralis.
12. Posterior staphyloma is a feature of pathological myopia.
13. Bull's eye maculopathy is seen in both toxicity of chloroquine and hydroxy-chloroquine.
14. A patient of CRAO retains the central vision and a small amount of visual field, due to the presence of cilioretinal artery also supplying the macula. Ciliorctinal artery is a branch of short posterior ciliary artery.
15. Putschers retinopathy is a feature of acute pancreatitis.
16. Most common type of staphyloma is posterior.
17. Splashed sauce appearance is a feature of CRVO.
18. Cherry-red spot is a feature of CRAO.
19. Dry ARMD is more common than wet ARMD.
20. Most important factor for occurrence of ROP is prematurity.
21. Prophylaxis of ROP is vitamin E therapy.
22. Most important factor for occurrence of retinopathy in a diabetic patient is duration and second most important is glycemic control.
23. Treatment of ROP is NOT PRP. It is laser photocoagulation of ONLY hypoxic part.
24. Fluid accumulation in CSR is in the subretinal space.
25. The most common retinal detachment is Rhegmatogenous.
26. The most radioresistant layer of the retina is Ganglion cell layer.
27. The most radiosensitive layer of the retina is photoreceptor layer.

MULTIPLE CHOICE QUESTIONS

1. All are used in the treatment of diabetic retinopathy except:

A. Removal of epiretinal membrane
B. Vitrectomy
C. Retinal reattachment
D. Exo photocoagulation

2. Which of the following is best to differentiate CRVO from carotid artery occlusion?

A. Dilated retinal vein
B. Retinal artery pressure
C. Tortuous retinal vein
D. Ophthalmodynamometry

3. ICG angiography is primarily indicated in:

A. Minimal classical CNV
B. Occult CNV
C. Angioid streak with CNV
D. Polypoidal choroidal vasculopathy

4. In the fetus Angiogenesis in eye all are involved except:

A. TNF α B. IL-8
C. BFGF D. VEGF

5. True about juxtafoveal telangiectasia is all except:

A. Variant of Coats' disease
B. Macular telangiectasia
C. Peripheral telangiectasia
D. Stuctural abnormality seen in vessels

6. All are true about Lambert-Eaton syndrome except:

A. Spares ocular muscle
B. Tensilon test positive

C. Proximal muscle involvement

D. Repeat nerve stimulation improve muscle strength

7. All are true about visual cycle except:

A. Condensation of opsin with aldehyde of retinal

B. NADP is reduced

C. NAD is reduced

D. Opsin combines with retinal to from visual purple

8. Which of the following conditions have autosomal dominant inheritance?

A. Gyrate atrophy

B. Best disease

C. Lawrence-Moon Biedl syndrome

D. Bassen-Kornzweig syndrome

9. Cherry-red spot is seen in all of the following conditions except:

A. GM1 gangliosidosis

B. Niemann-Pick disease

C. Krabbes disease

D. Sandoff's disease

10. A case of non-insulin dependent diabetes mellitus with a history of diabetes for one year should have an ophthalmic examination:

A. As early as feasible

B. After 5 years

C. After 10 years

D. Only after visual symptoms develop

11. Which drug can cause macular toxicity when given intravitreally?

A. Gentamycin

B. Vancomycin

C. Dexamethasone

D. Ceftazidime

12. The average distance of the fovea from the temporal margin of the optic disc is:

A. 1 disc diameter

B. 2 disc diameter

C. 3 disc diameter

D. 4 disc diameter

13. The retina receives its blood supply from all except:

A. Posterior ciliary artery

B. Central retinal artery

C. Retinal artery

D. Plexus of Zinn and Haller arteries

14. In Von Hippel-Lindau syndrome, the retinal vascular tumours are often associated with intracranial hemangioblastoma. Which one of the following regions is associated with such vascular abnormalities in this syndrome?

A. Optic radiation

B. Optic tract

C. Cerebellum

D. Pulvinar

15. A 25-year-old male gives history of sudden painless loss of vision in one eye for the past 2 weeks. There is no history of trauma. On examination the anterior segment is normal but there is no fundal glow. Which one of the following is the most likely cause?

A. Vitreous haemorrhage

B. Optic atrophy

C. Development cataract

D. Acute attack of angle closure glaucoma

16. Photodynamic therapy is used in the eye for the following disease:

A. Cataract

B. Glaucoma

C. Uveitis

D. Wet AMD (Age-Related—Macular—Degeneration)

17. All are ocular emergencies except:

A. Angle-Closure glaucoma

B. Central-serous retinopathy

C. Retinal detachment

D. Central retinal arterial occlusion

18. All are fundus findings of diabetic retinopathy except:

A. Microaneurysms

B. Retinal haemorrhages

C. Arteriolar dilatation

D. Neovascularisation

19. A 66-year-old elderly male presents with heart disease and has sudden loss of vision in one eye, examination reveals a cherry red spot over the fundus; the likely diagnosis is:

A. Central retinal vein occlusion

B. Central retinal artery occlusion

C. Amaurosis fugax

D. Acute ischemic optic neuritis

20. Cause of acute loss of vision in a patient of alcoholic pancreatitis is:

A. Purtscher's retinopathy

B. Sudden alcohol withdrawal

C. Acute congestive glaucoma

D. Central retinal artery obstruction

21. Cherry-red spot is seen in:

A. CRVO

B. Blunt trauma

C. Diabetes mellitus

D. Retinitis pigmentosa

22. For fluorescein angiography of retina, dye is injected in:

A. Femoral artery

B. Antecubital vein

C. Ophthalmic artery

D. Internal carotid artery

23. Retinitis pigmentosa is not associated with:

A. Ushers syndrome

B. Kornzweig syndrome

C. Kearn-Sayre syndrome

D. Marfan's syndrome

24. Choroidal neovascularisation is seen in all except:

A. Hypermetropia

B. Myopia

C. Trauma

D. Angiod streaks

25. Diabetic macular edema is due to all except:

A. Disruption of retinal pigment epithelium

B. Oxidative stress

C. Increase VEGF

D. Increase expression of protein kinase C

26. A 30-year-old patient with history of recurrent headache was sent for fundus examination. He was found to be having generalized arterial attenuation with multiple cotton-wool spots and flame shaped haemorrhages in both eyes. The most likely cause is:

A. Diabetic retinopathy

B. Hypertensive retinopathy

C. Central retinal artery occlusion

D. Temporal arteritis

27. Angiod streaks in the eyes are seen in:

A. Pseudoxanthoma elasticum

B. Tendinous xanthoma

C. Xanthelesma

D. Eruptive xanthoma

28. A 35-year-old insulin dependent diabetes mellitus (IDDM) patient on insulin for the past 10 years complains of gradually progressive painless loss of vision. Most likely he has:

A. Cataract

B. Vitreous haemorrhage

C. Total rhegmatogenous retinal detachment

D. Tractional retinal detachment not involving the macula

29. An 18-year-old girl who was using spectacles for last 10 years, came with the history of photopsia and sudden loss of vision in right eye. Which one of the following clinical examination should be performed to clinch the diagnosis?

A. Cycloplegic refraction

B. Indirect ophthalmoscopy

C. Schiotz tonometry

D. Gonioscopy

30. During the dark phase of visual cycle, which form of vitamin A combines with opsin to make rhodopsin?

A. All trans-Retinaldehyde

B. All trans-Retinal

C. 11-cis-Retinaldehyde

D. 11-cis-Retinal

31. A 25-year-old executive presents with metamorphopsia in his right eye. On examination the fundus shows a shallow detachment at the macula. The fluorescein angiography shows a "smoke stack" sign. Which of the following management should be given?

A. Topical antibiotic corticosteroid

B. Systemic corticosteroid for two weeks and then taper

C. Pulse methyl prednisolone for three days and then taper

D. Just wait and watch for spontaneous recovery

32. Relative colour and luminosity of photoreceptive input under changing light conditions are regulated and maintained by:

A. Muller cells

B. Amacrine cells

C. Ganglion cells

D. Retinal astrocytes

33. While working in the neonatal ICU, your team delivers a premature infant at 27 weeks of gestation and weighing 1500 gm. How soon will you request fundus examination by an ophthalmologist?

A. Immediately

B. 3–4 weeks after delivery

C. At 34 weeks gestational age

D. At 40 weeks gestational age

34. Significant loss of vision in a patient with hypertension can occur due to all of the following except:

A. Occipital infarct

B. Anterior ischemic optic neuropathy

C. Papilloedema

D. Retinal haemorrhage

35. In fluorescein angiography of the eye, all of the following structures can be examined except:

A. Lens B. Retina
C. Iris D. Uveal tissue

36. What is the most important factor for development of retinopathy of prematurity?

A. Low birth weight
B. Prematurity
C. Sepsis
D. Congenital anomalies

37. What is represented by ETDRS in a diabetic vision chart?

A. Early treatment for diabetic retinopathy study
B. Extended treatment for diabetes review study
C. Extensive therapy for diabetes research study
D. Eye test drum review study

38. Retinal detachment is seen in:

A. Diabetes
B. High myopia
C. Malignant melanoma
D. All of the above

39. Most common cause of blindness in non-proliferative diabetic retinopathy is:

A. Subretinal haemorrhage
B. Macular edema
C. Retinal detachment
D. Vitreous haemorrhage

40. All are true regarding retinitis pigmentosa, except:

A. Early treatment prevents progression of disease
B. Visual acuity remains till late
C. X-linked inheritance
D. Associated with somatic abnormalities

41. All of the following are ocular features of epidemic dropsy except:

A. Tortuosity of vessels
B. Optic disc oedema
C. Pre-retinal haemorrhage
D. Hard exudates

42. Diabetic retinopathy is common in:

A. NIDDM of 2 years duration
B. IDDM of 2 years duration
C. Juvenile onset diabetes before puberty
D. Pregnancy induced gestational diabetes

43. Lattice degeneration is seen in:

A. Myopia
B. Hypermetropia
C. Presbyopia
D. Rheumatoid arthritis

44. Most sensitive part of retina is:

A. Optic disc
B. Fovea centralis
C. Macula lutea
D. Peripheral retina

45. Neovascularisation is seen in:

A. Central retinal vein obstruction
B. Branch retinal artery obstruction
C. Branch retinal vein obstruction
D. All of the above

46. Cherry-red spot over retina is seen in all, except:

A. Tay-Sachs disease
B. Niemann-Pick disease
C. CRAO
D. Battern Mayo syndrome

47. Ring scotoma is feature of:

A. Embryonal nuclear cataract

B. Diabetic retinopathy

C. Blue dot cataract

D. Retinitis pigmentosa

48. Floaters can be seen in all, except:

A. Uveitis

B. Acute congestive glaucoma

C. Retinal detachment

D. Vitreous haemorrhage

49. Treatment of diabetic retinopathy:

A. Phacoemulsification

B. Retinal laser photocoagulation

C. LASIK

D. Pars plana vitrectomy

50. Diabetic retinopathy is treated by:

A. Strict glycemic control

B. Panphotocoagulation

C. Antihypertensive

D. Antioxidants

E. Cyclophotocoagulation

51. Snow ball opacity in vitreous is seen in:

A. Pars planitis B. Sarcoidosis

C. Juvenile RA D. Toxoplasmosis

E. Fuch's lesion

52. RD is diagnosed by:

A. + 90 D

B. Hruby lens

C. 3 mirror contact lens

D. Direct ophthalmoscopy

E. Indirect ophthalmoscopy

53. In a young patient presenting with recurrent vitreous haemorrhage, diagnosis is:

A. Eales' disease

B. CRVO

C. Proliferative retinopathy

D. Coats' disease

E. Episcleritis

54. Eye changes in diabetes mellitus include:

A. Paralysis of 3rd, 4th, 6th nerve palsy

B. Rubeosis iridis

C. Proliferative retinopathy

D. Subconjunctival haemorrhage

E. Hypermetropia

55. Periphery of retina is visualized by:

A. Indirect ophthalmoscope

B. Direct ophthalmoscope

C. Gonioscopy

D. Contact lens

56. Regarding fovea, which of the following statement is true?

A. Has the lowest threshold for light

B. Contains only cones

C. Contains only rods

D. Maximum visual acuity

E. Is located at apex of optic nerve

57. Cotton-wool spots are commonly seen in:

A. AIDS B. DM

C. Hypertension D. CMV

58. Black floaters in a diabetic patient indicate:

A. Vitreous haemorrhage

B. Maculopathy

C. Vitreous infarction

D. Posterior vitreous detachment

59. Amsler grid is used in:

A. Detecting maculopathy

B. Optic disc examination

C. Squint

D. Retinal examination

60. Retinopathy in neonate is due to:

A. Prematurity < 1500 gm

B. O_2 toxicity

C. Trauma

D. Diabetes

61. In Retinitis pigmentosa, following are true except:

A. Pigment present

B. Pale waxy disc

C. Narrowing of vessel

D. ERG–normal

62. Rubeosis iridis is not seen in:

A. CRVO

B. CRAO

C. Diabetic retinopathy

D. Neovascularization

63. Enlarging dot sign in fundus fluorescein scanning is seen in:

A. Cystoid macular edema

B. Central serous retinopathy

C. Significant macular edema

D. Coats' disease

64. Bull's eye retinopathy is seen in:

A. Chloroquine B. Methanol

C. Ethambutol D. Steroids

65. Following are seen in CRA occlusion except:

A. Gradual loss of vision

B. Headache

C. Sudden loss of vision

D. Retained central vision

66. Cherry-red spot is seen in:

A. Retinitis pigmentosa

B. Retinopathy of prematurity

C. Metachromatic leukodystrophy

D. CRVO occlusion

67. Visual loss in DR is due to:

A. Cataract formation

B. Background diabetic retinopathy

C. Proliferative diabetic retinopathy

D. Vitreous haemorrhage

68. Ultrasound is used in the eye for:

A. Orbital tumours

B. Endophthalmitis

C. Retinal detachment

D. Vitreous haemorrhage

69. Treatment of choice in proliferative diabetic retinopathy is:

A. Pan-retinal photocoagulation

B. Shift the patient to insulin

C. Scleral buckling operation

D. Vitrectomy

70. Most characteristic retinal feature of diabetic retinopathy is:

A. Cotton-wool spots

B. Neovascularization

C. Soft exudates

D. Microaneurysms

71. All of the following changes are seen in eclamptic retinopathy except:

A. Cotton-wool spots

B. Flame-shaped haemorrhages

C. Microaneurysms

D. Neovascularization

72. Most common cause of vitreous haemorrhage is:

A. Coats' disease

B. Eales' disease

C. Retinal detachment

D. Cataract

73. Which of the following is investigation of choice in a 50 years old male diabetic presenting with sudden appearance of black floaters in the eye?

A. Retinoscopy

B. Fluorescein angiography

C. Direct ophthalmoscopy

D. Indirect ophthalmoscopy

74. Cotton-wool spots are seen in all except:

A. Diabetes mellitus

B. Hypertension

C. Polyarteritis nodosa

D. Coats' disease

75. All are indications for pan-retinal laser photocoagulation in diabetic retinopathy except:

A. Optic disc neovascularisation

B. Pre retinal haemorrhage

C. Retinal neovascularisation

D. More than 10 cotton-wool spots

76. Most significant risk factor in retinal vein occlusion is:

A. Hypertension

B. Diabetes mellitus

C. High cholesterol levels

D. Smoking

77. Moderate loss of vision in diabetes mellitus is due to:

A. Vitreous haemorrhage

B. Presenile cataract

C. Arterio sclerotic retinopathy

D. Background retinopathy

78. Retinal changes in diabetes are due to:

A. Sorbitol

B. Glucose

C. Glycosylated end products

D. Aldol condensation

79. Cystoid macular edema not seen in:

A. Aphakia

B. CSR

C. Diabetic retinopathy

D. Retinitis pigmentosa

80. Following is pathognomic finding of retinal detachment:

A. Fluid shift B. Black shadow

C. Line D. Hole

81. Angiography is diagnostic in:

A. Retinoschisis

B. Rhegmatogenous retinal detachment

C. Central serous retinopathy

D. Vitreous detachment

82. Sudden increase in blood sugar in diabetics cause:

A. Myopic shift

B. Hypermetropic shift

C. Presbyopia

D. Anisometropia

83. Differential diagnosis of night blindness is all except:

A. Vitamin A deficiency

B. Retinitis pigmentosa

C. High myopia

D. Peripheral lenticular opacity

84. Following are seen in degenerative myopia except:

A. Lattice degeneration of retina

B. Foster-Fuch's spot

C. Lacquer cracks

D. Gyrate atrophy

85. Watered silk appearance of fundus is seen in:

A. Hypermetropia
B. Myopia
C. Astigmatism
D. Presbyopia

86. In deuteranopia there is defect of:
A. Red colour B. Green colour
C. Blue colour D. All

87. In retina, the ratio of artery to vein is:
A. 1:3 B. 2:3
C. 3:2 D. 3:1

88. Sudden loss of vision is seen in:
A. Eales' disease
B. Coats' disease
C. Papilloedema
D. Age related macular degeneration

89. In hypertension, loss of vision occurs due to:
A. Optic atrophy
B. Vascular accidents
C. Macular oedema
D. Vitreous haemorrhage

90. Projection of light is interfered in:
A. Morgagnian cataract
B. Acute congestive glaucoma
C. Macular degeneration
D. Retinitis pigmentosa

91. Rhegmatogenous retinal detachment is seen in all except:
A. Old age B. High myopia
C. Aphakia D. Eales' disease

92. Neovascularisation of the iris can be seen frequently in all, except:
A. Fuch's heterochromic cyclitis
B. Diabetic retinopathy
C. CRVO
D. Congenital cataract

93. Fundal picture in myopia:
A. Soft exudates
B. Hard exudates
C. Flame-shaped haemorrhages
D. Cystoid degeneration

94. Pars plana vitrectomy is done in all except:
A. Retinal detatchment
B. Vitreous haemorrhage
C. Removal of foreign bodies
D. Chorioretinitis

95. All are seen in diabetic retinopathy except:
A. Choroidal neovascular membrane formation
B. Rubeosis iridis
C. Preretinal bleed
D. Retinal detatchment

96. True about ARMD are all except:
A. Drusens are seen
B. Retinal degenerations
C. Choroidal neovascularization
D. Intravitreal Anti-VEGF is the treatment of choice

97. Cherry-red spot due to gangliosidosis is seen in:
A. Berlin's oedema
B. Niemann-Pick disease
C. Tay-Sachs disease
D. Batten Mayou disease

98. Visible retinal arterial pulsation is seen in:
A. CRVO B. CRAO
C. Raised IOT D. Normal eye

99. 'a' wave in ERG corresponds to activity of:
A. Ganglion cell layer
B. Pigment epithelium

C. Nerve bundle layer

D. Rods and cones

100. Resuscitation time of the human retina following ischemia is:

A. 30 minutes B. 45 minutes

C. 1–2 hours D. 15 to 20 minutes

101. Exudative retinal detachment is seen in:

A. Proliferative retinopathy

B. Toxaemia of pregnancy

C. Tumour of choroid

D. Hypertension

102. Purtscher's retinopathy results from:

A. Head injuries

B. Chest injuries

C. Pancreatitis

D. All of the above

103. In laser therapy for retinal disease, laser affects which layer of retina?

A. Layer of rods and cones

B. Pigment layer

C. Inner plexiform layer

D. Nerve fibre layer

104. For prevention of retrolental fibroplasias oxygen should be:

A. 30–40% B. 20–30%

C. 50–60% D. 70–80%

105. Retinal detachment is seen in all except:

A. Senile retinoschisis

B. Diabetic retinopathy

C. Lattice degeneration

D. Climatic droplet dystrophy

106. The superficial retinal haemorrhages are situated in:

A. Nerve fibre layer

B. Outer plexiform layer

C. Inner nuclear layer

D. Inner plexiform layer

107. The most frequent cataract seen in adult retinitis pigmentosa patient is:

A. PSC B. Anterior polar

C. Cortical D. Mixed

108. Lattice degeneration is associated with retinal detachment in approximately what percentage of patients?

A. 20% B. 30%

C. 10% D. 6%

109. Lebers congenital amaurosis is characterized by all except:

A. Bulls eye maculopathy

B. Reduced visual acuity

C. Salt and pepper fundus

D. Hamarlopia

110. Presence of papilloedema signifies the following stage of hypertensive retinopathy according to K.W. classification:

A. 1 B. 2

C. 3 D. 4

111. Short posterior ciliary arteries are about .... in number.

A. 10 B. 20

C. 30 D. 40

112. Retinal blood vessels are developed from:

A. Surface ectoderm

B. Paraxial mesoderm

C. Endoderm

D. Neuroectoderm

113. Earliest fundus abnormality seen in pregnancy-induced hypertension is:

A. Macular star

B. Flame-shaped haemorrhages

C. Cotton-wool spots

D. Narrowing of nasal arterioles

114. Most diagnostic test for Best disease is:

A. Dark adaptation

B. ERG

C. EOG

D. VEP

115. The electroretinogram may assist in the diagnosis of all of the following except:

A. Retinitis pigmentosa

B. Progression of retinal disease

C. Clinically unsuspected disease in familial retinal degenerations

D. Complications of glaucoma

116. Roth's spots in the fundus are seen in:

A. Diabetes

B. Chorioretinitis

C. Bacterial endocarditis

D. Retinoblastoma

117. All are seen in Albinism except:

A. Nystagmus

B. Glaucoma

C. Photophobia

D. Refractive error

118. Essential atrophy of choroid is due to inborn error of metabolism of amino acid?

A. Cystine B. Arginine

C. Ornithine D. Lysine

119. Which of the following is the most common ocular complication with renal transplantation?

A. Cataract

B. Glaucoma

C. CMV retinitis

D. Candida endophthalmitis

120. Ocular manifestation of Sturge-Weber syndrome is:

A. Hemangioma of face and glaucoma

B. Leisch nodules

C. Pulsating exophthalmos

D. Retinal haemorrhage

121. Treatment of choice for carotico-cavernous fistula:

A. Internal carotid artery ligation

B. Balloon embolisation

C. Resection

D. Conservative treatment

122. Argon laser is used in all except:

A. Retinal detachment

B. Retinal vein occlusion

C. Retinitis pigmentosa

D. Eales' disease

123. In PRP of the retina which quadrant is first coagulated?

A. Temporal B. Nasal

C. Superior D. Inferior

124. Photopsia is a characteristic of:

A. Rubeosis iridis

B. Retinal detachment

C. Chronic simple glaucoma

D. Optic neuritis

125. Which of the following PFCL has the highest molecular weight?

A. Perfluoro-n-octane

B. Perfluoro decalin

C. Perfluoro phenanthrene

D. Perfluoro-propane

126. Rods and cones differ in all except:

A. Intensity

B. Sensitivity

C. Signal transduction

D. Type of light

127. A patient presented with sudden onset of floaters and sensation of falling of a curtain in front of the eye. Which one of the following is the appropriate diagnosis?

A. Retinal detachment

B. Eales' disease

C. Vitreous haemorrhage

D. Optic neuritis

128. Which of the following is the most probable diagnosis in a patient with loss of central vision and a normal ERG with no family history?

A. Best's disease

B. Stargardt's disease

C. Retinitis pigmentosa

D. Macular hole

129. Retinitis pigmentosa is a feature of all except:

A. Refsum's disease

B. Kearn Sayre

C. NARP

D. Abetaglobulinemia

130. A 25-year-old male presents with painless sudden loss of vision, ocular and systemic examination is not contributory. What is the most probable diagnosis?

A. Retinal detachment

B. Eales' disease

C. Glaucoma

D. Cataract

131. Treatment for threshold retinopathy is:

A. Deoxygenation

B. Panretinal photocoagulation

C. Laser photocoagulation

D. Wait and watch

132. 60-year-old man, both HTN and DM for 10 years, there is reduced vision in one eye, on fundus examination there is a central bleed and the fellow eye is normal, the diagnosis:

A. Diabetic retinopathy

B Retinal tear

C. Optic neuritis

D. Hypertensive retinopathy

133. A young patient complaining with recurrent vitreous haemorrhage, diagnosis is:

A. Eales' disease

B. CRVO

C. Proliferative retinopathy

D. Coats' disease

134. A symptom of retinitis pigmentosa:

A. Coloured halos

B. Diplopia

C. Nyctalopia

D. Sudden loss of vision

135. Which is the most common complication of high myopia?

A. Glaucoma

B. Cataract

C. Haemorrhage

D. Retinal detachment

136. Which of the following is most radio-resistant structure in retina?

A. Pigment epithelium

B. Layers of rods and cones

C. Bipolar cell layer

D. Ganglion cell layer

137. Mizuo phenomenon is seen in:

A. Fundus albipathicus

B. Fundus flavimicetus

C. Oguchi's disease

D. Choroideremia

138. Most common cause of vitreous hemorrhage in diabetic retinopathy is:

A. CRVO

B. Posterior vitreous detachment

C. Neovascularization of disc

D. Trauma leading to rupture of central retinal artery

139. A 20-year-old male presents with a history of tennis ball injury to the right eye. On examination, a red spot is seen at macula. The most likely diagnosis is:

A. Macular hole

B. Berlin's edema

C. Macular bleed

D. Macular tear

140. Gyrate atrophy is a retinal degenerative disease involving deficiency of ornithine transcarbomylase enzyme. Such patients are likely to benefit from:

A. Ornithine free diet

B. Arginine free diet

C. Use of folic acid and pyridoxine

D. Use of B1, B6 and B12

141. The total area of the retina seen in direct ophthalmoscopy is:

A. 1 DD B. 2 DD

C. 3 DD D. 4 DD

142. CRAO may be seen in:

A. Diabetes mellitus

B. CMV retinitis

C. Panophthalmitis

D. Orbital mucormycosis

143. A 20-year-old male presents with night blindness and tubular vision. His IOP was 18 mm of Hg. Fundoscopy shows attenuation of arterioles and waxy pallor of optic disc. Ring scotoma seen on perimetry. ERG is subnormal:

A. Pigmentary retinal dystrophy

B. POAG

C. Lattice Degeneration of retina

D. Diabetic retinopathy

144. Three weeks following IOL implantation, a patient complains of diminished vision, on fundus fluorescein angiography, flower petal hyperfluorescence of macula is noted. Most likely diagnosis is:

A. CME

B. Central serous retinopathy

C. Macular dystrophy

D. ARMD

145. A young male presents with complaints of severe photophobia and loss of vision. Electrical examination reveals subnormal pattern, predominantly photopic pattern. The most probable diagnosis is:

A. Stargardt syndrome

B. Batten's syndrome

C. Cone dystrophy

D. Chloroquine toxicity

146. A 55-year-old diabetic patient presents with transient obscuration for 2–3 days followed by sudden diminution of vision. Which of the following would be the best test to evaluate his symptoms?

A. Serum ACE levels

B. Quantiferon-Gold TB test

C. Serum homocysteine levels

D. Serum creatinine levels

147. Calcification is seen in all of the following except:

A. Optic drusen

B. Retinoblastoma

C. Choroidal osteoma

D. PHPV

148. The risk of rhegmatogenous retinal detachment is increased in all of the following except:

A. Pseudophakia

B. Trauma

C. Hyperopia

D. Lattice degeneration

149. An infant weighing less than 1000 g is more likely to develop which of the following complications?

A. Glaucoma

B. Cataract

C. Severe ROP

D. Retinal detachment

150. 70 years old patient with NIDDM underwent macular dot laser surgery for mild non-proliferative retinopathy with macular edema, 8 weeks back, now complains of macular vitreal traction. Management would be:

A. Macular laser surgery

B. Pan endophotocoagulation

C. Pars plana vitrectomy

D. Intravitreal bevacizumab

151. A child born at 29 weeks and he was diagnosed zone 1 (grade 2) ROP in both eyes at post conceptional 33 weeks of age. What would be next treatment?

A. Urgent photocoagulation in both eyes to remove avascular peripheral retina

B. Follow up

C. Laser photocoagulation in worsen eye and follow up for other eye

D. Cryotherapy

152. The normal ratio of light peak and dark trough on an EOG:

A. 1

B. 1.5

C. More than 185%

D. Less than 185%

153. Regarding rhegmatogenous retinal detachment, all of the following are correct except:

A. There is abnormal pull on the retina due to changes in the vitreous

B. Anterior extent is up to ora serrata

C. Usually progresses rapidly

D. Management is usually surgical

154. A man presents with an iron foreign body in the eye. Which of the following is the best investigation to monitor the vision in him?

A. Serial arden ratio

B. Dark adaptometry

C. Serial visual evoked potentials

D. Serial electroretinogram

155. The development of subretinal demarcation lines (high water marks) in the retina is indicative of:

A. Longstanding retinal detachment

B. Fresh retinal detachment

C. Retinal tumour formation

D. Normal retinal finding

156. A 55-year-old diabetic patient presents with transient obscuration

for 2–3 days followed by sudden diminution of vision. Which of the following would be the best test to evaluate his symptoms?

A. Serum ACE levels

B. Quantiferon-Gold TB test

C. Serum homocysteine levels

D. Serum creatinine levels

157. A paediatrician in a district hospital with specialized neonatal care unit calls an ophthalmologist for consultation for which of the following?

A. A newborn with respiratory distress

B. A baby born at 28 weeks of gestation

C. A newborn with jaundice

D. A newborn with birthweight 2300 grams

158. Regarding myopic degeneration, which of the following is true?

A. It is seen more commonly in males than in females

B. Myopic degeneration can lead to retinal detachment

C. It is seen in < – 6 D myopia

D. Optic disc swelling is seen

159. A 7-year-old male child presents with normal vision 6/6 in the right eye and hand movement perception close to the face in the left eye. On fundoscopy, his right eye was normal and left eye showed retinal detachment, subretinal yellowish exudates and telangiectatic vessels. The most likely diagnosis is:

A. Coats' disease

B. Sympathetic ophthalmitis

C. Familial exudative vitreoretinopathy

D. Retinopathy of prematurity

160. A young male presents with central scotoma in left eye. His right vision showed 6/6 vision. On examination, in the left eye, there was focal foveal detachment. What would be the next step?

A. Examine retrolental cells

B. Inquire about the use of steroids

C. Ask for history of trauma in the other eye

D. Laser photocoagulation

161. A 28-week baby suffered from respiratory distress syndrome at birth. On day 14 of life, he developed sepsis. No other morbidity was seen. He should be evaluated for retinopathy of prematurity at what postnatal age?

A. 2 weeks B. 4 weeks

C. 6 weeks D. 8 weeks

162. A person is diagnosed to be a diabetic on his 45th birthday. You will recommend a dilated fundoscopic examination:

A. Immediately

B. Before his 50th birthday

C. When he turns 50 years of age

D. When he complains of dimness of vision

163. Microaneurysms are the earliest manifestation of diabetic retinopathy. Which of the following layer is involved in diabetic retinopathy?

A. Outer plexiform layer

B. Inner nuclear layer

C. Layer of rods and cones

D. Retinal pigment epithelium

164. Pneumorectopexy is an outpatient procedure in which retinal detachment is sealed with air insufflation?

Which of the following gas is used in pneumorectopexy?

A. Sulfur hexafluoride
B. Carbon dioxide
C. Nitrous oxide
D. Oxygen

165. Earliest feature of diabetic retinopathy is:

A. Microneurysms
B. Cotton-wool spots
C. Dot and blot haemorrhages
D. Hard exudates

166. All of the following cause visual loss of hypertension except:

A. Occipital infarct
B. Anterior ischemic optic neuropathy
C. Papilloedema
D. Hemorrhage

167. Extra retinal fibrovascular proliferation at ridge between normal and a vascular retina is which grade of ROP?

A. ROP 1 B. ROP 2
C. ROP 3 D. ROP 4

168. Cattle truck appearance in fundoscopy is due to:

A. CRAO
B. CRVO
C. Retinitis pigmentosa
D. Diabetic retinopathy

169. Waves present in electroretinogram are all except:

A. A wave B. B wave
C. C wave D. D wave

170. Which of the following is not an ophthalmic emergency?

A. Macular hole
B. Retinal detachment
C. CRAO
D. Acute primary angle closure glaucoma

171. The risk of rhegmatogenous retinal detachment is increased in all of the following except:

A. Pseudophakia
B. Trauma
C. Hyperopia
D. Lattice degeneration

172. Diffuse mottling of retina with focal areas of increased and decreased pigmentation between posterior pole and equator (Salt and pepper retinopathy) is observed in all of the following except:

A. Phenothiazine toxicity
B. Congenital rubella
C. Own settlement of retinal detachment
D. Fundus flavimaculatus

173. An infant weighing less than 1000 g is more likely to develop which of the following complications?

A. Glaucoma
B. Cataract
C. Severe ROP
D. Retinal detachment

174. Immediately after photodynamic therapy, color of the lesion becomes:

A. No change in color
B. Grey
C. Yellow
D. White

175. The normal ratio of light peak and dark trough on an EOG is:

A. 1
B. 1.5
C. More than 185%
D. Less than 185%

176. Regarding rhegmatogenous retinal detachment, all of the following are correct except:
A. There is abnormal pull on the retina due to changes in the vitreous
B. Anterior extent is up to ora serrata
C. Usually progresses rapidly
D. Management is usually surgical

177. The development of subretinal demarcation lines (high water marks) in the retina is indicative of:
A. Longstanding retinal detachment
B. Fresh retinal detachment
C. Retinal tumour formation
D. Normal retinal finding

178. A man presents with an iron foreign body in the eye. Which of the following is the best investigation to monitor the vision in him?
A. Serial Arden ratio
B. Dark adaptometry
C. Serial visual evoked potentials
D. Serial electroretinogram

179. Cherry-red spot and Hollenhorst plaque are seen in:
A. CRAO
B. CRVO
C. Branch RAO
D. Branch RVO

180. Cherry-red spot after trauma is seen in children due to:
A. CRVO
B. CRAO
C. Berlin's edema
D. Niemann-Pick's disease

181. Multifocal ERG is useful to assess the function of:
A. RODS
B. Macular cones
C. Ganglion cells
D. Retinal pigment epithelium

182. True statement regarding direct ophthalmoscopy are all except:
A. 2 disk diameter field of vision
B. Image is virtual and erect
C. Magnification is 5 times
D. Self-illuminated device

183. Most common type of staphyloma:
A. Anterior
B. Intercalary
C. Equatorial
D. Posterior

ANSWER AND EXPLANATION

1.	d	We do endophotocoagulation and not exophotocoagulation.
2.	d	We have to exclude carotid artery occlusion and not central artery occlusion, hence, the definitive method is ophthalmodynamometry.
3.	b	Indocyanine Green is 98% bound to plasma proteins and hence stays for a longer time in the blood. Hence, it is more useful in detecting choroidal lesions.
4.	b	Interleukins and Interferons are mainly related to inflammation.
5.	c	Juxtafoveal means beside the fovea.
6.	a	Lambert-Eaton syndrome causes myogenic ptosis.
7.	c	In visual cycle NADP is reduced to NAD.
8.	b	Best disease is dystrophy of the RPE cells.
9.	c	"Cherry-red spot" is seen in type II gangliosidosis and not in type I.

10. a NIDDM is generally diagnosed late and hence, fundus examination should be done immediately.
11. a Both Gentamycin and Amikacin are toxic to the macula.
12. b 1 DD is 1.5 mm.
13. d Circle of haller and zinn is anastamosis between short posterior ciliary arteries and supplies peripapillary area of optic disc.
14. c Von-Hippel Lindau syndrome is also called Angiomatosis retinae and is characterized by hemangiomas on the retina and the optic disc.
15. a A young male with painless loss of vision and no fundal glow the most likely cause is vitreous haemorrhage probably due to Eales' disease.
16. d PDT, i.e., photodyanamic therapy is used if the choroidal neovascular membrane is either subfoveal or juxtafoveal.
17. b CSR is an insidious and self-limiting disease of young males.
18. c Arteries may be constricted if there is associated hypertension but are not dilated.
19. b CRAO generally occurs in patients of heart disease due to embolism.
20. a Putscher's retinopathy occurs due to air or fat embolism.
21. b It occurs due to Berlin's edema after blunt trauma.
22. b Fluorescein angiography helps to diagnose leakages and capillary blocks.
23. d Ushers syndrome is the most common systemic association of RP.
24. a Retinal and choroidal changes are common in myopia but not in hypermetropia.
25. a Retinal pigment epithelial changes are a feature of ARMD and not of DM.
26. b According to Keith-Wagner grading this patient is grade III HR.
27. a Angiod streaks are dehiscence in the Bruch's membrane in patients with collagenous disorders.
28. a Since the vision loss is gradually progressive it is due to cataract.
29. b This patient should be checked for any retinal detachment; hence we should do indirect ophthalmoscopy.
30. c See visual cycle.
31. d This patient is a case of CSR which is a self-limiting disease.
32. b Amacrine cells adjust the bipolar cells in the negative feedback arrangement.
33. c Ideal time of screening is 4 weeks to postnatal age or between 31 and 33 weeks.
34. c Visual acuity is normal in patients of papilloedema.
35. a Lens is an avascular structure.
36. b In premature infants there is a free radical injury to the developing blood vessels leading to the retinopathy.
37. a See studies done in DR.
38. d DM can lead to tractional RD, high myopia causes rhegmatogenous RD and malignant melanoma will lead to exudative RD.
39. b Chronic CMEs can damage the macula.
40. a RP is a genetic disease and there is no effective treatment of retinitis pigmentosa.

41.	c	Epidemic dropsy occurs due to Sanguanarine toxicity.
42.	a	NIDDM is diagnosed late and hence history of 2 years may not mean 2 years.
43.	a	Lattice degeneration is a feature of pathological myopia.
44.	b	The thinnest part of the retina is ora serrata.
45.	a	Neovascularisation is not a feature of CRAO.
46.	d	Batten-Mayo syndrome is a cerebromacular degeneration characterized by Bull's eye maculopathy.
47.	d	RP in the initial stage involves the midperiphery of the retina and hence is characterized by ring scotoma.
48.	b	Floaters are opacities in the vitreous cavity.
49.	b	Photocoagulative lasers turn hypoxia into anoxia and hence the neovascularisation is prevented.
50.	a,b, d	Cyclophotocoagulation is done in absolute glaucoma and not in retinopathy.
51.	a,b	Snow-ball opacities are white exudates in the vitreous cavity.
52.	c,d, e	+90 D and Hruby lens are used to visualize the central retina.
53.	a	This is a typical presentation of Eales' disease, i.e., periphlebitis retinae. Coats' disease is a disease of children.
54.	a,b, c	Subconjunctival haemorrhage is a feature of hypertension.
55.	a,d	Here by contact lens we mean Goldmann three-mirror contact lens.
56.	a,d	At the centre of the fovea there are only cones, but whole fovea has both rod and cones.
57.	a,b, c	CMV retinitis presents as "Sauce and Cheese retinopathy".
58.	a,d	Floaters, i.e., opacity in the vitreous cavity is generally visualized as black.
59.	a	Amsler-Grid test is a method of charting 10 degree of the visual field.
60.	a,b	ROP is an oxidative damage to the developing blood vessels of the retina.
61.	d	ERG is subnormal in RP.
62.	b	CRAO is not characterized by neovascularisation as the condition is not hypoxic but anoxic.
63.	b	FFA findings of CSR are Enlarging Ink-Blot and Smoke-Stack appearances.
64.	a	Other causes of Bull's eye retinopathy are–cone dystrophy and Batten-Mayo syndrome.
65.	a,b	Central vision may be retained in CRAO in patients who have dual blood supply to the macula. It occurs in 14% of the population and the other artery is the cilio-retinal artery.
66.	c	See D/D of cherry-red spot.
67.	a,c, d	In BDR, vision can be affected only if there is CSMO, i.e., clinically significant macular edema.
68.	c,d	USG eye will diagnose intraocular lesions and not intraorbital tumours.
69.	a	Scleral buckling is the procedure to treat a rhegmatogenous RD. Vitrectomy and sclera buckling operations are done to manage the

complications which can occur after neovascularisation.

70. d Microaneurysms are less than 100 microns.

71. c Eclamptic retinopathy presents as hypertensive retinopathy and hence microaneurysms are not seen as they are a feature of DR.

72. b The next common cause of vitreous haemorrhage is trauma.

73. d The presentation is typical of vitreous haemorrhage.

74. c Cotton-wool spots or soft exudates are axonal debris.

75. b Preretinal haemorrhage impairs proper visualization of the retina and hence laser cannot be done.

76. a Other risk factors of CRVO are high IOP, hypermetropia and blood viscosity syndromes.

77. a Ideally the answer should be macular edema but as that is not the option the next best option is partial vitreous haemorrhage.

78. c Cataract is due to sorbitol and not the retinal changes.

79. b CSR is a shallow RD at the macula.

80. b Retina appears red when attached due to choroid. In RD it appears grey.

81. c CSR as mentioned has typical FFA findings.

82. a Increase in sugar will lead to swelling of the lens and hence increase in the refractive power of the eye.

83. d All other options are important causes of nyctalopia. Central lenticular opacities cause day blindness.

84. d Gyrate atrophy is a choroidal dystrophy due to deficiency of enzyme ornithine aminotransferase.

85. a Watered-silk appearance is a sharp foveal reflex on the macula.

86. b See color blindness.

87. b Normal V:A is 3:2.

88. a ARMD presents as gradual loss of vision. There is no visual loss in papilloedema.

89. c Macular edema will affect the vision.

90. d Projection of light is affected if large part of the retina is involved.

91. c Aphakia is absence of lens and is not related to retinal detachment.

92. d Any hypoxic condition of the retina can cause rubeosis iridis.

93. d Pathological myopia presents with degenerative changes.

94. d Chorioretinitis is an inflammatory condition and is not an indication for Vitrectomy.

95. a DR presents as retinal neovascularisation and not as choroidal neovascularisation.

96. b ARMD is a disease of choroid, also involving the RPE cells.

97. c Niemann-Pick disease is a sphingolipidosis and not gangliosidosis.

98. c Visible venous pulsations are normal but visible arterial pulsations are seen when IOP is markedly increased.

99. d Wave 'a' indicates photoreceptor activity whereas wave 'b' indicates the activity of bipolar cells.

100. c There will be permanent damage of the retina after this critical period.

101. c Any pathology of the choroid which percolates into the subretinal space will lead to exudative retinal detachment.

102. d All are the causes of putscher's retinopathy which is due to air or fat embolism.

103. b Laser treatment affects the RPE cells.

104. a ROP is mainly an oxidative injury due to oxygen inhalation; hence the concentration of oxygen needs to be guarded.

105. d Climatic droplet dystrophy is a corneal dystrophy.

106. a Superficial haemorrhages are at the level of NFL and deep haemorrhages are between outer plexiform and inner nuclear layer.

107. a Cataract associated with RP is most commonly posterior subcapsular (PSC).

108. b Any lattice degeneration can lead to hole formation causing rhegmatogenous retinal detachment.

109. d Lebers congenital amaurosis will lead to total loss of vision.

110. d See Keith-Wagner grading.

111. b Long posterior ciliary arteries are two in number whereas short are 20–30.

112. b Retina develops from neuroectoderm whereas the blood vessels develop from paraxial mesoderm.

113. d Attenuation of arteries is the first change in retina due to hypertension.

114. c Best disease is a dystrophy of RPE cells.

115. d ERG tells the activity of Photoreceptors and bipolar cells. Glaucoma involves the optic nerve and hence ERG does not help.

116. c Haemorrhage with a white pale centre is called Roth's spot and is a feature of endocarditis.

117. b Glaucoma is not a feature of albinism. Foveal development is impaired in albinism leading to decreased visual acuity, nystagmus, squint. Photophobia is due to decreased iris pigments or absence of melanin pigments in the iris.

118. c It is also called gyrate atrophy.

119. c Immunosuppression leads to candida infections.

120. a Sturge-Weber syndrome is a triad of hemangioma of the face called naevus flammeus, intracranial hemangioma and glaucoma.

121. b Balloon embolisation is done these days to treat C-C fistula.

122. c RP is a dystrophy of photoreceptors and has no effective treatment.

123. a In PRP we first give laser barrage around the macula so that we do not hit the fovea accidentally.

124. b Photopsia is flash of light seen by the patient of RD due to traction of the photoreceptors cells.

125. c PFCL is a vitreous substitute used in RD surgeries.

126. c Signal transduction occurs in the same way in both rods and cones by the method of hyperpolarisation.

127. a The history of falling of curtain and sudden onset of floaters is suggestive of retinal detachment.

128. d ERG is abnormal in RP, whereas Best disease and Stargardts disease are familial. Therefore we will mark the answer as Macular Hole.

129. d RP is associated with abetalipoproteinaemia.

130. b The history is suggestive of Eales' disease.

131. c Threshold retinopathy is ROP, i.e., retinopathy of prematurity.

132. a Retinal tears are commonly peripheral whereas HR is always bilateral. DR in the initial stages can present in one eye first.

133. a Eales' disease present as recurrent vitreous haemorrhage and are a disease of young males.

134. c RP is dystrophy of photoreceptor cells and primarily affects the rods, hence the patient complains of nyctalopia.

135. d Lattice degeneration in patients of high myopia can lead to hole formation causing rhegmatogenous retinal detachment.

136. d Ganglion cell layer is most radioresistant. In eye the most radioresistant structure is sclera and the most radiosensitive is lens.

137. c This disease is a congenital night blindness, hereditary in nature, with a discoloured posterior pole. It is characterised by Mizuo phenomenon where sitting for 1 hour in darkness leads to relieve of symptoms of night blindness and the fundus picture becomes normal. The basic pathophysiology includes lack of activity of rods.

138. c In DR, it is the neovascularisation that bleeds due to leaky blood vessels and leads to vitreous haemorrhage. It could be NVD, i.e., neovascularisation at disc or NVE, i.e., neovascularisation elsewhere.

139. b Red spot at macula after blunt trauma, most probable diagnosis is Berlin's edema, i.e., commotion retinae.

140. b Gyrate atrophy patients are of two types, those who respond to vitamin B6 have a better prognosis and those who do not have a worst prognosis. But arginine free diet help all patients, hence we mark it as the answer.

141. b Area of the fundus visualized by direct ophthalmoscope at any given focus, i.e., field of view is 2 DD (whereas with indirect it is 8DD) and by tilting the angle of the instrument we can visualize till the equator.

142. d Orbital mucormycosis causes vasculitis leading to CRAO. Other causes are:
   A. Vasculitis due to varicella infection.
   B. Optic neuritis.
   C. Local trauma which lead to damage to the blood vessel.
   D. Radiation retinopathy.
   E. Optic disc drusen.
   F. Depot medication around the eye.

143. a The history strongly suggests that the patient has retinitis pigmentosa, which is a dystrophy of photoreceptors, i.e., rods and cones (primarily rods are involved), with typical triad of pale waxy disc, attenuated arteries and bony spicules which is a form of pigmentary change. In the initial stage of the disease there is ring scotoma and in the late stage of the disease there is tubular vision.

144. a Flower petal pattern in the FFA is diagnostic of cystoid macular edema and is a known complication after cataract surgery.

145. c The patient is presenting with photophobia with abnormal photopic ERG response, the diagnosis is cone dystrophy.

146. c Homocysteine is a very important biomarker for vascular damage and a high level of homocysteine is related to vision loss in patients of type 2 diabetes.

147. d In all the three options, calcification is a very prominent feature.

148. c Retinal degenerations like lattice degenerations are common in myopes and hence rhegmatogenous retinal detachment is a common occurrence in pathological myopia, but not in hyperopia.

A complicated cataract surgery can be a risk factor for RD.

149. c Prematurity and low birth weight in an infant, given oxygen inhalation can lead to retinopathy of prematurity which occurs due to free radical injury to the developing blood vessels.

150. c Since in this patient, there is a vitreomacular traction, the treatment has to be pars plana vitrectomy. There is no role of lasers to manage tractions which need to be cut surgically. Bevacizumab is an anti-VEGF agent which regresses and prevents new blood vessels.

151. b Treatment in ROP is indicated only when the disease is "threshold disease" which is defined as five contiguous clock hours or eight non-contiguous clock hours, of stage III disease (i.e., with extra-retinal neovascularisation), in zone I or zone II associated with plus disease (i.e., tortuosity of veins and arterioles). In the above question, the patient is suffering from stage II disease in both eyes; hence we should keep the patient on a regular follow-up.

152. c This ratio of light peak, i.e., maximum potential in light divided by dark trough, i.e., lowest potential in dark, this is called Arden Ratio.

153. c Progression depends on the site of RD. If it's inferior, progression is slow whereas if it's superior it is fast.

154. d Initially in the first week after the injury the ERG shows hypernormal a and b waves. This is due to recovery after the initial trauma and later due to metallic ion injury to muller cells and outer retina, there is gradual dimunition of b wave in one to two years.

155. a Demarcation line is seen due to retained fluid in the subretinal space, which causes friction leading to secondary proliferation changes in the RPE, leading to fibrous metaplasia of RPE. This line can be pigmented or non pigmented.

156. c Homocysteine enhances blood clotting and atherosclerotic changes, and in eye mainly it is associated with CRAO, CRVO and non-arteritic AION. It is also raised in patients of type 2 diabetes specially in proliferative stage.

157. b The child has to be checked for ROP, i.e., retinopathy of prematurity. Prematurity is more important

factor than low birth weight, hence we answer B.

158. b Degeneration in peripheral retina in myopes are most commonly lattice degeneration, which can lead to hole formation and rhegmatogenous retinal detachment.

159. a Since the patient is a MALE CHILD of 7 years, presenting with telangiectasia, the most probable diagnosis is Coats' disease.

Coats' usually affects only one eye (unilateral) and occurs predominantly in young males. Peak age of onset is between 6–8 years of age. Coats' disease is thought to result from breakdown of the blood-retinal barrier in the endothelial cell, resulting in leakage of blood products containing cholesterol crystals and lipid-laden macrophages into the retina and subretinal space. Over time, the accumulation of this proteinaceous exudate thickens the retina, leading to massive, exudative retinal detachment.

160. b YOUNG MALE, presenting with focal foveal detachment, most probably is a case of CSR, i.e., CENTRAL SEROUS RETINOPATHY. In CSR steroids are contraindicated, as it aggravates the condition.

161. b Ideal time of screening is 4 weeks to postnatal age or between 31 and 33 weeks.

162. a Type 2 diabetes is usually diagnosed late, hence fundus examination should be done at the time of diagnosis.

163. b Capillaries are present between OP and IN layer.

164. a The other gas that can be used is C3F8 (per fluorocarbons).

165. a Microaneurysms.

166. c Visual acuity is normal in papilloedema.

167. c ROP3.

168. a It is the interrupted blood column in veins due to CRAO.

169. d *a wave* : activity of rods and cones.

b wave : activity of bipolar and muller cells.

c wave : activity of RPE.

170. a Macular hole is not an ocular emergency.

171. c Risk factors for retinal detachment include pathological myopia, retinal tears, trauma, family history, as well as complications from cataract surgery.

172. c Since the question mentions between posterior pole and equator, the best possible option is C. Otherwise all options are correct.

173. c Retinopathy of prematurity (ROP), previously known as retrolental fibroplasias (RLF), is a *disease* of the *eye* affecting *prematurely-born babies* generally having received *intensive neonatal care*. All preterm babies are at risk for ROP, and very low birthweight is an additional risk factor. Both *oxygen toxicity* and relative *hypoxia* can contribute to the development of ROP.

174. d PDT or photodynamic therapy is used to cure wet ARMD. We inject a dye called verteporfin, which collects in the the new blood vessels below the macula, and next we apply diode laser (not in photo-

coagulative mode), this causes blood clotting in these blood vessels, hence managing the neovascularisation.

175. c **Electro-oculography**

- In this technique, changes in the resting ocular potential are picked up by electrodes placed at the inner and outer canthi when the eyes are moved from side to side.
- Changes in the potential thus obtained with changes of illumination are indicative of the activity of the pigmentary epithelium and the outer segments of the visual receptors.
- These changes are often diminished or absent in retinal dystrophies and degenerations before visual symptoms are evident.
- The ratio of the light peak over the dark trough is known as *Arden Index.*
- *A value above 185 is normal*, below 150 abnormal and 150–185 borderline.

176. c Rhegmatogenous retinal detachment occurs due to full thickness break in the retina. Rapid progression is generally not a rule.

177. a Demarcation line is seen due to retained fluid in the subretinal space, which causes friction leading to secondary proliferation changes and fibrous metaplasia of RPE. This line can be pigmented or non-pigmented.

178. d Initially after injury, the ERG shows hyper normal a and b waves. This is due to recovery after the initial trauma and later due to metallic ion injury to muller cells and outer retina, there is gradual dimunition of b waves in one or two years.

179. a Hollenhorst plaques are cholesterol emboli causing central retinal artery occlusion.

180. c Berlin's edema is edema at the macula due to blunt trauma and is morphologically described as cherry-red spot.

181. b Multifocal ERG allows the local ERG responses to be recorded from many regions of the retina. An abnormal multifocal ERG indicates that the foveal cones or bipolar cells are dysfunctional and a source of vision loss. It also indicates precise distribution of retinal dysfunction and can be correlated with field testing. It is particularly useful in:

1. Unknown visual loss with normal appearing retina.
2. Distinguishing between optic nerve and retinal disease.
3. Diagnosis of focal cone dystrophy where multifocal ERG is the only diagnostic test.

182. c The magnification of direct ophthalmoscope is 15 times.

183. d Most common site of posterior staphyloma is temporal to the disc.

RECENTLY ADDED QUESTIONS

1. **"Silent choroid" on FFA is feature of:**
   A. Best's disease
   B. Age related macular degeneration
   C. Stargardt's disease
   D. Cystoid macular edema
2. **All are manifestation of dengue virus infection in eye except:**
   A. Cataract B. Maculopathy
   C. Vitreous haemorrhage D. Optic neuritis
3. **Immediately after photodynamic therapy, color of the lesion becomes:**
   A. No change in color
   B. Grey
   C. Yellow
   D. White
4. **The Following device shown in the figure is used for indirect ophthalmoscopy. What is the power of the lens that should be used with it to visualize the retina?**

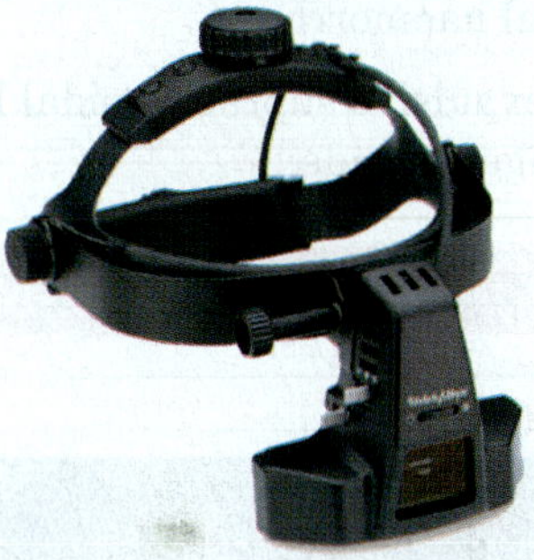

   a. +90 D b. –58 D
   c. +60 D d. +20 D
5. **Which of the following will not cause hypotonic maculopathy?**
   A. Suprachoroidal haemorrhage
   B. Cyclodialysis of uvea
   C. Corneal perforation
   D. Filtration site leak

ANSWERS OF RECENTLY ADDED QUESTIONS

1. c Silent choroid also called dark choroid sign, is a FFA finding where due to heavy deposition of lipofuscin granules, the choroidal fluorescence is not seen and it looks dark. It improves the visualisation of the small retinal capillaries that becomes easily evident in the dark background.

   Stargardt's disease: It is the most common macular dystrophy. About 80% cases show silent choroid in early stage. **Inheritance:** Autosomal recessive trait very common typical form (STGD1) caused by mutations involving the ABCA4 gene, multiple maps to the short arm of chromosome 1.

   An accumulation of discrete "pisciform" flecks at the level of the RPE is a hallmark of the disease happens due to accumulation of lipofuscin throughout RPE.
2. a Cataract. Anterior segment features are: Subconjunctival haemorrage and anterior uveitis.
3. d Photodynamic therapy is done in wet ARMD where we use VERTEPORFIN as photosensitizer and specific wavelength of diode.
4. d The lenses used for indirect ophthalmoscopy can range from +13 D to +30 D. Most commonly used is +20 D.
5. a Suprachoroidal haemorrhage involves bleed into suprachoroidal space from

ruptured posterior ciliary vessels. Patient agitation and pain followed by an extremely firm globe with increased IOP suggest suprachoroidal haemorrhage.

S/o expulsive suprachoroidal haemorrhage include:

- Darkening of the red reflex
- Incision gape
- Progressive shallowing of the AC, increased IOP
- Iris prolapsed
- Expulsion of the lens, vitreous, and bright red blood

IMAGE-BASED QUESTIONS

1. The diagnosis is:

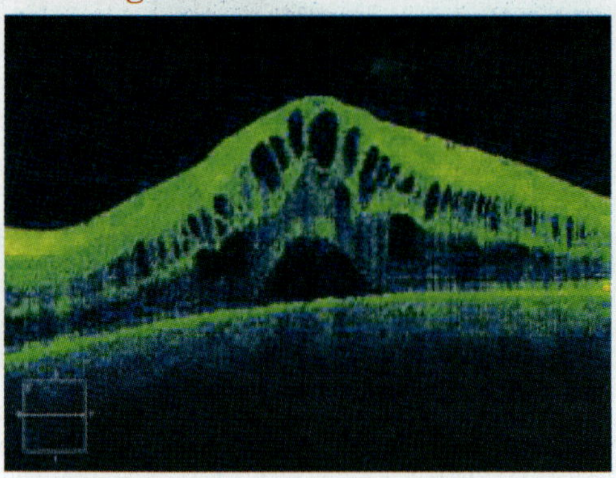

A. CME
B. CSR
C. Retinal detachment
D. ARMD

2. The diagnosis is:

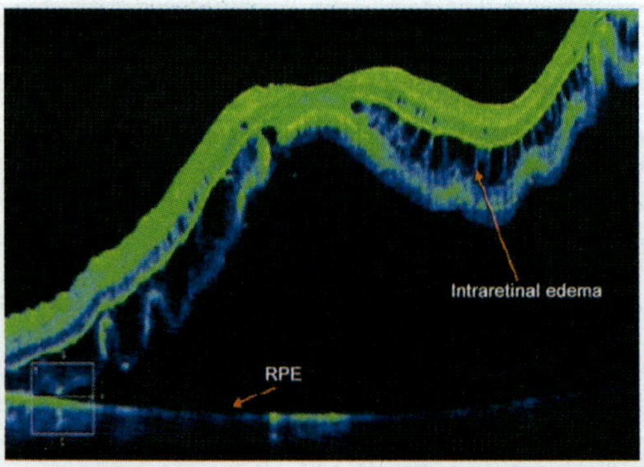

A. CME
B. CSR
C. Retinal detachment
D. ARMD

3. The diagnosis is:

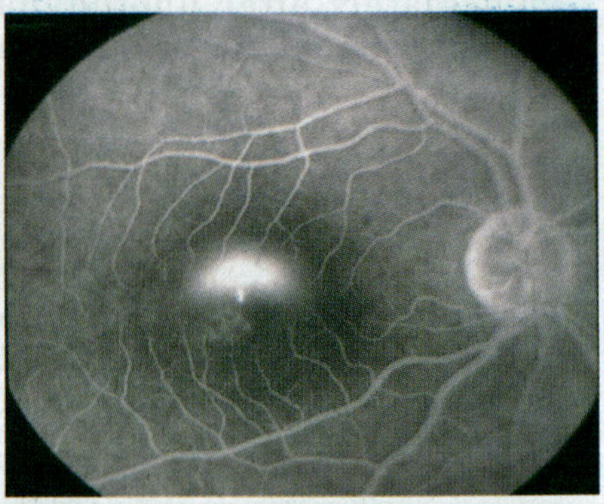

A. CSR
B. CME
C. Macular hole
D. Macular haemorrhage

4. The diagnosis is:

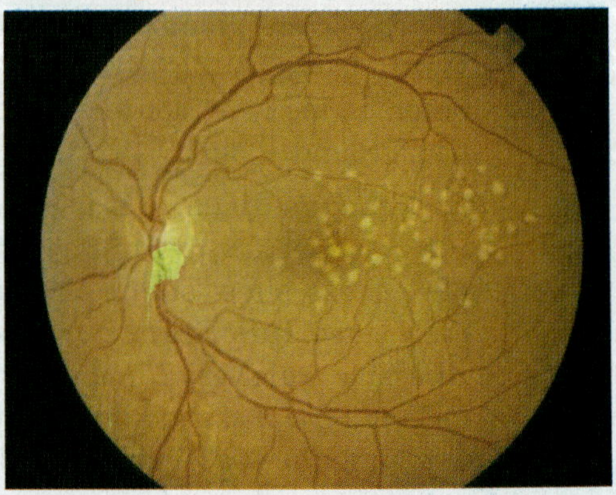

A. Macular edema
B. Dry ARMD
C. Wet ARMD
D. Macular hole

5. The diagnosis is:

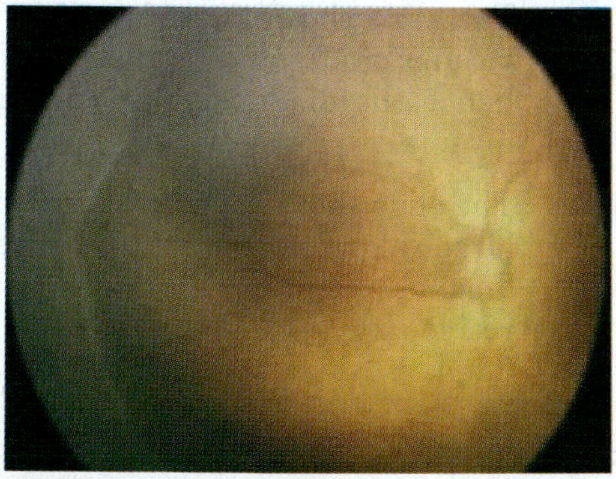

A. Retinal detachment
B. Retinopathy of prematurity
C. Retinoschisis
D. Vitreous detachment

6. The diagnosis is:

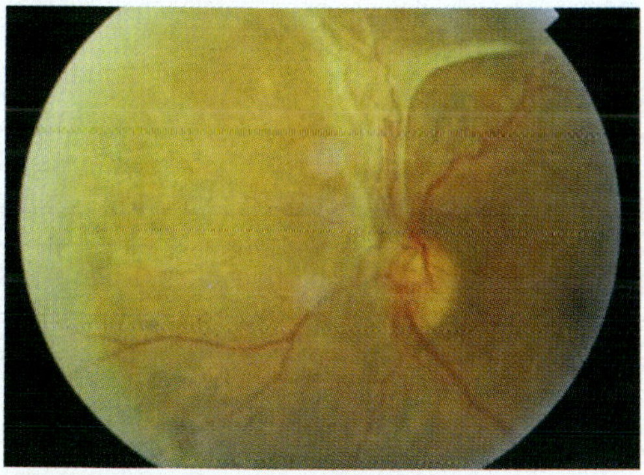

A. Exudative retinal detachment
B. Tractional retinal detachment
C. Rhegmatogenous retinal detachment
D. Vitreous detachment

7. The diagnosis is:

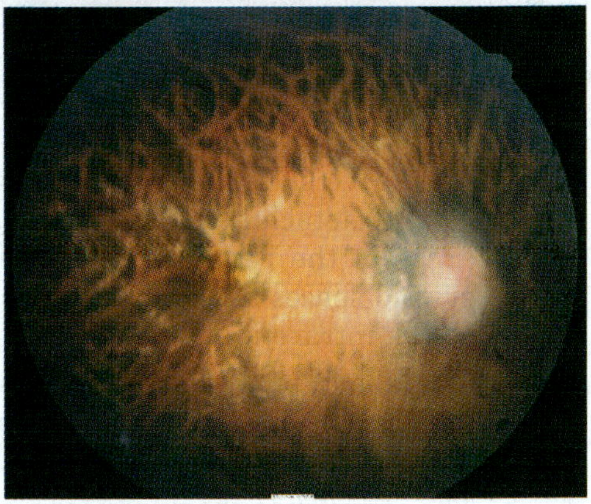

A. Pathological myopia
B. Pseudoxanthoma elasticum
C. Osteogenesis imperfecta
D. Ehlers-Danlos syndrome

8. The diagnosis is:

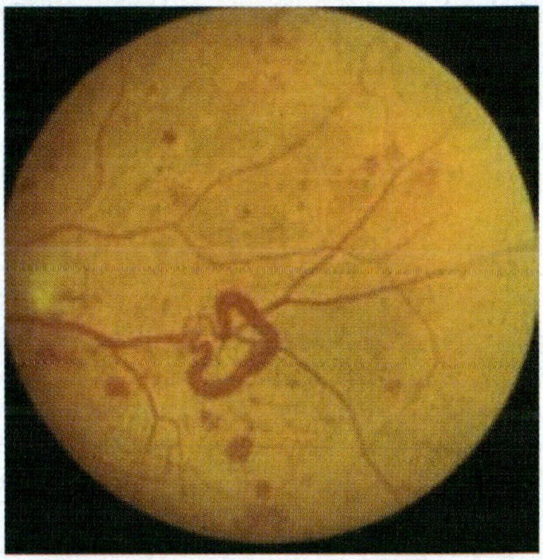

A. Background diabetic retinopathy
B. Preproliferative diabetic retinopathy
C. Proliferative diabetic retinopathy
D. Hypertensive retinopathy

ANSWERS OF IMAGE-BASED QUESTIONS

1. a The above is an OCT slide where we see cystoid spaces filled with fluid, hence the diagnosis is CME.
2. c The above slide shows OCT showing retinal detachment involving large areas of the retina. Also there are cystoid spaces filled with fluid which shows intraretinal edema.
3. a The above slide shows fluorescein angiography indicating smoke-stack pattern, hence diagnosis is CSR.
4. b The above slide shows drusens which is a feature of dry ARMD.
5. b The slide shows ridge formation of retinopathy of prematurity.
6. b The slide shows traction bands leading to retinal detachment.
7. a The slide shows tigroid fundus with lacquer cracks and annular crescent, hence the diagnosis is pathological myopia.
8. b The slide shows looping of veins with large blot haemorrhages, hence the diagnosis is preproliferative diabetic retinopathy.

GUIDANCE

Adversity gives birth to greatness. The greater the challenges and difficulties we face, the greater opportunity we have to grow and develop as people. A life without adversity, a life of ease and comfort produces nothing and leaves us with nothing. This is one of the indisputable facts of life.

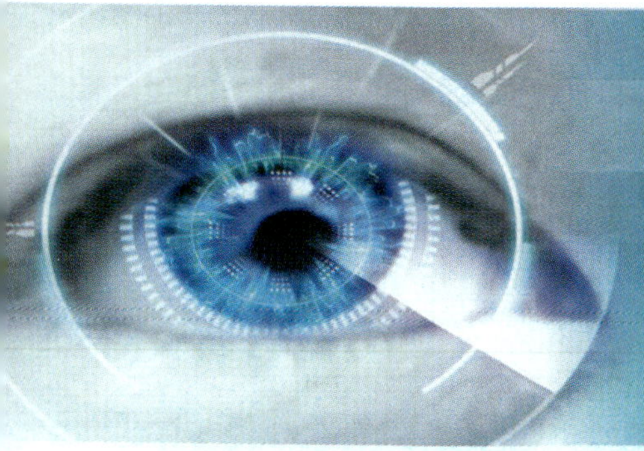

CHAPTER 12

Vitreous

VITREOUS

It primarily constitutes of type 2 collagen fibres and hyaluronic acid.

Vitreous humour: It is the largest and simplest connective tissue present as a single piece in the human body. It is divided into three parts:

a. **Hyaloid layer or membrane:** They are not true membranes but condensed outermost cortical vitreous.
   - Anterior hyaloid membrane.
   - Posterior hyaloid membrane.

b. **Cortical vitreous:**
   - Entire peripheral zone of main vitreous mass.
   - Represents only 2% of total vitreous volume.
   - Contains:
     – Collagen II fibrils interspersed with sodium hyaluronate.
     – Vitreous cells (hyalocytes): **Hence it is the metabolic center of vitreous body.**

c. **Medullary vitreous:**
   - Major part.
   - Less fibrillar and no hyalocytes.

- **Cloquet's canal:** Also called hyaloid canal runs from optic disc to posterior lens surface. Down this canal runs hyaloid artery of fetus. It is 1–2 mm in width. Its walls are formed by vitreous condensation.

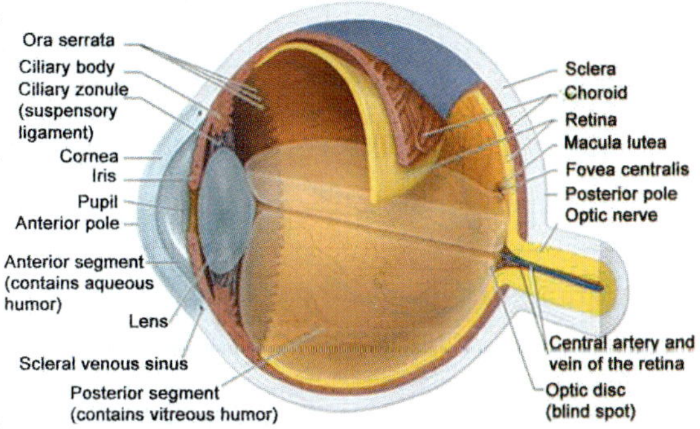

Fig. 12.1: Diagrammatic view: The vitreous humor is illustrated only in the bottom part of the eyeball

FLOATERS

Floaters are opacities in the vitreous humour. Patient complains of floating object in front of eye.

Causes of Floaters

1. *Muscae volitantes:* Physiological opacities representing the residue of primitive hyaloid vasculature.

2. *Asteroid hyalosis:* Small white, round bodies suspended in the vitreous gel. They are formed due to accumulation of **calcium and lipids.**
3. *Synchysis scintillans:* Vitreous is laden with small, white, angular and crystalline bodies formed of **cholesterol.**
4. *Red cell opacities:* Due to small vitreous haemorrhage or left out of large vitreous hemorrhage.
5. *Tumour cell opacities:* May be seen as free-floating opacities in some patients with retinoblastoma and reticulum cell sarcoma.
6. *Inflammatory cells:* In case of intermediate and posterior uveitis.

Vitreous Haemorrhage

It occurs from the retinal vessels and may be preretinal or intragel.

Etiology:

1. Spontaneous due to retinal break after PVD.
2. Trauma.
3. Inflammatory disease, e.g., chorioretinitis and periphlebitis retinae.
4. Vascular disease: Hypertensive retinopathy, CRVO.
5. Metabolic: DR.
6. Blood dyscrasias and bleeding disorders.

Clinical Features:

1. Sudden development of floaters if the haemorrhage is partial.
2. Sudden painless loss of vision if the haemorrhage is total.
3. Black shadow against the red glow when seen on distant direct ophthalmoscopy or no red glow if the haemorrhage is total.

Diagnosis:

B scan helps in the diagnosis.

Sequelae:

1. Complete absorption within 4–8 weeks.
2. Organisation in the recurrent bleeding.
3. Ghost cell glaucoma.
4. Vitreous degeneration.
5. Retinitis proliferans leading to tractional retinal detachment.

Treatment:

1. *Bed rest* with elevation of the patients head followed by treatment of the cause.
2. *Vitrectomy:* It may be anterior, core or subtotal and total. It can be done by two techniques, either open sky vitrectomy which is done through limbus or large corneal section, or pars plana vitrectomy.

NEET DRILL

1. Primary vitreous develops from mesoderm.
2. Secondary and tertiary vitreous develops from neuroectoderm.
3. Strongest attachment of vitreous to retina is at vitreous base near ora serrata.
4. Synchysis scintillans are floaters composed of cholesterol.
5. Asteroid bodies are floaters composed of calcium and lipids.
6. Vitreous : plasma ratio of ascorbate is 9 : 1.
7. Muscae volitantes are floaters, which are remnants of hyaloid tissue.
8. Mittendorf dots are remnants of hyaloid tissue seen behind the lens.
9. Bergmeister papilla are remnants of hyaloid tissue near the optic disc.

MULTIPLE CHOICE QUESTIONS

1. **Mucopolysaccharide hyaluronic acid is present in:**
   A. Vitreous humour
   B. Synovial fluid
   C. Cartilage
   D. Cornea
2. **The most common cause of vitreous haemorrhage in adults is:**
   A. Retinal hole B. Trauma
   C. Hypertension D. Diabetes
3. **A vitreous aspirate has been collected in an emergency at 9 pm. What advice would you like to give to the staff on duty regarding the overnight storage of the sample?**
   A. The sample should be kept at 4 degree centigrade
   B. The sample should be incubated at 37 degree C
   C. The sample should be refrigerated at in deep freezer
   D. The sample should be refrigerated for the initial 3 hours and then at 37 degree C
4. **Which one of the following statements concerning persistent hyperplastic primary vitreous (PHPV) is not true?**
   A. It is generally unilateral
   B. Visual prognosis is usually good
   C. It may calcify
   D. It is most easily differentiated from retinoblastoma by the presence of exophthalmos or cataract
5. **Snowball opacity in vitreous is seen:**
   A. Pars planitis B. Sarcoidosis
   C. Juvenile RA D. Toxoplasmosis
   E. Fuch's lesion
6. **Vitreous opacities may be due to:**
   A. Herpetic keratouveitis
   B. Posterior uveitis
   C. Hyaloid asteroids
   D. High myopia
7. **Vitreous haemorrhage in young adult indicates:**
   A. Retinal detachment
   B. Glaucoma
   C. Eales' disease
   D. Chorioretinitis
8. **Vitreous haemorrhage is not seen is:**
   A. Hypertension
   B. Eales' disease
   C. Trauma
   D. Diabetes mellitus
   E. Vitreous degeneration
9. **Vitreous haemorrhage is seen in:**
   A. Coats' disease B. Eales' disease
   C. CRVO D. CRAO
10. **Examination of vitreous is best done by:**
    A. Direct ophthalmoscope
    B. Indirect ophthalmoscope
    C. Slit lamp with contact lens
    D. Oblique illumination
11. **Volume of the vitreous:**
    A. 2 ml B. 3 ml
    C. 4 ml D. 6 ml
12. **Most common complication of lens surgery in a case of persistent hyperplastic primary vitreous (PHPV) is:**
    A. Orbital cellulitis
    B. Retinal detachment
    C. Vitreous haemorrhage
    D. Keratitis

13. Secondary vitreous develops from:
A. Ectoderm B. Endoderm
C. Mesoderm D. All

14. When compare to blood vitreous humor has high concentration of:
A. Glucose B. Sodium
C. Potassium D. Ascorbate

15. The strongest attachment of vitreous to retina:
A. Posterior pole
B. Optic disc
C. Vitreous base
D. Along blood vessels

ANSWER AND EXPLANATION

1.	a	Secondary and Tertiary vitreous is composed of hyaluronic acid and Type II collagen.
2.	d	Diabetes is the most common pathology among the four mentioned in the question.
3.	a	Just like any other sample, it should be stored at 4 degrees.
4.	d	PHPV is always associated with microphthalmos. Regarding prognosis, it is good in case of anterior PHPV and poor in posterior PHPV.
5.	a,b	Snow ball opacities are the inflammatory exudates floating in the vitreous. JRA and Fuch's heterochromic cyclitis is anterior uveitis. In toxoplasmosis there is intense vitritis but snowballs are not the feature.
6.	b,c, d	Herpetic keratouveitis leads to anterior uveitis hence vitreous opacities are not the feature.
7.	c	Eales' disease is periphlebitis retinae seen in the young males due to hypersensitivity to tubercular antigen.
8.	e	Haemorrhage is not a feature of degeneration.
9.	b	CRVO in later case can complicate as vitreous haemorrhage but the most common cause is Eales' disease so we answer that.
10.	b	I/O is the best method to visualize the vitreous.
11.	c	Total volume of the eye is 7 ml and out of this 4 ml is of the vitreous.
12.	c	In patients with PHPV which is a vascular hyaloid tissue of primary vitreous, lensectomy with vitrectomy is done and the biggest challenge is the intraoperative bleeding from this vascular tissue.
13.	a	It develops from neuroectoderm. Secondary vitreous is adult vitreous composed of type 2 collagen and hyaluronic acid.
14.	d	High level of ascorbate, helps to protect the retina from oxidative damage.
15.	c	The strongest attachment of vitreous is at vitreous base at Ora Serrata.

GUIDANCE

When your determination changes, everything else will begin to move in the direction you desire. The moment you resolve to be victorious every nerve and fibre in your being will immediately orient itself towards your success. On the other hand, if you think "This is never going to work out", then at that instant every cell in your being will be deflated and give up the fight, and then everything really will move in the direction of failure.

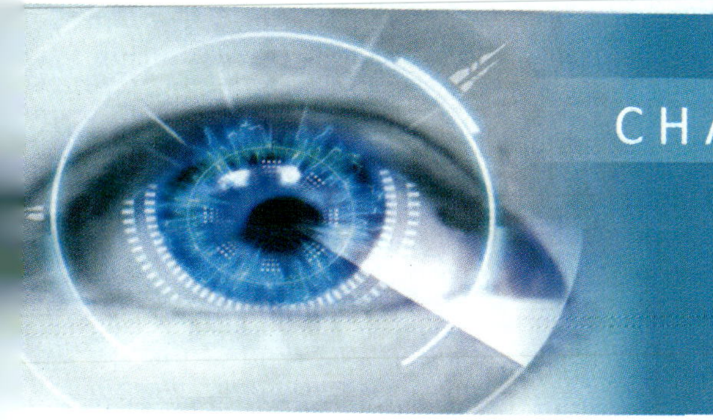

CHAPTER 13

Squint and Optics

GROSS ANATOMY OF EXTRAOCULAR MUSCLES

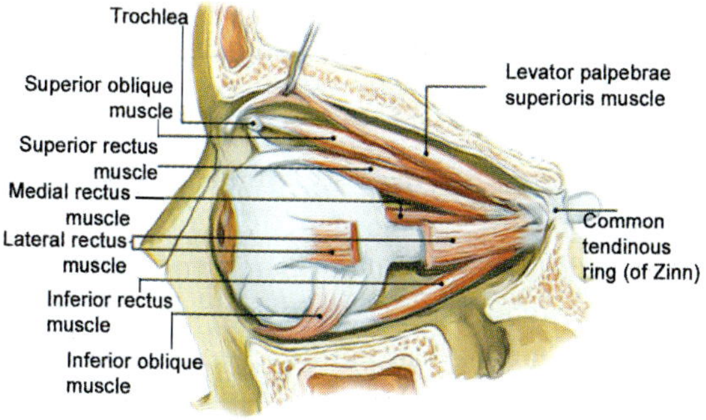

Fig. 13.1

Origin of Extraocular Muscles

Five of the six extraocular muscles (except inferior oblique) originate at the orbital apex.

1. All four recti originate from Annulus of Zinn, an oval fibrous ring at the orbital apex.
2. Superior oblique arises just above the Annulus of Zinn.
3. Sixth extraocular muscle, the inferior oblique, originates from the maxillary bone, adjacent to the lacrimal fossa, posterior to the orbital rim.

Insertion of Extraocular Muscles

1. The rectus muscle inserts into the sclera via their tendons, ANTERIOR TO THE EQUATOR of the globe. The spatial formation created by connecting their insertions is called SPIRAL OF TILLAUX. The medial rectus tendon inserts closest to the limbus, followed by inferior, lateral and superior rectus, in that order (can learn as MILS).
2. The oblique muscles insert into the sclera posterior to the equator of the globe.

SUPERIOR OBLIQUE

It inserts into the posterior, superolateral sclera in a broad fan-like fashion, under the superior rectus muscle. The tendon insertion is functionally separated into two parts:

Anterior one third of the tendon functions almost exclusively to incyclotort the globe. The posterior two thirds of the tendon functions to depress and abduct the globe.

INFERIOR OBLIQUE

It has almost no tendon, at its insertion, and inserts into posterior inferolateral sclera.

Squint and Optics

- **Total diopteric power of eye (Reduced eye) is 58D to 60D.**

  Reduced eye: Simplified form of the complicated refractive system of the eye is referred as reduced eye.

  Refractive power of cornea: 45D.

  Refractive power of lens: 16D–17D.

  Refractive index of cornea: 1.37.

  Refractive index of lens: 1.39.

  Refractive index of aqueous and vitreous humour: 1.33.

- Though the refractive index of the cornea is less than the lens, its refractive power is more. Hence, it is the **curvature of the cornea which plays the major part in the refraction**.
- 1 mm change in axial length leads to 3 D change in the refractive power.
- Eyeball is a cystic structure with a volume of 6.5 ml and weight of 7 gm. Its circumference is 75 mm. AP diameter is 24 mm, lateral diameter is 23.5 mm and vertical diameter is 23 mm.
- In direct ophthalmoscope the magnification is 15 times. The image formed is virtual and erect.
- In indirect ophthalmoscope the magnification is 5 times. The image formed is real and inverted.

Can be Remembered as:

- Direct, i.e., Everything Visualized Straight.
- Indirect, i.e., Everything Visualized Inverted.

Indirect Ophthalmoscope

- Indirect ophthalmoscope provides a stereoscopic view of the fundus with low magnification (5 times) enabling a good overall view of the retina to be obtained. Hence it is not useful to visualize the fovea which is better seen with either direct ophthalmoscope or with slit-lamp bimicroscopy.
- Relatively high light source so used, will make a view of retina possible even if there are severe media opacities like – cataract and vitreous haemorrhage.
- **Scleral indentation:** It enables the visualization of peripheral retina anterior to the equator and to perform a kinetic evaluation of the retina.
- Though a variety of aspheric condensing lenses are used; but + 20D is most useful for general purpose examinations.
- When retina is being examined by a small pupil, +30D lens (low magnification and large field) is used.
- **Principle of this method** is to make the eye highly myopic by placing a strong convex lens in front of it. This forms a real, inverted image of the fundus in the air between the lens and the observer which can be studied.

Direct Ophthalmoscope

In this method the emergent rays from the patients eye are parallel and brought to focus on the retina of emmetropic observer when the accommodation is relaxed. The image formed is erect and virtual. Magnification is 15 times. It is more in myopes and less in hypermetropes.

Goldmann's three mirror contact lens: It helps to visualize the whole of the retina as well as the angle of the anterior chamber.

It has 3 mirrors, which are angled and a central part which acts as a contact lens and helps to visualize the central fundus. The three mirrors are inclined at 59°, 67° and 73°.

A. Central contact lens, to see posterior pole (Central 30°).

B. Smallest, at 73° to visualize anterior chamber angle and far periphery.

C. Middle size at 67°, to visualize mid periphery and region anterior to equator.

D. Largest at 59°, to visualize equator and regions posterior to equator.

Hruby lens: It is a planoconcave lens of –58.6D. It is used for slit-lamp bimicroscopy.

Amblyoscope or Synaptophore: It is an instrument in which there are two eye pieces (+ 6.5D lens in each eye piece) situated at the end of two adjustable tubes which can be altered in angulation and position to suit a squint of any angle of deviation. Position of each eye piece is so adjusted that each eye looks directly into it and can see a picture projected into it from a slide placed in the illuminated slide carrier.

Uses of Amblyoscope:

1. Estimation of the state of binocular vision – i.e., grade I, II and III.
2. Estimation of angle of deviation of the squint.
3. For detection of ARC—Abnormal retinal correspondence.
4. For detection of EF, i.e., Eccentric fixation.

Refraction by a prism: In prism, while the light ray is deviated towards the base, the image is displaced towards the apex of the prism. By utilizing this phenomenon, we are able to detect the presence of a prism in an optical system. We hold the glass up between the eye and any object which forms a straight line, and if the continuity of the straight line is broken, we know that a prism is present and since the line appears to be deviated towards the apex, we know in which direction the apex of the prism lies.

This method helps us to assess the optical centre of the specks glasses.

Pin-hole Vision

- Pin-hole allows only the monochromatic ray of light hence in cases of refractive error, the vision improves. Size of pin-hole is –1 mm.
- In macular hole and central cataract, pin-hole will worsen the vision.
- In glaucoma, vision is unaffected by pin-hole.

Biometry

It is the process of calculating the IOL power. To calculate the IOL power, SRK I and II are commonly used.

SRK I–P = A-2.5 L–0.9 K

A is a constant depending on style of IOL design.

L is axial length.

K is keratometric reading.

P is required power.

SRK II – Modification of SRK I, according to the axial length.

Short Eye:

- Axial length 21–22 mm, add 1 to A constant.
- Axial length 20–21 mm add 2 to A constant.
- Axial length is less than 20 mm add 3 to A constant.

Long eye: Axial length greater than 24.5 mm subtract 0.5 from A constant.

For very long eye (> 24.5 mm) SRK/T formula is used.

Where T stands for retinal thickness correction factor.

Going by the rules of affectivity, powers of standard lenses increased according to their position.

Anterior chamber lens – + 17D
Pupil supported lens – + 19D
Posterior chamber lens – + 20D or +21D

Visual Angles

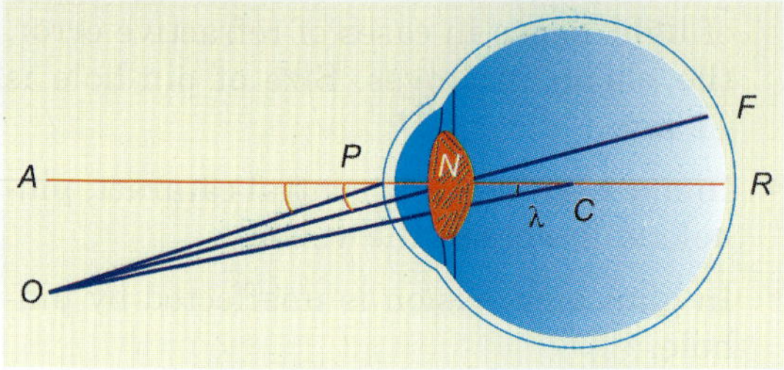

Fig. 13.2: Axes of the eye

a. **Angle alpha (α):** It is the angle between optic axis (APR) and visual axis (FNO) at the nodal point, i.e., Angle ANO.

b. **Angle gamma (γ):** It is the angle between optic axis (APR) and fixation axis (CO) at the centre of rotation (C), i.e., angle ACO.

c. **Angle kappa (κ):** It is the angle between pupillary line and visual axis at the cornea. Pupillary line is the line passing through the centre of the pupil, and visual axis is the line passing through the fovea. In the above figure pupillary line coincides with the optic axis (line passing through the centre of the cornea) and hence angle kappa is angle APO.

   The centre of the pupil is somewhat nasal to the centre of cornea, but for clinical purpose the optic axis and pupillary line can be considered coincident, and the angle formed at the cornea (APO) is considered equal to that subtended at the nodal point (ANO).

Pseudoexotropia

It is due to large positive angle kappa, which is seen in Hypermetropes.

Pseudoesotropia

It is due to large negative angle kappa, which is seen in Myopes.

Errors of refraction: These are as follows:

1. **Myopia:**
   - Myopia is an error of refraction where the light rays are focused in front of the retina due to more axial length of eye and hence the refractive power in the eye is more than what is required. Therefore, it is corrected by concave lens.
   - In high myopes there is an increased risk of retinal detachment hence an indirect ophthalmoscopy is a must in these cases to scan the retina.
   - A child with myopia generally presents with history of difficulty in seeing the blackboard and squeezing his eyes while doing so. The squeezing of eyes causes a pin-hole effect which increases the depth of vision in myopes.

2. **Hypermetropia:**
   - It is an error of refraction where the light rays are focused behind the retina due to short axial length and hence the refractive power in the eye is less than what is required. Therefore, it is corrected by convex lens.
   - An infant is physiologically hypermetrope by 2.5 to 3.0 diopters and eyeball is short, i.e., 17 mm.
   - The effective power of a plus lens increases as it moves away from the eye whereas in case of a minus lens it decreases.

3. **Astigmatism:** It is a refractive condition where the refractive power of the two principal axes is different. It is classified in the following ways:

   First

   a. *Simple myopic:* When one axis is emmetropic and the other axis is myopic.

b. *Simple hypermetropic:* When one axis is emmetropic and the other axis is hypermetropic.

c. *Compound myopic:* When both the principal axes are myopic.

d. *Compound hypermetropic:* When both the principal axes are hypermetropic.

e. *Mixed:* When one axis is myopic and the other axis is hypermetropic.

Second

a. *Oblique:* When the principal axis is not at 180 and 90, but the angle between the two axis is 90 degree.

b. *Bioblique:* When the principal axis is not at 180 and 90 degrees and also the angle between the two axis is less than 90 degrees.

Third

a. *Regular:* When the refractive power is same along the single axis.

b. *Irregular:* When the refractive power varies even in the same axis.

Fourth

a. *With the rule:* When power of vertical axis is more than horizontal axis.

b. *Against the rule:* When power of horizontal axis is more than vertical axis.

4. **Anisometropia:** In this condition the difference between the refractive powers of the two eyes is more than +2.5D.

5. **Aniseikonia:** It is a condition where size and shape of the images in two eyes are unequal.

Etiology:

a. *Optical phenomenon:* Different dioptric images due to difference in refraction of two eyes (some degree of anisometropia).

b. *Anatomical:* Difference in distribution of retinal elements.

- Slight change in size and shape of ocular images is responsible for stereoscopic binocular vision–upto 5%.
- Maximum aniseikonia occur in case of unilateral aphakia–upto 30%.
- Aniseikonia may be:

  a. Symmetrical.

  b. Asymmetrical.

Degree of aniseikonia is measured by–**Space Eikonometer.**

Treatment:

1. *Correction by iseikonic lenses:* It causes magnification without introducing any appreciable refractive power.
2. *Contact lenses:* With contact lens use, less problem of aniseikonia.

6. **Abberopia:** It refers to wavefront aberrations or higher order aberrations which causes the decrease in the quality of vision. It is measured by abberometer and corrected by C-Lasik.

Aphakia: Absence of lens is called Aphakia.

- Eye becomes highly hypermetropic.
- Total power of eye is reduced to + 44 D from + 60 D.
- Total loss of accommodation:

  Note: Accommodation is lost even in IOLs as the artificial lens is not attached to suspensory ligaments and cannot change its curvature as a natural lens.

- **Best available treatment for aphakia is posterior chamber (in the bag) intraocular lens.**

  Intraocular lens has advantage over glasses in better field of vision, better underwater vision and no chromatic aberration.

- **Other modalities:**

A. Spectacles: It's a cheap and easy method.

Disadvantages:

1. *Image magnification is by 25%–30%* so not useful in unilateral aphakia (will cause diplopia).
2. *Spherical and chromatic aberrations* (due to thick lens).
3. *Limited field of vision* and poor eccentric acuity.
4. **Roving—Ring scotoma** causing **"Jack-in-box phenomenon"** owing to prismatic effect of the peripheral part of thick convex lens. In aphakia, with the eye in primary position there is a ring scotoma of approximately 15°. Ring scotoma is due to prismatic deviation at periphery of strong lens. When the eye moves to the side of scotoma, the scotoma moves in opposite direction (i.e., towards the fixation point). The objects tend to appear and disappear in the most disconcerting way, hence called **"Jack-in-box phenomenon"**.
5. **Pin-cushion effect** due to spherical aberrations. In this condition the straight lines become curves and linear becomes converted into parabolas which change their shape with each movement of the eye. Pin-cushion effect is due to spherical aberration induced by strong convex lens.
6. Cosmetic blemish in young aphakes.

B. Contact lens:

Advantages:

1. Causes less magnification—5–6%.
2. Elimination of aberrations and prismatic effect of thick glasses.
3. Wider and better field of vision.
4. Better for uniocular aphakia.

Disadvantages:

1. Costly.
2. Cumbersome.
3. Can lead to corneal complications.

C. Refractive corneal surgery:

1. *Keratophakia:* A lenticule from donor cornea is placed between the lamellae of patient's cornea.
2. *Epikeratophakia:* A lenticule from donor cornea is stitched over the surface of cornea after removing the epithelium.
3. *Hyperopic LASIK.*
4. *Hyperopic PRK* (Photorefractive keratectomy).

Accommodation: It is a reflex process, when a person sees at the near distance. It involves the contraction of ciliary muscles which causes relaxation of suspensory ligaments leading to increase in the curvature of the anterior surface of the lens causing an increase in the refractive power of the lens hence focusing the near.

Presbyopia:

- Presbyopia is not an error of refraction but physiological insufficiency of accommodation (after 40 years) leading to difficulty or failure of near vision.
- The treatment of presbyopia is prescription of convex lenses.

Rough guideline according to age in emmetrope

Age	*Power of convex lenses*
40–45 years	+1 DS
45–50 years	+ 1.5 DS
50–55 years	+ 2.0 DS
55–60 years	+ 2.5 DS

- Maximum correction is never > + 3.5D as this is the maximum accommodative power.

Pseudomyopia: It is an accommodation spasm (accommodative inertia) causing blurring of vision on looking at near in young individuals.

Purkinje Images

They are formed when a strong beam of light is projected on the eye. They are four in number:

- I and II image is formed on anterior and posterior surface of cornea.
- III and IV image is formed on anterior and posterior surface of lens.
- **IV image is inverted.**
- For measurement of corneal thickness, I and II Purkinje images are used.
- For measurement of AC depth, II and III Purkinje images are used.
- For measurement of lens thickness, III and IV Purkinje images are used.

Retinoscopy: It is also called **Skiascopy** or **Shadow test.** It is an objective method of finding out the error of refraction by the method of neutralisation. It can be done with or without a cycloplegic.

Principle of Retinoscopy

In retinoscopy, an illuminated area of the retina serves as an object, and the image at the far point of the eye is located by moving the illumination across the fundus and noting the behaviour of luminous reflex in the pupil. **If the image is formed between the patient and the observer, the movements of the reflex and the external light are in opposite directions; and if it falls outside this region, either behind the patients eye or behind the observers the two move in the same direction.** When far point of patient's eye corresponds to the nodal point of the observers' eye, a neutral point occurs. The rationale of the method is therefore to add lenses to the dioptric system of the patient's eye until the point of reversal is seen by the observer.

Observations

Depending upon the movement of red reflex, when a plane mirror retinoscope is used at a distance of 1 meter, the results are interpreted as below:

a. No movement of red reflex indicates myopia of 1D.

b. When red reflex moves along with the movement of the retinoscope, it indicates either emmetropia or hypermetropia or myopia of less than 1 dioptre.

c. When red reflex moves against the movement of the retinoscope, it indicates myopia of > –1D.

Cycloplegics and Mydriatics

- **The choice of cycloplegic for refraction (retinoscopy) in < 7 years of age is 1% Atropine eye ointment.**
- Tropicamide has the quickest (20–40 minutes) and briefest (3–6 hours) action but is an unreliable cycloplegic. Hence, it is satisfactory for refraction testing in adults and as a short mydriatic for fundoscopy.

- **Phenylephrine is the only drug that causes only mydriasis and no cycloplegia (paralysis of accommodation due to paralysis of ciliary muscles).** All the other mydriatics are also cycloplegics.
- Tropicamide and cyclopentolate are short-acting mydriatics whereas atropine and homatropine are long-acting mydriatics.

Calculations

The power with which the point of neutralization is attained is our retinoscopic reading for that axis. This is then corrected for the distance and the cycloplegic if used. For distance, if retinoscopy is done at 1meter then addition factor will be –1D and if done at 66 cm, i.e., 2/3 meter then addition factor is –1.5 D. For cycloplegic correction, if atropine is used then the correction factor is –1, for cyclopentolate it is –0.75 and with any other cycloplegic the correction factor is –0.5. We add all the factors to the retinoscopic reading to get the corrected retinoscopic reading. If phenylephrine is used then we will not add any correction factor as it is only a mydriatic and not a cycloplegic.

CONTACT LENS

Definition

Contact lens is a small polymer wafer designed to rest on the cornea or sclera and is generally used to correct refractive errors.

Types:

1. Hard: Gas-impermeable lenses.
2. RGP: Rigid gas-permeable lenses.
3. Soft lenses:
   - Low water content.
   - High water content.

LENS MATERIALS

Soft Contact Lens

a. Hydrogel—PHEMA (Poly-Hydroxy-Ethyl-Methacrylate).

b. Elastomer—Silicon rubber.

- **Hydrogel lenses with high water content are:**

a. Permalens perfilcon-A – 71%

b. Sauflon PW

c. Lidofilcon-B – 79%

} Extended wear lenses

Semi-Soft Contact Lenses or RGPs

a. CAB-Cellulose Acetate Butyrate.

b. Styrene.

c. Siloxane-methacrylate.

d. Fluoro based or fluorinated components:
   1. Fluoro-siloxane-acrylate.
   2. Polyperfluoroether.

Hard Lens

PMMA–Polymethylmethacrylate.

Note:

- **Patients using soft contact lens (if use tap water for cleaning the lens) are at increased risk of Acanthamoeba keratitis, whereas the most common infection after contact lens use is pseudomonas.** A soft contact lens user presenting with pain, watering, photophobia and blepharospasm with a white spot at the centre of the cornea, the most probable diagnosis is pseudomonas infection.
- **DK:** Symbolises oxygen permeability of contact lens; where **D** is diffusion coefficient and **K** is solubility coefficient.
- **DK/t:** Denotes oxygen transmissibility, where t is the thickness of the contact lens.
- **Fluorescein:** It is not used in soft lens fitting evaluation as it stains the lens.

(Except for large molecules fluorescein like **Fluorexon**).

- Benzalkonium chloride should never be used for disinfecting *soft* contact lens.
- **Toric lenses** are used for correcting cylinder power. Astigmatic correction can be achieved with rigid spherical (upto 4D of astigmatism), rigid toric and soft toric lenses.

  Spherical lenses have single radius of curvature at the central anterior and posterior surface whereas toric lenses have different radii of curvature at the two principle meridians and so theoretically, can correct any amount of astigmatism.
- **X-Chrom lenses:** These lenses transmit light in red part of the spectrum and are useful to patients with red-green defective vision.
- Cornea obtains its glucose supply from aqueous humour and limbal vessels. Hence use of contact lens will not decrease its glucose supply.
- Cornea obtains its O_2 supply from atmosphere. Hence use of contact lens decreases O_2 supply from atmosphere. Therefore high water content contact lenses are preferred as its oxygen transmissibility is more than low water content.
- The primary metabolism in cornea is aerobic, hence if oxygen supply is decreased (as in contact lens users). The utilization of glucose is decreased.

Complications of Soft Contact Lenses

A. *Hypoxia.*

B. *Mechanical*

1. Corneal wrinkling specially with tight lens.
2. Superior epithelial arcuate lesion commonly called "corneal split".
3. Abrasions.

C. *Toxic*

- With preservatives in contact lens solution.
- SPK—Superficial punctate keratitis is the hallmark.

D. *Inflammation*

1. CLARE (contact lens induced acute red eye).
2. CLPC (contact lens induced papillary conjunctivitis).
3. CNPC (culture negative peripheral ulcer).
4. Neovascularization of cornea.

E. *Infective:* Infective keratitis.

Bandage Contact Lens

Bandage contact lenses are therapeutic devices that are used to treat a range of external ocular surface disorders primarily affecting the cornea and adjacent ocular tissues.

Types:

1. Hydrogel contact lens: Made of cross linked HEMA. It may be:

a. *High water content*
   - In epithelial defects and anterior segment pathology.

b. *Medium water content*
   - For drug delivery.
   - Severe corneal thinning and perforation.

c. *Low water content*
   - In dry eye states.
   - As an adjunct in cases of cyanoacrylate tissue adhesive.

2. Collagen shields:

- For drug delivery—mainly in early cases of bacterial ulcers.

- For damaged epithelium after radial keratotomy, penetrating keratoplasty, epikeratophakia.

3. High DK gas permeable lenses:

- For cases of deviant corneal topography where soft contact lenses may not stabilize.
- In high regular or irregular astigmatism.

Hence mainly the bandage lenses used in anterior segment pathology are soft contact lenses.

APPLICATIONS OF THERAPEUTIC CONTACT LENSES (BANDAGE CONTACT LENSES)

A. Eyelid/Tarsal abnormalities:

- Entropion.
- Trichiasis.
- Ectropion, anatomic abnormalities or lagophthalmos.
- Upper palpebral conjunctival abnormalities such as concretions.

B. Ocular surface abnormalities:

- Cicatrizing conditions.
- Dry eye.
- Chemical injuries.

C. Corneal surface abnormalities:

- Recurrent erosion syndrome.
- Trophic keratitis.
- Traumatic epithelial abnormalities.

D. Corneal thinning disorders:

Descematocele.

E. Endothelial decompensation:

Bullous keratopathy due to either surgery or Fuch's dystrophy.

F. Drug delivery.

AMBLYOPIA

It is defined as deficiency of form sense resulting in reduction in visual acuity of greater than two lines between the eyes or an absolute reduction in acuity below 6/9.

Pathophysiology

Cell shrinkage in parvocellular layers of lateral geniculate body.

Signs and Symptoms

1. Decreased visual acuity, in spite of giving best corrected vision.
2. Decreased accommodation ability.
3. Afferent pupillary defect (in severely affected eye).
4. Eccentric viewing.
5. Enhanced crowding phenomenon.
6. Defect in hyperacuity.
7. Light sense is diminished (sunglasses effect).
8. Neutral density filters, when placed over amblyopic eye may not degrade acuity in contrast to normal eye where visual acuity is degraded.

CLASSIFICATION OF AMBLYOPIA

a. **Congenital amblyopia:** Color blindness, Nystagmus, Albinism.

b. **Strabismic amblyopia:** Due to squint, the squinted eye is not able to maintain the foveal centration, hence becomes amblyopic.

c. **Form deprivation amblyopia:** It occurs in case of hazy media like congenital cataract, keratitis etc. In such a situation macula is not formed as the light rays do not reach the macula, hence the visual reflexes are not developed. This leads to amblyopia.

d. **Refractive amblyopia:**

1. *Anisometropic amblyopia:* Anisometropic amblyopia occurs due to suppression in the eye with higher error. This is more common in hypermetropes, than in myopes. It was found that there is 100% prevalence of amblyopia in myopes with anisometropia > 6.5 D and hypermetropes with anisometropia of > 3.5 D.
2. *Ametropic amblyopia.*
3. *Meridional amblyopia.*

Treatment

Patients with strabismic amblyopia demonstrate the best response to treatment compared to the other types of amblyopia.

1. **Refractive correction.**
2. **Occlusion:** The concept of occlusion is to occlude the sound eye and to force use of the amblyopic eye. **Occlusion is the most effective treatment of amblyopia.**

   It may be:

   i. *Total:* To occlude both form sense and light sense (if vision < 6/18).

   ii. *Partial:* To occlude only form sense.

   If no improvement has occurred after 6 months, further occlusion is unlikely to be fruitful.

   The rule for occlusion is as follows:

   - In 1 year old child the duration of occlusion is 1 day and then open it for one day, i.e., the ratio is 1:1.
   - In 2 years old child this ratio is 2:1, i.e., two-day occlusion and one day no occlusion.
   - In 3 years old–3:1, 4 years old–4:1, 5 years old–5:1, 6 years old–6:1.

   After 6 years of age occlusion is not of much help.
3. **Penalisation:** It is a form of occlusion in which atropine is given in the eye to be occluded.
4. **CAM stimulator:** It constitutes high contrast square wave gratings of different frequency. It is used to stimulate the amblyopic eye.
5. **Pleoptics:** It constitutes the stimulation of fovea by means of **after-images** in case of eccentric fixation. The principle of pleoptic therapy is the creation of a situation in which the fovea is shielded and the perifoveal area (used by the patient for fixation) is temporarily blinded by a bright flash of light. The shield is then removed and the patient is asked to fixate with the shielded fovea so that fixation becomes central.

   This treatment is considered only when patient is suffering from eccentric fixation (EF) and is done between 6 years and 9 years of age.
6. **Drug therapy:** *Levodopa/Carbidopa:*

   Dopamine has been demonstrated to be a neurotransmitter in retinal amacrine and interplexiform cells and is important in information processing in the brain. It couples and uncouples the horizontal cells of the retina. Levodopa is a precursor of dopamine and carbidopa prevents the breakdown of levodopa. The greatest advantage of pharmacological therapy includes the potential of treating older amblyopes where the conventional modalities have high failure rates.

Binocular Vision

It is defined as state of simultaneous vision with two seeing eyes that occurs when an individual fixes his visual attention on an object of regard.

- Fixation of visual reflex in infant starts developing at < 1 month of age and is completed by 5–6 months of age (Hence, the full development of fovea and macula is accomplished by 5–6 months).
- Binocular function fully develops by 5 years and orthoptic exercises are most useful till 5 years of age, though improvement can be seen till 8 years to 9 years.
- **Grades of Binocular Vision:**

  Grade I: Simultaneous perception.

  Grade II: Fusion.

  Grade III: Stereopsis.

  Stereopsis in true sense is possible only binocularly and occurs due to 5% of aniseikonia that we have in our eyes. But uniocularly also we get some hint of stereopsis. These are:

  1. **Linear perspective.**
  2. **Overlay of contours.**
  3. **Motion parallax.**
  4. **Dimunition of color with distance.**
  5. **Dimunition of texture with distance.**
- **Horopter:** It is the sum total of points in physical space, that stimulate **corresponding retinal elements of the two eyes.**
- **Panum's Area:** The field in front of and behind the horopter in which the expected diplopia does not occur is known as **"Panum's fusional space".**

1. Diplopia (Double vision)

It is not a presenting feature in latent squint or anisometropia.

Classification:

A. **Horizontal:** Images are side by side. It is due to involvement of horizontal muscles.
   - **Uncrossed:** Homonymous.
   - **Crossed:** When false image is on opposite side of deviating eye (Heteronymous).

Convergent Squint:
Uncrossed diplopia
Divergent Squint:
Crossed diplopia

} To remember crossed diplopia in divergent squint

B. **Vertical:** Images are up and down, due to the involvement of vertical muscles.

C. **Torsional:** It is due to the involvement of oblique muscles.

2. Uniocular/Binocular

Causes of Uniocular Diplopia

- Subluxated lens.
- Double pupil.
- Incipient cataract.
- Keratoconus.

Causes of Binocular Diplopia

- Paralytic squint.
- Myasthenia gravis.
- Diabetes mellitus.
- Thyroid disorders.
- Blow out fractures.
- Anisometropic glasses (uniocular aphakic glass).
- After squint correction.

ACTION OF EXTRAOCULAR MUSCLES

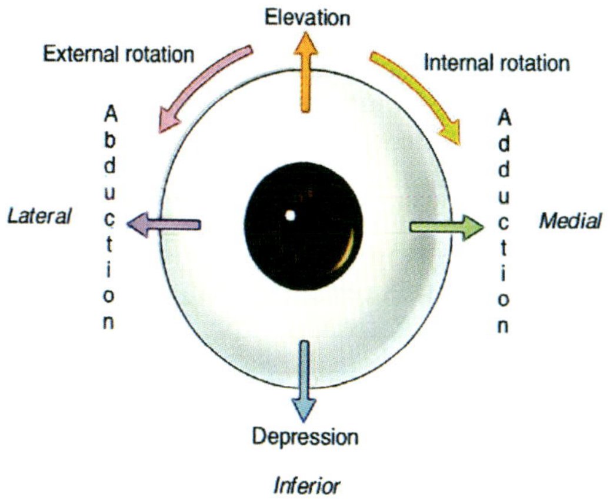

Fig. 13.3

1. **Horizontal Recti:**
   a. Lateral rectus–Abduction.
   b. Medial rectus–Adduction.
2. **Vertical Recti:**
   a. *Superior Rectus*
      – Elevation.
      – Intorsion.
      – Adduction.
   b. *Inferior Rectus*
      – Depression.
      – Extorsion.
      – Adduction.
3. **The Obliques:**
   a. *Superior Oblique*
      – Intorsion.
      – Depression.
      – Abduction.
   b. *Inferior Oblique*
      – Extorsion.
      – Elevation.
      – Abduction.

To Remember:

- Superiors are intorters **(IS).**
- Recti are adductors **(RAD).**
- Obliques are abductors.

Squint

It is the misalignment of the visual axis of the two eyes.

CLINICAL EVALUATION

1. **Visual acuity.**
2. **Hirschberg test:** It is also called corneal reflex test (CRT), where light is shown in front of the eyes and should be symmetrically seen slightly (0.5 mm) nasal to the centre of the pupil. The amount of deviation of 1 mm corresponds to 7 degrees, i.e., 15 prism diopters. If light reflex is at the border of the pupil it corresponds to 15 to 18 degrees of squint and if it is at the limbus, it corresponds to 45 degrees of squint.
3. **Prism test/krimsky's test:** It is a modification of Hirschberg test where we place prisms in front of the deviated eye, until the corneal light reflexes are symmetrical.
4. **Cover tests:**
   a. *Cover test:* It is a monocular test designed to test for the presence of heterotropia. It should be performed for both near and distance. If the left eye shows displacement of corneal reflex, the examiner should cover the opposite right eye and search for movement of the left eye. A nasal movement to take up fixation indicates exotropia, a temporal movement esotropia, a downward one hypertropia and upward one hypotropia.
   b. *Alternate cover test:* It is used to test heterophoria. It is done ONLY IF cover uncover test is normal. One eye is covered for 2 secs and then the

cover is quickly shifted to another eye. At this moment, the examiner notes any movement of uncovered eye as it assumes fixation. If no movement occurs patient is orthophoric. A nasal movement indicates exophoria and temporal movement indicates esophoria. A downward movement indicates hyperphoria and vice versa.

We can place prisms to know the amount of phoria. The base is placed opposite to the direction of squint, e.g., in a convergent squint the prism is placed base out, the alternate test is then performed, and the end point reached when the prism negates ocular movements. The angle of deviation is read from strength of the prism.

5. **Dissimilar image tests:**

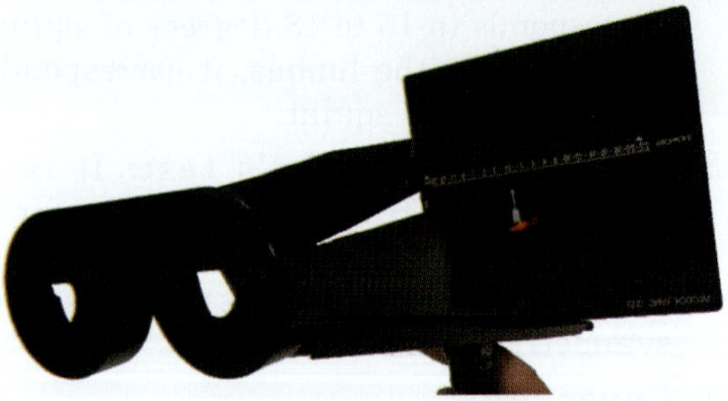

Fig. 13.4

a. *Maddox wing:*

It dissociates the two eyes for near fixation (one third of a metre) and measures the amount of heterophoria. The right eye sees only a white vertical arrow and red horizontal arrow whereas left eye sees only horizontal and vertical row of numbers. The odd numbers are on the right side and even on left side in the horizontal row, and for vertical row odd numbers are down and even numbers are upwards. The horizontal deviation is measured by asking the patient which number the white arrow points to. The odd numbers point to esodeviations, whereas even numbers indicate exodeviations. The vertical deviation is measured by asking the patient, which number the red arrow intersects. Odd numbers indicate right hyperdeviations whereas even numbers indicate left hyperdeviations. The third arrow is below and right of horizontal white scale to measure cyclophoria. The amount of cyclophoria is determined by asking the patient to move this red torsion lever so that it is parallel to the horizontal row of numbers or the red arrow.

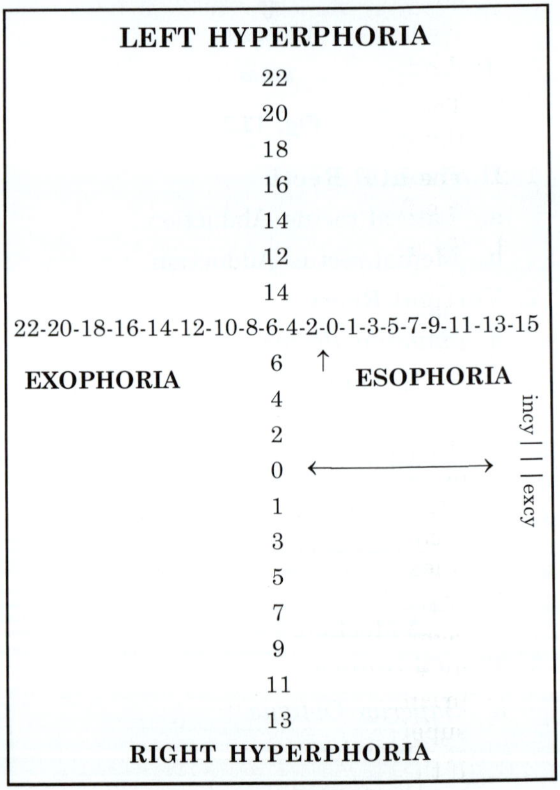

Fig. 13.5

b. *Maddox rod:*

The test is based on diplopia projection. The dissociation of the deviation is brought about by presenting a red light image to one eye and a white light to other eye, while prisms are used to superimpose these. It tests and effectively measures the angle of deviation (horizontal and vertical). The strength of prism is increased, until the streak of light passes through the centre of light source, the strength of prism indicates the amount of deviation present.

Instrument: MADDOX rod is a handheld instrument composed of red parallel planoconvex cylinder lenses which refracts light rays, so that a point source of light is seen as a line or streak of light. Due to optical properties, the streak of light is seen perpendicular to the axis of the cylinder.

Method:

1. The patient is instructed to fixate on the light source with both eyes open.
2. The MADDOX rod is then placed over the fixating eye (right side).
3. To measure the horizontal deviation, the MADDOX rod is placed horizontally making the red line to be vertical, the patient is then asked if the red line superimposes the white light, or it is to the left or right of the light.
4. If patient sees the red line to the left of the light, patient has exotropia or exophoria, and Base in (BI) prism of increasing strength are used until the lines are superimposed.
5. If the patient sees the red line to the right of the light, patient has esotropia or esophoria, and Base out (BO) prisms are used, until the lines are superimposed.
6. If the line is below the light there will be hyper-deviation, in which base down prisms are used to measure and correct deviation.
7. If the line appears above the light, there will be hypo-deviation and base up prisms are used to measure and correct deviation.

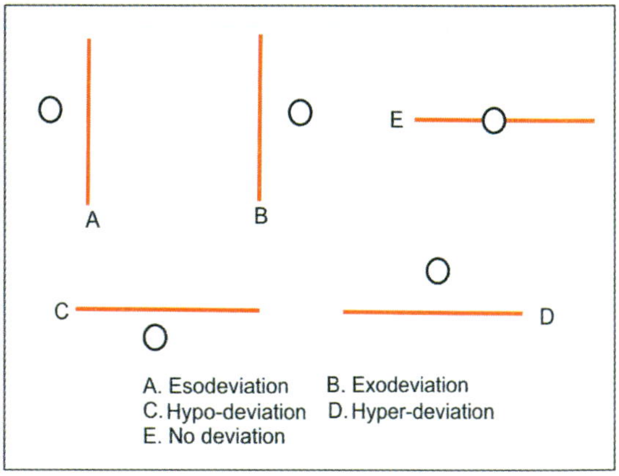

Fig. 13.6

c. *Hess test:*

It is a dissimilar image test for paralytic squints. The technique is as follows:

1. The patient wears red green goggles, with the red filter in front of the right eye.
2. The patient holds a green light projection and the examiner the red one.
3. The examiner projects the red light onto the screen and asks the patient to superimpose his green light on it. Then this is repeated, with red filter in patients left eye.

Interpretations:

If the patient has right lateral rectus palsy and fixates with right eye (red glass), excessive innervation will flow to left normal medial rectus (Hering's law), as a result the patients green marker will indicate a point on the screen which is beyond the correct alignment. If the patient now fixates with left normal eye (red filter), normal amount of fixation is required to take up fixation. However, right lateral rectus is paralytic, hence, the patients green marker will indicate a point short of correct alignment.

When the test has been completed, the relative positions are connected by straight lines.

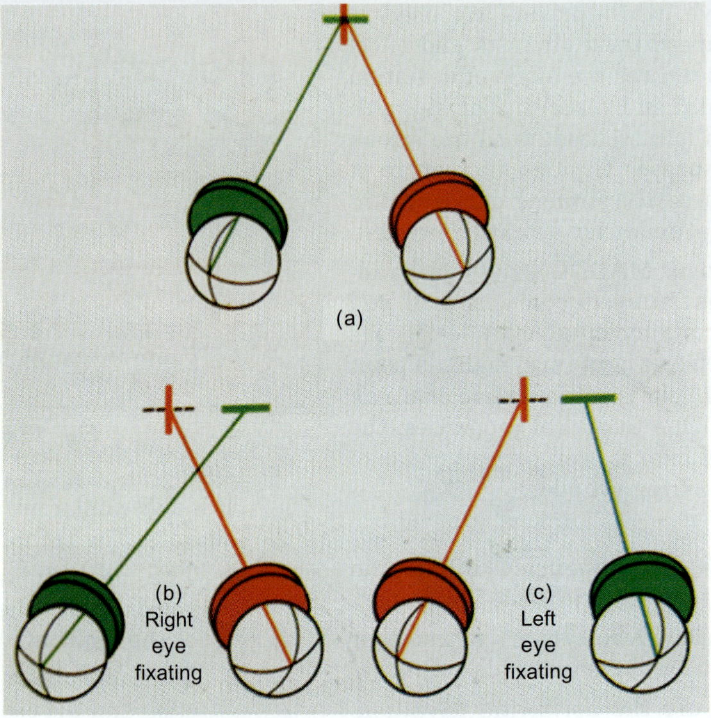

Fig. 13.7: Principles of Hess test

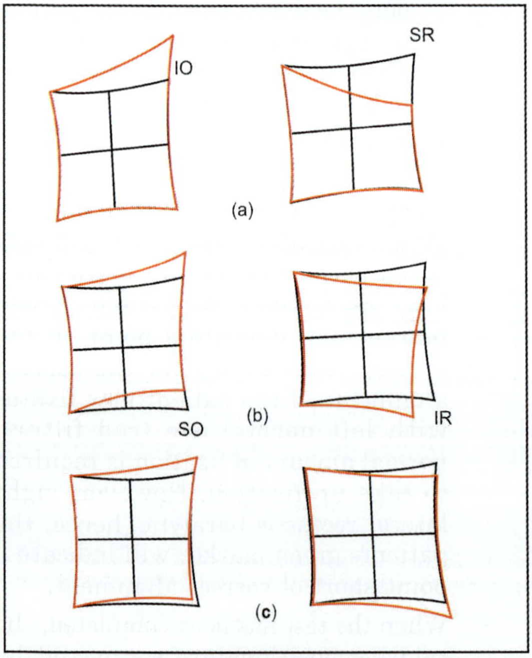

Fig. 13.8

d. *The Lees screen:*

This is similar to Hess test but dissociation is carried out using a mirror, not red green goggles. The apparatus consists of two glass screens at right angles to each other, bisected by two sided plane mirror.

e. The Lancaster Red Green test is similar to HESS test.

TESTS OF BINOCULAR CO-OPERATION

1. The base-out prism test:

It is also known as 4 prism diopter base out test, or 4 prism diopter reflex test (PRT) is an objective non-dissociative test to prove the presence of binocular single vision by assessing motor fusion.

Through the use of 4 prism diopter, retinal image is displaced and diplopia is induced, which is the driving force of the eye, to change fixation and thereby regain bifoveal fixation, meaning they overcome that amount of power. It is used to detect microtopia, l (less than 10 Prism diopters). It is used to test if patient has bifoveal fixation or there is monofixation. In spite of normal looking alignments. It is a sensitive test to check for presence of binocular single vision in presence of small scotoma.

Method: Patient is asked to fixate on a target, while examiner places the 4 prism diopter in front of one eye and observes the response.

Normal Eye:

The shifting of image caused by the prism, will produce a movement towards apex of the prism (of eye under the prism), and the fellow eye will have a outward movement in the same direction, of the same magnitude, due to Hering's law. Simultaneously the fellow eye produces a fusion convergence movement as there is no central suppression of that fellow eye. This is the result of overcoming the diplopia experienced.

2. **Worth's four-dot test:**

It is performed with the patient wearing red lens in front of right eye which filters all light except red and green lens in front of left eye which filters all light except green. The patient then views a box with four lights, one red, two green and one white. The results are as follows:

1. If all four lights are seen its normal fusion.
2. If four lights are seen in presence of manifest squint, there is ARC.
3. If only two red lights are seen there is left suppression.
4. If three green lights are seen, it's right suppression.
5. If two red and three green lights are seen, there is diplopia.
6. If green and red lights alternate, there is alternating suppression.

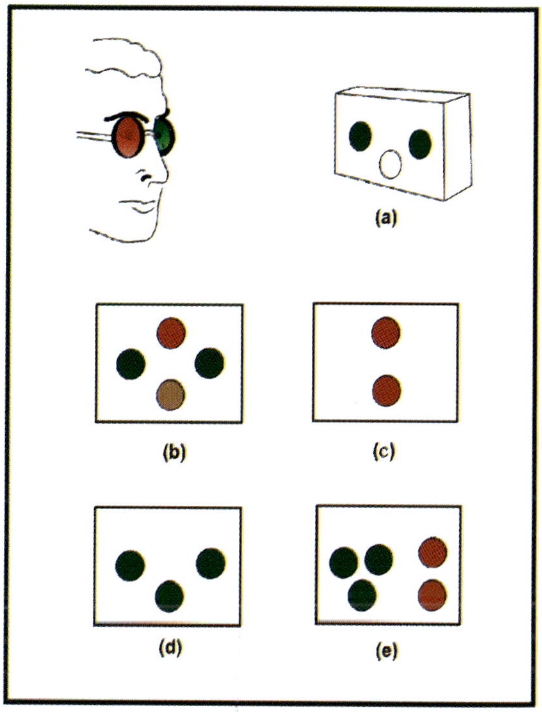

Fig. 13.9: Worth's four-dot test

3. **The bagolini striated glasses:** It consists of fine striations, which convert a light point into a line (similar to maddox rod). The two lenses are placed in a trial frame at 45 and 135 degrees in front of each eye. This enables dissimilar images to be presented to each eye under natural conditions. In the normal and patients of ARC, the two lines will intersect at the point of light in form of a cross.

When interpreting results, the line associated with each eye is the line perpendicular to the lens in front of that eye. If the lens in front of the right eye is at 135 degrees, then the line on the results representing the right eye will be at 45 degrees.	Suppression responses 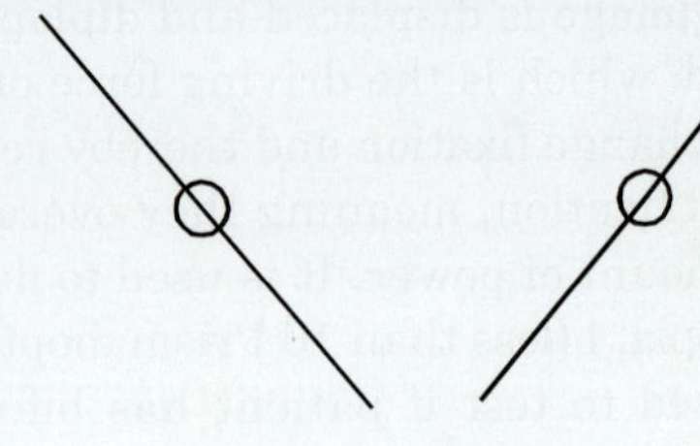
One light: If the patient sees one light, that means that either they have fused the two images from each eye together, or are suppressing of one of the images. **Two lights:** If the patient sees two lights, this is indicative of diplopia as the patient has an image from each eye but is unable to fuse the two. **One line:** If only one line is seen, this means one eye is suppressing. The eye that is suppressing is the eye which the corresponding line is not seen.	Binocular single vision responses 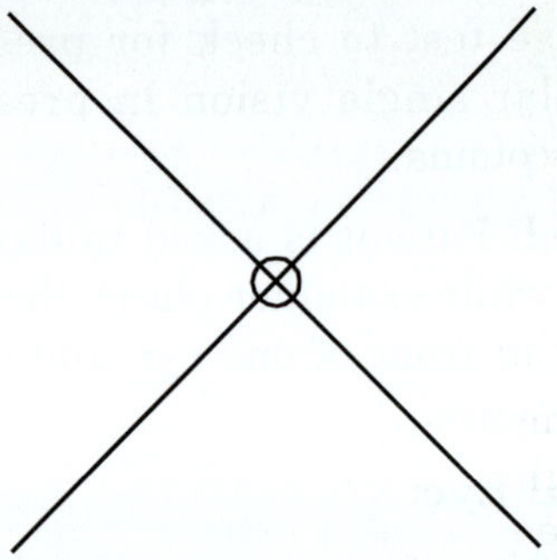
Two lines: If the patient sees two lines, this means that there is no suppression of either eye. **Disappearing line:** The patient may report that they see one line, then the lines switch and they can only see the other line. This is the case in an alternating deviation, where there is always one eye suppressing, however the fixing eye is switching.	A possible microtropia response 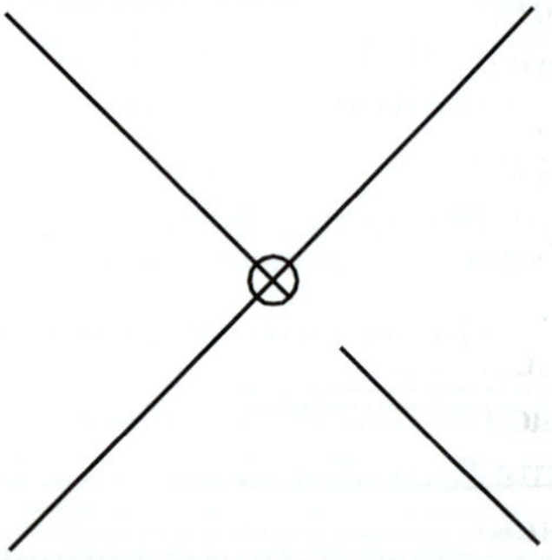
Broken line: If a line has a break in it, this means that there is a scotoma somewhere on the retina. **Normal binocular single vision (BSV)** In a patient with normal binocular functions, the expected results would be a cross with the light where the two lines intersect.	Possible manifest strabismus responses 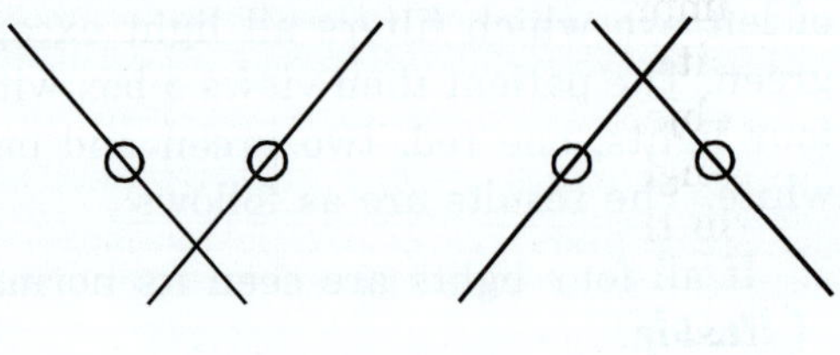

Fig. 13.10

4. The synaptophore:

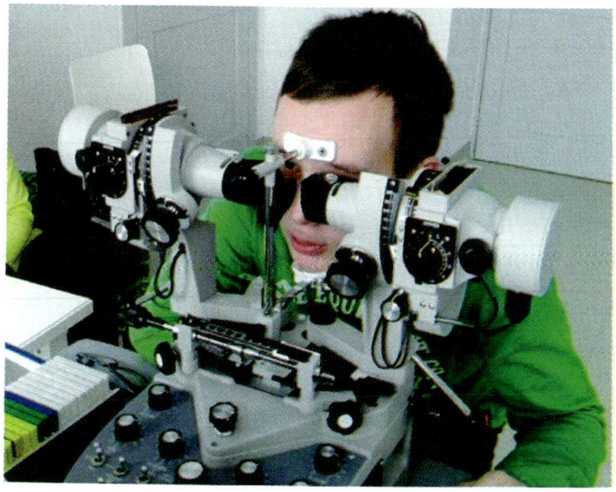

Fig. 13.11

It consists of two cylindrical tubes, with a mirrored right angled bend and a + 6.5D lens in each eyepiece. Pictures are inserted in a slide carrier, situated at the end of each tube. It can determine the three grades of binocular single vision as follows:

A. *Simultaneous perception:* It is determined by presenting two dissimilar but not mutually antagonistic pictures, such as BIRD AND A CAGE.

B. *Fusion:* It implies the ability of the two eyes to produce a composite picture, from two similar pictures, each one of which is incomplete in one small detail. E.g.: Two rabbits each lacking, either a tail or a bunch of flowers.

C. *Stereopsis:* Ability to obtain an impression of depth by the superimposition of two pictures of the same object taken from slightly different angles. E.g.: Bucket that is appreciated in three dimensions.

Classification:

1. **Pseudostrabismus:** Ocular alignment is normal and the patient is misdiagnosed as squint. It may be eso or exo. **Pseudosquint can be differentiated from true squint by Hirschberg's test.**

   Causes of Pseudoesotropia

   1. Wise flat nasal bridge.
   2. Broad epicanthic folds.
   3. Close-set eyes.
   4. A negative angle Kappa-Angle between visual axis and optical axis.

   Causes of Pseudoexotropia

   1. A large positive angle kappa.
   2. Hypertelorism.

2. **Latent squint or heterophoria:** The tendency of the eyes to deviate is kept latent by fusion. It may be eso, exo, hyper or cyclo.

3. **Manifest squint or heterotropia:** It may be concomitant or inconcomitant.

Concomitant squint: When the amount of deviation in the squinting eye remains constant in all directions of gaze.

Etiology:

It occurs due to any obstacle to the development of binocular single vision which may be due to sensory, motor or central cause.

Sensory: When a clear image is not formed on retina due to refractive errors or hazy media.

Motor:

1. Abnormality of shape and size of orbit.
2. Abnormality of extraocular muscles.
3. Abnormality of accommodation or convergence.

Central: Due to cortical abnormalities.

TYPES OF CONCOMITANT SQUINT

1. **Esotropia.**
2. **Exotropia.**
3. **Hypertropia.**

Esotropia: It may be unilateral or alternating. It is broadly classified as accommodative, non-accommodative or secondary (i.e., due to sensory deprivation).

Childhood Esotropia

Childhood esotropia can be classified as:

- Infantile esotropia—It presents within 6 months of age.
- Accommodative esotropia.
- Non-accommodative esotropia.

Infantile Esotropia

1. Presents within first 6 months of birth.
2. The angle of deviation is usually large (30D).
3. Nystagmus, if present is usually horizontal.
4. Refractive error is usually normal for the age.
5. Fixation is alternating in the primary position and cross-fixating in side-gaze.

Accommodative Esotropia

It is associated with activation of accommodation reflex.

The three main forms are:

1. **Refractive:**
   - Normal AC/A ratio (Accommodation Convergence/Accommodation).
   - Excessive hypermetropia (+4D to+7D).
2. **Non-Refractive:**
   - High AC/A Ratio.
   - Refraction normal for age of child.
   - Little or no deviation for distance.
3. **Mixed:** It is caused by combination of hypermetropia and high AC/A ratio.

Children having mild hypermetropic refractive error are prone to exert more accommodative power, in order to compensate for the mild hypermetropia. On the other hand, accommodation is one of the most important factors which stimulate convergence, termed as accommodative convergence. The relation between the two is expressed by the ratio AC/A. *This is the magnitude of change in convergence (in prism dioptres) caused by an increase in accommodation (expressed in dioptres).* Hence excessive accommodation exerted may lead to convergent squint in children known as accommodational squint. Therefore, its first line of treatment is correction of refractive error.

Miotics are used as a treatment modality for accommodative esotropia with high AC/A ratio (i.e., accommodation convergence/accommodation ratio). They are used as short term measure in children who will not wear spectacles and have high AC/A ratio.

Mode of action: The miotic therapy works through production of peripheral accommodation so that less accommodative effort is required by the patient for near vision and thereby less accommodative convergence is induced.

Dose: 0.125% Ecothiophate (Phospholine iodide) once daily or 4% pilocarpine four times daily for 6 weeks.

Non-accommodative Esotropia

It can be of following types:

1. *Stress-induced esotropia:* Breakdown of efficient fusional mechanisms through emotional or physical stress.
2. *Sensory-deprivation esotropia:* It is caused by monocular organic lesion like cataract or optic atrophy.

3. *Divergence-insufficiency esotropia:* It is characterized by greater deviation for distance than for near.
4. *Spasm of near reflex:* It is characterized by intermittent episodes of sustained convergence associated with spasm of accommodation and miosis. It is treated with cycloplegics.
5. *Consecutive esotropia:* Esotropia due to surgical overcorrection of Exotropia.
6. *Due to sixth nerve palsy:* Paralytic squint.

Exotropia: It may be of the following types:

1. **Congenital exotropia:** It occurs from birth and is very rare.
2. **Primary:** It occurs from two years of age. It may be intermittent or constant.
3. **Secondary:** It occurs due to sensory deprivation in adults.
4. **Consecutive:** It occurs due to surgical overcorrection.

Treatment of Concomitant Squint

1. Spectacles with full correction.
2. Occlusion therapy.
3. *Preoperative orthoptic exercises:* This is given after the correction of amblyopia to overcome suppression.
4. Squint surgery.
5. Postoperative orthoptic exercises to improve fusional range and maintain binocular single vision.

Incomitant squint: It is a type of heterotropia in which the amount of deviation varies in different directions of gaze. It includes:

1. Paralytic squint.
2. A and V pattern heterotropias.
3. Restrictive squint.

Paralytic squint: It may be neurogenic, myogenic or due to lesion of neuromuscular junction.

Features:

1. *Diplopia:* It is more marked towards the action of paralysed muscle.
2. Confusion.
3. Nausea and vertigo.
4. *Ocular deviation:* It may be primary or secondary. Primary deviation is the deviation of the squinted eye and secondary deviation is of the normal eye during cover-uncover test. Primary deviation is less than secondary deviation **according to Hering's Law.** In restrictive squint-primary deviation > secondary deviation.
5. Restricted ocular movements.
6. Compensatory head posture.
7. False projection or orientation.

Hering's Law states that during any conjugate eye movement, equal and simultaneous innervation flows to the yoke muscles.

Sherrigton's Law

Sherrington's law of reciprocal innervation states that increased innervation and contraction of a muscle is automatically associated with a reciprocal decrease in innervation and relaxation of its antagonist.

Pathological Sequelae of Extraocular Muscle Palsy

1. Overaction of contralateral synergist.
2. Contracture of direct antagonist.
3. Secondary inhibitional palsy of the contralateral antagonist muscle.

CLINICAL VARIETIES OF PARALYTIC SQUINT

1. **Isolated muscle paralysis:** It is most commonly of fourth and sixth nerve.

A. **Fourth Nerve:** Fourth nerve is the only cranial nerve which is crossed, i.e., has contralateral innervation, and emerges from the dorsal aspect of the brain. It is the most slender and longest cranial nerve.

Clinical Features of 4th Nerve Palsy:

1. *Hyperdeviation of the involved eye:* This hyperdeviation increases when the head is tilted to the ipsilateral shoulder; termed as **Bielchowskys test.**
2. *Excyclotorsion:* It is compensated by head tilt to opposite shoulder.
3. Limited depression in adduction.
4. Vertical diplopia which is worse on looking down.

B. **Sixth Nerve:** An isolated sixth nerve nucleus is never nuclear in origin as its nucleus is closely related to the fasciculs of seventh nerve.

Clinical Features of 6th Nerve Palsy:

1. Defective abduction of the affected side.
2. Convergent squint in the primary position.
3. Horizontal diplopia which is worse in the field of paralysed muscle.
4. Face turn in the field of paralysed muscle.

2. **Paralysis of third nerve:** It may be external ophthalmoplegia when only the extraocular muscles are paralysed, internal ophthalmoplegia when only the internal muscles are paralysed or total ophthalmoplegia when all the muscles supplied by the third nerve are paralysed.

Clinical Features of Total Ophthalmoplegia:

1. Ptosis.
2. *Deviation:* Eye is down and out and slightly intorted.
3. Restricted ocular movements.
4. Pupil is fixed and dilated.
5. No accommodation.
6. Crossed diplopia.
7. Head posture.

Treatment

1. **Medical treatment** for six months, i.e., B-complex for neurotonics and systemic steroids for non-specific inflammations.
2. **Surgery:** It is indicated after six months. The principle is either strengthening (by resection) the paralytic muscle or weakening (by recession) of the overacting muscle.

A and V pattern: This term is used when the amount of deviation in squinting eye varies by more than 10 prisms in upward gaze and 15 prisms in downward gaze.

Special Ocular Motility Defects

1. **Duane's Retraction Syndrome:** It is a congenital defect occurring due to fibrous tightening of lateral or medial or both rectus muscle.

   Features:

   1. Limitation of abduction, adduction or both.
   2. Retraction of the globe and narrowing of the palpebral fissure on attempted adduction.
   3. Eye in primary position may be orthotropic, esotropic or exotropic.

2. **Brown's Superior Oblique Tendon Sheath Syndrome:** It is a congenital motility defect due to fibrosis of superior oblique tendon. It is characterized by limitation of elevation in adduction with

normal elevation in abduction. There is a positive forced duction test on attempts to elevate the eye in adduction.

3. **Strabismus Fixus:** It is rare disorder. There is bilateral fixation of eyes in convergence position due to fibrous tightening of the medial recti.

Strabismus Surgery

1. *Muscle weakening procedures:* Recession, marginal myotomy and myectomy.
2. *Muscle strengthening procedures:* Resection, tucking and advancement.
3. *Procedures that change direction of the muscle:*
   A. Vertical transposition of horizontal recti to correct A and V patterns.
   B. Transplantation of muscles in paralytic squint.

Refractive Surgeries

These are the surgeries to change the refractive power of eye.

Pre-requisites of Refractive Surgery

1. **Age above 18 years:** Refractive surgery should not be done under 18 years of age as the refraction is not stable.
2. Stable refractive error for one year.
3. Normal anterior segment with no pathologies.
4. Normal retina with no pathologies.
5. Normal pachymetry reading of at least 490 microns.

Refractive surgeries are classified as:

A. Incisional Refractive Surgeries:

i. Radial keratotomy.

ii. Astigmatic keratotomy.

B. Lamellar Refractive Surgeries:

PRK–Photo-refractive Keratectomy.

LASIK–Laser-in-situ Keratomileusis.

C-LASIK.

LASEK or Epilasik.

Femtosecond laser ablation.

C. Newer Refractive Procedures:

i. Phakic Intraocular Lens or ICLs, i.e., implantable contact lens.

ii. Clear lens extraction.

D. Refractory Surgery for Presbyopia:

1. **Conductive Keratoplasty.**
2. **Prelex.**

Radial Keratotomy

- Done for the treatment of myopia.
- Procedure involves giving deep radial corneal stromal incisions in the periphery. This weakens the paracentral and peripheral cornea (causing bulging) and hence central cornea is flattened.
- Low and moderate degrees of myopia (upto 5 D) achieve the best results.
- Stability of refraction is lower compared to other refractive procedures.
- Shorter incision—**Mini-radial keratotomy** indicates promising stability outcome.

Astigmatic Keratotomy

- It involves making transverse (Also called tangential, or T) cuts in an arcuate or straight fashion perpendicular to the steep meridian of the cornea.
- This produces localised ectasia of the peripheral cornea and central flattening of the incised meridian and thereby decreasing the amount of astigmatism.
- Due to "**Coupling Effect**", corneal meridian 90° away from transverse incision becomes steeper.
- The change in pre-operative spherical equivalent is close to zero.

Photo-Refractive Keratectomy (PRK)

- The procedure involves, removal of corneal epithelium and use of excimer laser (193 μm) to reprofile the anterior curvature of the cornea which changes its refractive power (by changing its radius of curvature).
- Treatment zone is 6.0 mm to 6.5 mm, this is large so as to avoid halos and edge glare.
- It can correct myopia, hyperopia and astigmatism.
- Results are best for low myopia (up to 5D).

This is because:

a. High myopic patients often regress 6–12 months after surface PRK because of stromal regeneration and/or epithelial hyperplasia which causes the ablated zone to steepen again.

b. Sub-epithelial haze is more in high myopes.

The patient with a nebular opacity involving the superficial corneal stroma should best be treated by this method as it will help the patient to get rid of this opacity during the correction of his refractive error.

LASER-IN-SITU—KERATOMILEUSIS (LASIK)

Procedure

See Figure 13.12.

A flap with parallel sides is lifted using the microkeratome.

↓

The excimer laser is used to remove a lenticule of pre-determined power from the exposed corneal stroma.

↓

The flap with its intact epithelium is then folded back and as it drapes over the modified stromal surface, the refractive power of anterior corneal surface is modified.

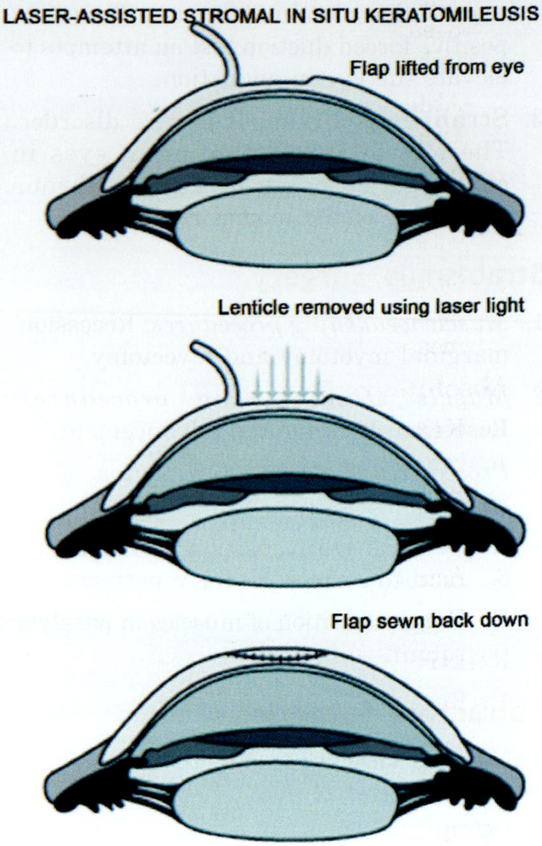

Fig. 13.12: (Q.No. 5) Procedure of LASIK

- It corrects – High myopia up to –25D.
  Hypermetropia.
  Astigmatism up to 8D.
- It is a better alternative than PRK for correcting high myopia and hypermetropia whereas in low myopes PRK is a better choice.
- **Preoperative Evaluation**
  a. Refraction.
  b. **Ultrasonic Pachymetry**—It is done to evaluate the central corneal thickness to assess the safe limits of corneal stroma removal with laser ablation.

The "**Munnerlynn formula**" can be used to predict the amount of stroma to be removed.

Ablation depth = (Optical zone)^2 × Diopters/3

At least 250 microns of stromal bed should be left to prevent corneal ectasia.

c. Detailed slit-lamp examination, retinal evaluation, eye dominance testing and measuring of IOP.

- **Absolute contraindications of LASIK**
  1. Keratoconus and other ectatic conditions.
  2. Central corneal thickness of < 500 microns.
  3. Active ocular disease.
  4. Pregnant and lactating mother.
- **Relative contraindications of LASIK**
  1. Recurrent erosion syndromes.
  2. Large pupillary size.
  3. Small palpebral fissure.
- **Complications:**
  1. Decentered ablation leading to irregular astigmatism (due to improper centered laser beam or poor homogeneity).
  2. **Central island formation:** It is a small steep area in the central cornea formed due to fluid accumulation or delayed clearance of debris. It generally regresses over time.
  3. Irregular flap, displaced/dislodged flap.
  4. Dry eye – **It is the most common postoperative complication**.
  5. DLK–Diffuse lamellar keratitis also known as **"Sand of Sahara Syndrome"**.
  6. Interface contamination.
  7. Epithelial ingrowth.
  8. Interface infection.

C-LASIK

- Also called **Customized-LASIK.**
- **C-LASIK** or **Zyoptix** is the new generation of excimer laser used for the treatment of refractive disorders. This technique takes into account the patient's:
  1. Subjective refraction.
  2. Ocular optical aberrations (these are higher order aberrations called **"Wave Front Aberrations"** broadly described as **"Aberropia"**).
  3. Corneal topography to design a personalized treatment based on total structure of the eye.
- Improving the optics of eye by removing aberration increases the contrast and spatial detail of retinal image.
- **Hence this technique is superior to LASIK.**

Lasek Or Epi-Lasik

- It stands for Laser Sub-Epithelial Keratomileusis.
- The procedure involves raising of a superficial flap, containing only epithelial cells and use of excimer laser to reprofile the anterior curvature of cornea. After this, the flap is draped back on the modified stromal surface.

Femtosecond Laser Ablation: In this procedure the flap during the LASIK process is raised by the femtosecond laser and not the microkeratome. Femtosecond laser is a Nd: Glass laser with the wavelength in infrared region (1053 nm). Femtosecond lasers are defined as lasers emitting pulses between few to hundreds of femtoseconds (1 femtosecond = 10–15 seconds). These flaps have the advantage over microkeratome flaps that they are more uniform in thickness, better stability and is a bladeless procedure.

Phakic Intraocular Lens Implantation Or Implantable Contact Lens

It is the implantation of another lens in a phakic eye.

- Its advantage over clear lens extraction is–preservation of patient's accommodative ability.
- Lenses may be implanted:
  a. Iris—claw lenses.
  b. Posterior chamber plate haptic lenses—It is placed between crystalline lens and iris.

Clear-Lens Extraction (CLE)

It is the extraction of a clear lens, i.e., which is still not cataratous in cases of high myopia. The main disadvantage of this procedure for correction of high myopia is the risk of surgically induced retinal detachment (RD).

Refractive Surgery for Presbyopia

Conductive Keratoplasty: It is a procedure in which heat from radiofrequency waves are used to shrink the collagen of the peripheral cornea hence leading to central steepening. It helps to correct mild hypermetropia and presbyopia. If the patient is hypermetropic then we treat both the eyes but if only presbyopia has to be dealt then we treat only one eye. This monovision so created helps the patient to see near from the treated eye and far and intermediate from the untreated eye. Induction of myopia in the treated eye is in the range of –1D to –2D. The disadvantage of the procedure is that it can be done only in patients who can adjust with the monovision and also it may prove to be a temporary correction with regression of number with time.

PRELEX

Prelex stands for presbyopic lens exchange. It corrects vision by replacing the eyes natural lens which has wrong focusing power with artificial multifocal intraocular lens implant that has the correct focusing power for the eye. Multifocal IOL heps to see the near, intermediate and far distance.

NEET DRILL

1. Longest extraocular muscle is SO, i.e., superior oblique.
2. Smallest extraocular muscle is IO, i.e., inferior oblique.
3. In pseudophakia all four Purkinje images are present.
4. Angle α: Angle between optic axis and visual axis at the nodal point.
5. Angle κ: Angle between pupillary line and visual axis at the cornea.
6. Yoke muscles are contralateral synergists, e.g., yoke muscle of LIR, i.e., RSO (just make every word opposite).
7. Eyeball is an ablate sphere with: AP diameter–24 mm/Lateral diameter–23.5 mm/Vertical diameter—23 mm/circumference—75 mm.
8. Volume of the eyeball is 6.5 ml.
9. Weight of the eyeball is 7 gm.
10. Total refractive power of the eye is 58–60D.
11. Total refractive power of the reduced eye is the same, i.e., 58–60D.
12. Reduced eye is a simplified refractive system of the eye.
13. Magnification of direct ophthalmoscope is 15 times.

14. Magnification of the indirect ophthalmoscope is 5 times.
15. Image formed by direct ophthalmoscope is virtual and erect.
16. Image formed by indirect ophthalmoscope is real and inverted.
17. Distant direct ophthalmoscope is done at 25 cm.
18. Periphery of the retina is visualized by indirect ophthalmoscope whereas centre of the retina is visualized by direct ophthalmoscope.
19. Distant direct ophthalmoscope is done to see the media of the eye.
20. The total area of the retina seen at one time by direct ophthalmoscope is 2DD.
21. The total area of the retina seen at one time by indirect ophthalmoscope is 8DD.
22. Nodal point is the optical centre of the eye situated just behind the lens.
23. High myopia is >6D.
24. Treatment of choice of amlyopia is occlusion of the normal eye.
25. Amaurosis is complete loss of vision whereas amblyopia is partial loss of vision.
26. Amaurosis fugax is transient loss of vision in a curtain like manner.
27. Fixation reflex develops by 5–6 months of age.
28. Binocular single vision develops by 5–6 years of age.
29. Every change of diopters leads to 2% of either minification or magnification. If we are using convex lens it is magnification and if concave it is minification.
30. Light passing through the prism deviates towards the base and image towards the apex.
31. Visual acuity is a measure of FORM SENSE.
32. Crossed diplopia is a feature of exotropia whereas uncrossed in esotropia.
33. Superiors are intorters whereas Recti are adductors.
34. Using atropine as a means of occlusion is called Penalisation.
35. Fourth Purkinje image is inverted.
36. In mature cataract, we see three purkinje images, fourth is absent.
37. Infant is hypermetropic by 2.5D to 3.0D.

MULTIPLE CHOICE QUESTIONS

1. A 30-year-old man has 6/5 vision each eye, unaided. His cycloplegic retinoscopy is + 1.0 D sph at 1 metre distance. His complaints are blurring of newsprint at 30 cm, that clears up in about two minutes. The most probable diagnosis is:

A. Hypermetropia

B. Presbyopia

C. Accommodative inertia

D. Cycloplegia

2. Left sided lateral gaze is affected in lesion of:

A. Right frontal lobe

B. Left occipital lobe

C. Right occipital lobe

D. Left frontal lobe

3. A lady wants LASIK surgery for her daughter. She asks for your opinion. All the following things are suitable for performing LASIK except:

A. Myopia of – 4 diopters

B. Age of 15 years

C. Stable refraction for 1 year

D. Corneal thickness of 600 microns

4. A patient using contact lens develops corneal infection. Laboratory diagnosis of acanthamoeba keratitis was established. The following is the best drug for treatment:

A. Propamidine

B. Neosporin

C. Ketoconazole

D. Polyhexamethylene biguanide

5. A 30-year-old man came to the outpatient department because he had suddenly developed double vision. On examination it was found that his right eye, when at rest, was turned medially. The most likely anatomical structures involved are (See Fig. 13.12):

A. Medial rectus and superior division of oculomotor nerve

B. Inferior oblique and inferior division of oculomotor nerve

C. Lateral rectus and abducent nerve

D. Superior rectus and trochlear nerve

6. A 35-year-old hypermetrope is using 1.50 D sphere both eyes. Whenever his glasses slip downwards on his nose he will feel that his near vision:

A. Becomes enlarged

B. Becomes distorted

C. Becomes decreased

D. Remains the same

7. A 12-year-old child complains of headache and decreased vision. On examination he has a visual acuity of 6/36 in the right eye and 6/6 in the left eye. On retinoscopy at 66 cms, the left eye showed correction of 1.5 D and the right eye of 5 D. The anterior chamber and fundus of eye were normal. What may be the cause of decreased vision in the right eye?

A. Amblyopia

B. Occipital lobe infarct

C. Optic neuritis

D. Refractive error

8. Function of superior oblique muscle is:

A. Elevation with eye rotated outwards

B. Elevation with eye rotated inwards

C. Depression with inward rotation

D. Depression with outward rotation

9. Direct distant ophthalmoscopy is done at a distance of:

A. 10 cm B. 25 cm

C. 50 cm D. 1 meter

10. In a 3-year-old child mydriatic used for refraction is:

A. 1% atropine drops

B. 1% atropine ointment

C. 1% homatropine drops

D. Tropicamide drops

11. Treatment of choice in aphakia:

A. Contact lens B. Spectacles

C. IOL D. Laser therapy

12. True regarding lateral rectus palsy is:

A. Crossed diplopia

B. Uncrossed diplopia

C. Divergent squint

D. Pupillary dilatation

13. Which of the following causes exclusively mydriasis?

A. Atropine
B. Cyclopentolate
C. Phenylephrine
D. Tropicamide

14. Most important factor to focus rays on retina:

A. Lens
B. Corneal curvature
C. Axial length
D. Media of globe

15. The refractive power of eye is:

A. 15 D B. 29 D
C. 58 D D. 100 D

16. Fixation of visual reflex is accomplished by:

A. 6 months B. 1 year
C. 2 years D. 3 years

17. A 12-year-old boy comes into room with left sided head tilt, on correcting that he has right sided hypertropia, which increases on left gaze and tilting the head towards right, which muscle is affected?

A. Right superior oblique muscle
B. Left superior oblique muscle
C. Right superior rectus muscle
D. Left superior rectus muscle

18. Equal and opposite innervation is explained by which law?

A. Herring's law
B. Sherrington's law
C. Donder's law
D. Hutchison's rule

19. Magnification obtained with direct ophthalmoscope for an emmetropic patient is:

A. 5 times B. 10 times
C. 15 times D. 20 times

20. A 20-year-old student has a myopia of 2.0 D and a post-traumatic nebular corneal opacity in her right eye. Which of the following is the best refractive surgery option for her?

A. Photorefractive keratectomy
B. LASIK
C. Radial keratotomy
D. Epikeratoplasty

21. On performing refraction using a plane mirror on a patient who has a refractive error of –3 diopter sphere with –2 diopter cylinder at 90° from a distance of 1 m under no cycloplegia, the reflex would be seen to move:

A. With the movement in the horizontal axis and against the movement in the vertical axis
B. With the movement in both the axes
C. Against the movement in both the axes
D. With the movement in the vertical axis and against the movement in horizontal axis

22. A soft contact lens user presents to you with pain, watering, photophobia and a white spot in the center of the cornea. What will be your initial management?

A. Start frequent antibiotic eye drops after discontinuing the contact lens
B. Pad and bandage the eye for 12 hours
C. Frequent instillation of artificial tears
D. Topical non-steroidal anti-inflammatory drugs (NSAID)

23. A 3-year-old child presents with a right convergent squint of 6 months duration. What is the appropriate management?

A. Immediate surgical correction followed by amblyopia therapy

B. Proper refractive correction, amblyopia therapy followed by surgical correction

C. Prescribe spectacles and defer surgery until the child is 5 years old

D. Botulinum toxin injection followed by occlusion therapy

24. Aniseikonia means:

A. Difference in the axial length of the eyeballs

B. Difference in the size of corneas

C. Difference in the size of pupils

D. Difference in the size of images formed by the two eyes

25. A friend of yours has a spectacle correction of –6.0 and –8.0. He telephones you one morning and tells that he has started seeing some opacities floating in front of his eye and that his vision has decreased slightly over the last few days. As an intern in the ophthalmology section, what would you do?

A. Reassure

B. Refraction and prescribe a new spectacle

C. Direct ophthalmoscopy

D. Indirect ophthalmoscopy

26. Change in length of eyeball by one millimeter causes how much myopia?

A. 3 dioptres B. 1 dioptre

C. 2 dioptres D. 4 dioptres

27. A 16-year-old boy complains of pain in the right eye. After refractometry, he was prescribed a + 3.5 D sphere lens. The cover test is normal. There is no heterophoria. The diagnosis is:

A. Organic amblyopia

B. Anisometric amblyopia

C. Emmetropic amblyopia

D. Toxic amblyopia

28. A child was taken to the doctor by his mother, complaining that there is decrease in his school performance. His teacher says that he frequently squeezes his eyes and says that there is difficulty in seeing the blackboard. What is the most probable diagnosis?

A. Myopia

B. Hypermetropia

C. Presbyopia

D. Astigmatism

29. A lady using contact lens developed photophobia, blurred vision and watery discharge was diagnosed to be suffering from over wearing syndrome. Most appropriate management is:

A. Avoid use of lens for 48–72 hours

B. Antibiotic and cycloplegic

C. Change the contact lens

D. Send the lens for culture and sensitivity

30. After maximum correction, the vision of right eye is 6/36 and left eye is 6/6 and with 66 cm retinoscopy right eye is +4.5 D and left eye has +1.5 D with normal fundus. Most likely cause of defect in vision is:

A. Refractive error

B. Amblyopia

C. Optic neuritis

D. Anisometropia

31. The following are grades of binocular single vision except:

A. Simultaneous perception

B. Fusion

C. Retinal correspondence

D. Stereopsis

32. All of the following are associated with squint except:

A. Diplopia

B. Stereopsis

C. Confusion

D. Deviation

33. All are used for macular function test except:

A. Maddox rod test

B. Two-point discrimination test

C. Electroretinogram

D. Laser inferometry

34. Uncrossed diplopia is seen in:

A. Exotropia B. Exophoria

C. Esophoria D. Esotropia

35. Refractive index of cornea is:

A. 1.33 B. 1.37

C. 1.41 D. 1.43

36. Contact lens is best used in:

A. High myopia

B. Aphakia

C. Irregular astigmatism

D. High astigmatism

37. Indirect ophthalmoscopy is done for assessing all, except:

A. Ora serrata

B. Vitreous base

C. Retinal periphery

D. Fovea

38. Accommodative squint is managed by:

A. Correction of refractive error

B. Surgery

C. Occlusion of affected eye

D. Convergent exercises

39. Which muscle is intortor of eyes?

A. Superior rectus

B. Medial rectus

C. Inferior rectus

D. Inferior oblique

40. A 3-year-old child with 15 degree esotropia, the management of the child will be:

A. Refractive correction

B. Prism cover test

C. Surgical alignment

D. Wait and watch

41. True about amblyopia:

A. No organic cause

B. Correction should be done before 6 years

C. Spectacles

D. Exercise of affected eye

E. Surgery has a role

42. True about cross-cylinder:

A. Half of the curvature is cylindrical

B. Plus lens

C. Minus lens

D. Both plus and minus lens

43. In complete 3rd nerve palsy:

A. Eye deviated medially

B. Superior and inferior recti affected

C. Dilated pupil

D. Ptosis

E. Convergence/accommodation is lost

44. Amblyopia is treated by:

A. Optical correction

B. Occlusion

C. Orthoptic exercise

D. Pleoptic exercise

45. Refractive power of eye depends upon mainly following factor/ factors:

A. Lens

B. Cornea

C. Vitreous humour

D. Aqueous humour

E. Axial length of the eye

46. Treatment of presbyopia:

A. LASIK

B. Concave lens

C. Convex lens

D. Radial keratotomy

47. Refractive power of eye can be changed by:

A. Radial keratotomy

B. Keratomileusis

C. IOL

D. LASIK

E. Photocoagulation

48. Periphery of retina is visualized by:

A. Indirect ophthalmoscopy

B. Direct ophthalmoscopy

C. Gonioscopy

D. Contact lens

49. Treatment modalities for myopia are:

A. Radial keratotomy

B. Laser keratomileusis

C. Epikeratophakia

D. Laser keratoplasty

50. Image seen by indirect ophthalmoscopy is:

A. Inverted and virtual

B. Erect and virtual

C. Inverted and real

D. Erect and real

51. Complications of soft contact lens are all except:

A. Giant papillary conjunctivitis

B. Folliculosis

C. Corneal vascularisation

D. Corneal erosion

E. Acanthamoeba keratitis

52. Superior oblique is supplied by:

A. Upper branch of 3rd N

B. Lower branch of 3rd N

C. Trochlear

D. Abducens

53. In retinoscopy for refractive error at 1 m we add 1D; if done at distance of 66 cm, the addition factor will be:

A. –2 B. –1.5

C. –0.5 D. –5

54. Refractive condition of the eye at birth is:

A. Hypermetropia of 2D

B. Myopia of 2D

C. Hypermetropia of 5D

D. Myopia of 5D

55. Presbyopia is due to:

A. Loss of elasticity of the lens capsule

B. Weakness of ciliary muscles

C. Weakness of suspensory ligament

D. All of the above

56. Diplopia is not a presenting feature in:

A. Manifest squint

B. Paralytic squint

C. Latent squint

D. Anisometropia

57. Intraocular lens has advantage over glasses in:

A. Better field of vision

B. Better accommodation

C. Better under-water vision for swimmer

D. No chromatic aberration

E. All of the above

58. Radial keratotomy is used as treatment modality for:

A. Small degree in myopia

B. Progressive non-healing ulcer

C. High astigmatism

D. High hypermetropia

59. All are true about indirect ophthalmoscope except:

A. Image is real and inverted

B. Details of fundus can be seen even with slightly hazy media

C. Magnification is more than direct ophthalmoscope

D. Used for seeing periphery of fundus

60. All are features of paralytic squint except:

A. Unequal fixation

B. Vertigo

C. Amblyopia

D. Abnormal head position

61. Diplopia in paralytic squint is:

A. Uniocular

B. Binocular

C. Both of the above

D. No diplopia

62. Which of the following extraocular muscles does not have an adductor action?

A. Medial rectus

B. Superior recuts

C. Inferior oblique

D. Inferior rectus

63. Best treatment modality for astigmatism is:

A. Bandage contact lens

B. Soft contact lens

C. Toric contact lens

D. Hydrophilic contact lens

64. Soft contact lenses are made up of:

A. HEMA B. PMMA

C. PVC D. Glass

65. Most common infection in eye following use of soft contact lens is:

A. Acanthamoeba

B. Pseudomonas

C. Staphylococcus

D. Streptococcus

66. Shortest acting mydriatic is:

A. 1% Hyoscine

B. 1% Atropine

C. 1% Tropicamide

D. 1% Cyclopentolate

67. Power of lens used in emmetropic person for posterior chamber intraocular lens implant is:

A. + 13 D B. + 18 D

C. + 19.5 D D. + 24.5 D

68. Best line of treatment in a 3 years old child with 15° esotropia of recent onset is:

A. Orthoptic exercises

B. Relieving prisms

C. Refractive correction

D. Surgery

69. In retinoscopy at 1 meter, point of neutralization is achieved when far point of eye is:

A. 1 meter in front of eye

B. 6 meters in front of eye

C. At fovea

D. Behind the lens

70. Amblyoscope is used for:

A. Exophthalmos

B. Lens

C. Squint assessment

D. Field of vision

71. Power of lens used in indirect ophthalmoscopy is:

A. + 10 D B. + 20 D

C. + 15 D D. + 18 D

72. A child presents in the OPD with complaints of strabismus when he looks outward on either side; which of the conditions is associated with the above complaints?

A. Lateral rectus palsy

B. Infantile esotropia

C. Pseudoesotropia

D. Retraction syndrome

73. About concomitant squint which of the following is true?

A. Secondary deviation is greater than primary deviation

B. Secondary deviation is equal to primary deviation

C. Secondary deviation is less than primary deviation

D. None of the above

74. Maximum visual acuity occurs in:

A. Macula lutea

B. Macula densa

C. Fovea centralis

D. Optic disc

75. "Jack-in-box" phenomenon is due to:

A. Spherical aberration

B. Pin-cushion distortion

C. Roving ring scotoma

D. Aphakia

76. Optical aberration is reduced by:

A. Iris B. Lens

C. Cornea D. Aqueous

77. The red glow moves along with light when patient is having:

A. Myopia

B. Astigmatism

C. Hypermetropias

D. None

78. Crossed diplopia occurs in:

A. Exophoria B. Exotropia

C. Esophoria D. Esotropia

79. Distant direct ophthalmoscopy reveals all except:

A. Peripheral retinal changes

B. Detached retina

C. Iris hole

D. Media opacities

80. In concave mirror retinoscopy, if shadow moves in same direction as mirror, refractory error is:

A. Hypermetropia

B. Myopia of 1D

C. Myopia < 1D

D. Myopia > 1D

81. A prism deviates the light rays:

A. Towards the base

B. Towards the apex

C. No deviation

D. Irregularly in all directions

82. A 45-year-old patient with 6/36 vision improves to 6/9 on pin-hole test. The patient is most likely to have:

A. Central cataract
B. Macular hole
C. Refractive error
D. Glaucoma

83. A contact lens most suitable for a patient with keratoconus is:

A. Soft B. RGP
C. Toric D. Hard

84. A 45-year-old patient with increase in myopic error from 1D to 5D in last 6 months. He is most likely to have:

A. PSC cataract
B. Nuclear cataract
C. Cortical cataract
D. Mature cataract

85. Miotics are used in the treatment of:

A. Concomitant convergent squint
B. Glaucoma
C. Both
D. None

86. The angle between optical axis and line passing through pupil is:

A. Alpha B. Beta
C. Gamma D. Kappa

87. Action of superior rectus is:

A. Elevation, abduction, extorsion
B. Depression, abduction, extorsion
C. Elevation, adduction, intorsion
D. Depression, abduction, intorsion

88. The wavelength of ablation in LASIK is:

A. Ultraviolet
B. Infrared
C. Visible spectrum
D. Microwave

89. The recommended size of the pin-hole is:

A. 1 mm B. 2 mm
C. 1.2 mm D. 1.6 mm

90. The best modality of amblyopia management is:

A. Surgery B. Occlusion
C. Levodopa D. Penalisation

91. Binocular diplopia is seen in:

A. Aphakia
B. Subluxation of lens
C. Keratoconus
D. Polycoria
E. Intumescent cataract

92. Accommodation is maximum at the age of:

A. 25 years B. 5 years
C. 14 years D. 30 years

93. The most common cause of myopia is:

A. A-P diameter is increased
B. The thickness of lens is increased
C. The viscosity of aqueous humour is increased
D. The viscosity of vitreous humour is increased

94. Objective assessment of the refractive state of the eye is termed:

A. Retinoscopy
B. Gonioscopy
C. Ophthalmoscopy
D. Keratoscopy

95. Visual acuity in infants is tested with the help of:

A. Landolts rings

B. 4 dot test

C. Perimetre

D. Slit lamp

96. The refractory power of eye is normally 59 dioptres. Two thirds of this is contributed by:

A. Anterior surface of the lens

B. Posterior surface of the lens

C. Anterior surface of the cornea

D. Aqueous humor and vitreous humor combined

97. Yolk muscle of the right superior rectus muscle is:

A. Left superior rectus

B. Left inferior oblique

C. Left inferior rectus

D. Left superior oblique

98. Alpha angle is the angle between:

A. Pupillary axis and optical axis

B. Visual axis and optical axis

C. Centre of eyeball rotation and line of fixation

D. None of the above

99. Cylindrical lenses are used in:

A. Hypermetropia

B. Myopia

C. Astigmatism

D. Presbyopia

100. Facultative hypermetropes manage to see because of:

A. Pin-hole effect

B. Miosis

C. Accommodation

D. Convergence

101. Aniseikonia is corrected with:

A. Galleliotelescope

B. Prism

C. Cylindrical lenses

D. Contact lenses

102. Which is the most common complication of high myopia?

A. Glaucoma

B. Cataract

C. Haemorrhage

D. Retinal detachment

103. Anomaloscope is used to detect:

A. Squint

B. Simultaneous perception

C. Fusion

D. Stereopsis

E. All of the above

104. On retinoscopy at 1 mt distance there is no movement of the reflex. The patient is:

A. Emmetropic

B. 1 D myopic

C. 1 D hypermetropic

D. 2 D myopic

105. Amsler grid is used in:

A. Detecting color vision

B. Maculopathy

C. Retinal function

D. Refractive errors

106. Visual acuity test is a test of:

A. Light sense B. Contrast sense

C. Color sense D. Form sense

107. Defect in amblyopia lies in:

A. Lateral geniculate body

B. Optic tract

C. Rods and cones

D. Optic nerve

108. Soft contact lens leads to all of the following problem except:

A. Acanthamoeba keratitis

B. Corneal vascularisation

C. Papillae formation

D. Folliculosis

109. For a newborn baby with squint, surgery should be done at:

A. 3–4 years B. Immediately

C. 10–12 years D. 18–21 years

110. Compulsory head tilt is seen with the paralysis of:

A. Superior rectus

B. Inferior rectus

C. Superior oblique

D. Lateral rectus

111. Pseudoexotropia is a feature of:

A. High hypermetropia

B. High myopia

C. Epicanthus

D. High astigmatism

112. Action of left superior oblique muscle is:

A. Dextrodepression

B. Dextroelevation

C. Levodepression

D. Levoelevation

113. Treatment of concomitant squint is:

A. Surgery B. Spectacles

C. Exercises D. All

114. Hirschberg test is used to detect:

A. Squint B. Diplopia

C. Fusion D. Field defects

115. Physiological tone of the ciliary muscle is about:

A. 3 D B. 4 D

C. 5 D D. 1 D

116. Landolts broken ring test is used for:

A. Knowing the type of squint

B. Recording the visual acuity

C. Testing the power of extraocular muscles

D. Testing the binocular single vision

117. Damage to superior oblique muscle causes diplopia in which direction?

A. Horizontal and downward

B. Vertical and downward

C. Horizontal and upward

D. Vertical and upward

118. Snellen's chart is used to test:

A. Vision B. Refraction

C. Presbyopia D. Color blindness

119. Visual acuity of infants is best assessed by:

A. Visual evoked potential

B. E-Test

C. Snellen's chart

D. Sheridan-Gardiner test

120. Limited abduction and adduction is seen in:

A. Type 1 Duane's refraction syndrome

B. Type 2 Duane's refraction syndrome

C. Type 3 Duane's refraction syndrome

D. Double elevator palsy

121. Which of the following reflects wavelength (nanometers) of laser used for shaping cornea in refractive surgery?

A. 193 B. 451

C. 532 D. 1069

122. False about indirect ophthalmoscopy is:

A. Can be used in hazy media

B. Magnification is 4 to 5 times

C. Convex lens is used

D. Image formed is virtual and erect

123. The critical angle of cornea-air interface is:

A. 36 degrees B. 46 degrees

C. 56 degrees D. 66 degrees

124. A 59-year-old male presents with dimness of near vision. On examination, the media was clear in both the eyes. What would be the next step?

A. Refraction with near add

B. Refraction under atropine

C. Radial keratotomy

D. Cataract surgery

125. Miotics are used in:

A. Divergent squint

B. Convergent squint

C. Paralytic squint

D. All

126. A patient comes with recent onset paralytic squint. Which of this is true of paralytic squint?

A. Congenital

B. Amblyopa is present

C. Diplopia

D. Secondary deviation is equal to primary deviation

127. Maximum refraction takes place between:

A. Air tear film

B. Tear film and cornea

C. Cornea and aqueous

D. Aqueous lens

128. When water enters eye, blurring of vision due to:

A. Elimination of refraction through water

B. Extra refraction through water

C. Impurities of water

D. Speed of light is more through water

129. True about amplitude of accommodation is all except:

A. Is the difference between near point and far point

B. Is about 10 dioptres in emmetropic eye

C. Increases as age advances

D. Changes with spherical aberration

130. A 35-year-old male complains of vision distortion. The distortion increases progressively in both the meridians on wearing his spectacles. All of the following are correct regarding the patient's problem except:

A. It is also called pin-cushion distortion

B. It is due to wearing of cylindrical glasses

C. It is due to asymmetrical convex lenses in both the eyes

D. It is aniseikonia

131. Right trochlear nerve palsy can lead to:

A. Diplopia on upward gaze and adduction

B. Right head tilt

C. Exotropia

D. Hypertropia

132. Dissociated squint is common in:

A. Infantile esotropia

B. Infantile exotropia

C. Duanes retraction syndrome

D. Hypertropia

133. Extraocular muscle arising outside the orbit:

A. IO B. IR

C. SO D. SR

134. The power of lens used in indirect ophthalmoscopy is:

A. +20D B. +58D

C. +90D D. +60D

135. Maximum power is on:

A. Anterior surface of cornea

B. Posterior surface of cornea

C. Anterior surface of lens

D. Posterior surface of lens

ANSWER AND EXPLANATION

1.	c	Since his blurring of near vision clears with time it cannot be presbyopia and hence we answer accommodative inertia.
2.	a	Saccadic movement is controlled by the frontal lobe and its innervation is contralateral.
3.	b	Minimum age for any refractive surgery should be at least 18 years.
4.	d	PHMB is the first line of treatment and we can add propamidine isethionate or neomycin for synergistic effect.
5.	c	Convergent squint is a feature of lateral rectus palsy which is supplied by abducens nerve.
6.	a	The effective power of a plus lens increases with the distance.
7.	a	Since his best corrected visual acuity is only 6/36, he is a case of amblyopia.
8.	c	Superiors are intorters. SO depresses whereas SR elevates the eye.
9.	b	Distant direct ophthalmoscopy is used to see the media of the eye.
10.	b	The choice of cycloplegic in children within 7 years of age is atropine eye ointment.
11.	c	Aphakia is high degree of hypermetropia and the choice of treatment is IOL.
12.	b	LR palsy will lead to convergent squint. We get crossed diplopia in divergent squint and uncrossed in convergent squint.
13.	c	Phenylephrine is a mydriatic with no cycloplegic action.
14.	b	The more a surface is curved, the more is its refractive power.
15.	c	The refractive power is 58 D–60 D.
16.	a	Visual reflex formation occurs by 5–6 months.
17.	a	In SO palsy, the hypertropia increases on tilting the head on the side of the palsy. This is called Bielchowsky's sign.
18.	b	Sherrington's law states that there is equal but opposite innervation in the agonist and antagonist.
19.	c	Mx of direct ophthalmoscope is 15 times and indirect ophthalmoscope is 5 times.
20.	a	PRK deals with superior stroma and LASIK deals with deep stroma. Hence in case of Nebular CO, we should do PRK so that we get rid of this nebular opacity.
21.	c	The uncorrected retinoscopic reading is –2 and –4. Since both the readings are myopia of more than 1, we will

get against the movement in both the axes.

22. a The most common infection after contact lens use is pseudomonas.

23. b The sequence of managing a concomitant squint is refraction, amblyopia therapy, orthoptic exercises (if needed) and if no improvement then finally surgery.

24. d Anisekonia is measured by Eikonometre.

25. d High myopes are at an increased risk of developing retinal detachment; hence IO is done to screen it.

26. a Change of 1 mm axial length will cause change of 3 D, whether myopia or hypermetropia.

27. b Since the question mentions +3.5 D in only one eye, hence it is a case of anisometropia.

28. a The child has myopia and squeezing of the eyes causes a pin-hole effect leading to improvement of the vision due to this effect.

29. a Over-wearing syndrome indicates that we should avoid its use to get the relief of symptoms.

30. b Since in one eye the vision does not improve more than 6/36 even with the best possible correction, this is a case of amblyopia.

31. c Retinal correspondence means that every point in the retina has a corresponding point in the other retina. We all have corresponding retinal points.

32. b Stereopsis means depth perception.

33. c Actually all are the tests of macular function but since ERG is least commonly used for this purpose compared to the other options given, we mark this as the answer.

34. d Uncrossed diplopia is a feature of convergent paralytic squint.

35. b 1.33 is the index of the aqueous and vitreous humor.

36. c All are indications of contact lens use but the best is irregular astigmatism where specks do not help at all. We use RGPs in this case.

37. d IO is not useful to study the foveal details as its magnification is very less.

38. a Correction of high hypermetropia helps to correct the convergence by relieving the amount of accommodation exerted.

39. a Superiors are intorters and recti are adductors.

40. a,b,c See answer 23.

41. a,b,c Amblyopia is pathology of the LGB and hence there is no role of exercise or surgery in this case.

42. d Cross cylinders help to check the accuracy of the refraction and consist of both plus and minus lens.

43. b,c,d,e In third nerve palsy eye is down and out.

44. a,b,d Pleoptic exercises are used to treat eccentric fixation.

45. a,b,e The main refracting media of the eye are cornea and lens.

46. c Presbyopia is treated by plus lenses, i.e., convex lenses used only for near vision.

47. a,b,c,d Keratomileusis is changing the curvature of the cornea. Both

refractive surgeries and IOL can change the refractive power but not photocoagulation.

48. a,d We can see the peripheral retina with Goldmann three mirror contact lens.

49. a,b Epikeratophakia is a method of increasing the curvature of the cornea by putting a corneal lenticule from a donor cornea, and is a treatment modality of aphakia.

50. c In IO image is inverted and real.

51. b Contact lens incites only papillary reaction and no follicular reaction.

52. c LR_6SO_4, rest of the muscles are supplied by third nerve.

53. b For cycloplegic factor, if we use atropine, the correction factor is –1, for cyclopentolate it is –0.75 and if any other cycloplegic then the correction factor is –0.5.

54. a An infant is hypermetropic by 2.5–3.0 D.

55. d All these are age-related changes which lead to failure of accommodation, hence, causing presbyopia.

56. c,d Diplopia is a feature of paralytic manifest squint.

57. a,c,d IOLs cannot change their shape and hence accommodation is not possible. We need to use near glasses even after IOL surgery except if we use multi-focal IOLs.

58. a In RK, we give peripheral radial cuts on the cornea and hence there is flattening of the centre leading to decrease in refractive power. Hence, it corrects myopia.

59. c Magnification of IO is 5 times compared to DO which is 15 times.

60. c Amblyopia is a partial loss of vision with no organic cause. It occurs due to disuse of eyes and is not a typical feature of paralytic squint.

61. b See causes of binocular and uniocular squint.

62. c Obliques are abductors.

63. c Toric lenses are contact lenses with cylindrical correction.

64. a HEMA is hydrogel. Other material is Elastomer.

65. b Infection chances are always more in soft contact lens and the most common etiological agent is pseudomonas.

66. c Shortest acting is tropicamide and longest acting is atropine.

67. c IOL is calculated by biometry and the most common power for the emmetropic person is 19.5D to 20D.

68. c The first step for any concomitant squint is refraction.

69. a The point of neutralization is achieved when the far point of the patient corresponds to the nodal point of the examiner.

70. c Amblyoscope also called synaptophore is also used to see the grades of binocular function and for convergence exercises.

71. b Most common lens used is +20D. Other lens used is +13D.

72. c Since strabismus is perceived on looking both the sides, this is pseudostrabismus due to epicanthus.

73. b Primary deviation is deviation of the squinted eye and secondary deviation is that of the normal eye on cover-uncover test.

74. c Fovea centralis is the most sensitive part of the retina.

75. c Roving-Ring scotoma in aphakia is due to high prismatic effect of the thick plus lens. It is this scotoma which causes Jack-in-box phenomenon.

76. a Iris regulates the amount of light reaching the retina and hence helps reducing the aberrations.

77. c WITH THE MOVEMENT: Indicates that either the patient is emmetropic, hypermetropic or myopia of less than 1D.

78. b Crossed diplopia is a feature of divergent squint.

79. a Peripheral changes will be visible by indirect ophthalmoscope.

80. d The result of concave mirror retinoscopy is just the opposite of plane mirror retinoscope.

81. a The light is deviated towards the base of the prism whereas image is deviated towards the apex of the prism.

82. c Improvement on pin-hole indicates the best corrected vision which the patient can achieve on refraction.

83. b RGP semi-soft lenses replace the irregular surface of the cornea with a regular surface leading to the correction of the astigmatism.

84. b Nuclear sclerosis leads increased refractive index of the lens leading to lenticular myopia.

85. a Miosis, convergence and accommodation are components of the near reflex. Giving miotics leads to decrease amount of accommodation exerted leading to improvement of the convergence.

86. d Kappa is angle between optic axis and pupillary line.

87. c See action of muscles.

88. a Excimer lasers are ultraviolet radiations.

89. a Pin-hole is 1 mm in diameter.

90. b It is the normal eye which is occluded.

91. a A unilateral aphakia if corrected by specks will lead to diplopia as the specks causes the magnification of the image by 30%.

92. b Accommodation is maximum in children; hence we need atropine ointment as a choice of cycloplegia.

93. a The two main factors are axial length and corneal curvature.

94. a Retinoscopy is not a method to see the retina.

95. b Best method for evaluation of visual acuity in infants is Teller Acuity cards (which has pictures) based on FPL, i.e., Forced Preferential Looking.

96. c Major factor to focus the light rays on the retina is corneal curvature,

97. b Make all the three words, just the opposite, i.e., yoke muscle of right superior rectus is left inferior oblique.

98. b Angle alpha is around 5 degrees.

99. c Cylindrical lens gives power in a single axis and hence corrects astigmatism.

100. c Accommodation increases the refractive power of the eye by increasing the curvature of the anterior surface of lens and hence any patient with mild uncorrected hypermetropia will compensate by exerting more accommodation to make his vision clear.

101. d Anisekonia is corrected by isekonic lenses which cause magnification of the image without introducing any appreciable refractive power.

102. d RD is a complication of pathological myopia.

103. e It is the other name of synaptophore.

104. b If distance is 1 m then no movement is myopia is of 1D.

105. b Amsler grid is a method of assessing 10 degree of visual field surrounding fixation.

106. d There are three senses, i.e., light sense, contrast sense and form sense.

107. a Alongwith LGB there is involvement of the visual pathway till the visual cortex.

108. d There is no follicular reaction in the contact lens use.

109. b Visual reflex develops at 5–6 months and hence squint should be corrected as soon as feasible to avoid amblyopia.

110. c In superior oblique palsy, there is head tilt to the opposite side.

111. a Hypermetropes have a high positive angle alpha, which leads to pseudoexotropia.

112. a In an outward deviated eye the function of elevation and depression is of recti.

113. d All the three modalities are used for the treatment.

114. a Hirschberg test is based on the position light reflex in relation to the pupil, if at the border the squint is around 18 degree, if at the middle of pupillary border and limbus it is 35 degree and if the reflex is at the limbus, it is 45 degree.

115. d The basic tone is 1 D.

116. b It is useful for patients who are illiterate.

117. b Diplopia will occur in the direction of the action of the muscles.

118. a Snellen's acuity chart is used to check the visual acuity of the patient.

119. a Visual acuity assessment in such small children is done by either Teller acuity cards or electrophysiological test like VEP.

120. c Type 3 Duane's retraction syndrome.

The hallmark of Duane's retraction syndrome is retraction of the globe on attempted adduction caused by co-contraction of medial and lateral recti. Some children have associated congenital anomalies like deafness and speech disorder.

According to Hubler, it is divided into three types:

Type 1: This is most common. It is characterized by absence or limitation of abduction and normal adduction.

Type 2: This is least common. It is just the opposite, i.e., limited adduction with normal abduction.

Type 3: It is limitation of both adduction and abduction.

121. a The wavelength of Excimer laser used for refractive surgery is 193 nm. It is an ultraviolet laser. 1064 nm is the wavelength of NdYAG laser which is used for posterior capsulotomy and peripheral iridotomy.

122. d Image formed in indirect ophthalmoscope is real and inverted.

123. b Critical angle is the max angle for refraction after which there is total internal reflection. Gonioscopy is based on this principle. The angle is 46 degrees.

124. a 59 years patient with clear media means there is no cataract, and since there is difficulty in near vision, we should do refraction for both near and far. We do not use atropine in elderly patients as the ciliary muscles are already weak and we do not need cycloplegia for refraction. Radial keratotomy is a refractive surgery done for myopia.

125. b Miosis, convergence and accommodation are part of near reflex, giving miotics compensates for some accommodation leading to improvement of convergent squint.

126. c Paralytic squints are generally not congenital and hence amblyopia is not a problem. Secondary deviation is more than primary deviation.

127. a Tear film and cornea have the same refractive index.

128. a The medium for light becomes water and water instead of air and water hence there is less refraction.

129. c Amplitude of accommodation decreases with age.

130. a The description of the distortion is characteristic of **aniseikonia**, which is difference of image size between the two eyes which is **different from pin-cushion distortion.**

- **In pin-cushion distortion, refraction increases with the distance from the optical axis.**
- The visible effect is that lines that do not go through the centre of the image are bowed inwards, towards the centre of the image, like a pin-cushion.

131. d Superior oblique palsy will lead to diplopia in downgaze and adduction as diplopia occurs in the direction of action of the muscle. Since it is a depressor, the eye will be hypertropic.

132. a DVD is a condition where innervation of one eye causes it to move involuntarily and independent of the other, hence not following the Hering's and Sherrington's law. Some level of dissociative occlusion is required. To trigger the brain to suppress the vision in the eye. It is a feature of infantile esotropia.

133. a Inferior oblique arises from orbital surface of the maxilla lateral to the lacrimal groove.

134. a The condensing lens used for indirect ophthalmoscopy can vary from 14D, 20D, 28D, 30D. Most commonly used is 20D as it provides adequate magnification and field of vision.

135. a The power of anterior surface of cornea is 48D and posterior surface, it is –5D with a net power ranging from 42 to 45D.

RECENTLY ADDED QUESTIONS

1. Identify the below image and its use:

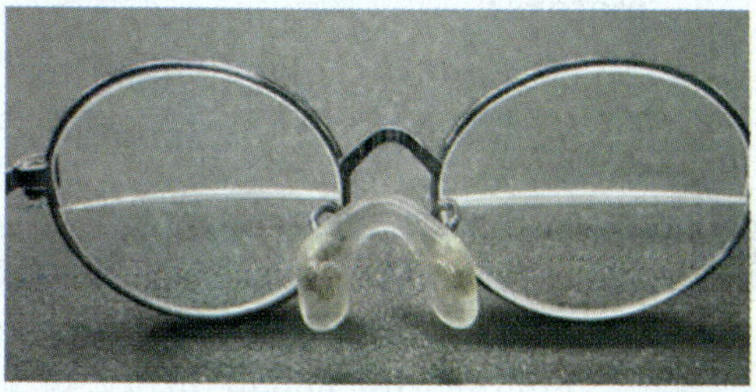

A. Progressive glasses for presbyopia
B. Bifocal glasses for Presbyopia
C. Executive bifocals for pediatric pseudophakia
D. Bifocals for aphakia

2. The image is shown depicting the refractory error of the patient. Identify the error.

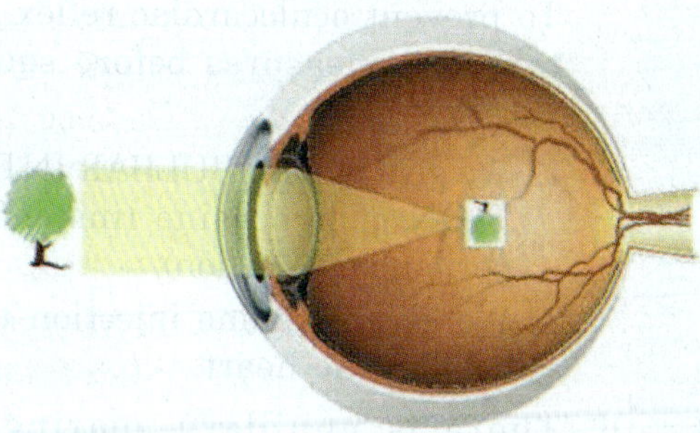

A. Presbyopia B. Hypermetropia
C. Myopia D. Astigmatism

3. For Presbyopia what number of spectacles are advised to a lady of 50 years?

A. 1D B. 2D
C. 3D D. 4D

4. A 50-year-old emmetropic patient needs what power of spectacles to correct his astigmatism?

A. +1 B. +2
C. +3 D. None

5. Which of the following is an example of simple myopic, with the rule astigmatism:

A. -2 D cylindrical at 180 degrees
B. -2 D spherical and +1 cylindrical at 90 degrees
C. +2 spherical and +1 cylindrical at 90 degrees
D. +2 D cylindrical at 180 degrees

6. In direct ophthalmoscopy:

A. The examiner uses right to see right eye of patient, patient looks in the light
B. The examiner uses his left eye for right eye of patient, patient looks straight
C. The examiner uses his left eye for left eye of patient, patient looks in the light
D. The examiner uses his right eye for right eye of the patient, patient looks straight

7. A surgeon was doing strabismus surgery on a child, when there was a severe decrease in heart rate, what immediate step you will take to manage?

A. Lessen the plain of anesthesia
B. Atropine
C. Stop surgery immediately
D. Glycopyrrolate

8. Third nerve palsy in diabetes mellitus presents with:

A. Pseudoptosis
B. Proptosis
C. Abnormal pupillary reflex
D. Normal pupillary reflex

9. What is the yoke muscle of right eye lateral rectus in dextroversion?

A. Medial rectus left eye
B. Superior oblique left eye
C. Inferior oblique left eye
D. Inferior recti left eye

10. What is the angle subtended by the largest letter in the Snellen chart on a person's eye who is reading it from a distance of 6 meters?

A. 60 minutes B. 10 minutes
C. 50 minutes D. 1 minute

ANSWERS OF RECENTLY ADDED QUESTIONS

1. c These are bifocals of paediatric age group.

2. c Myopia is a condition where total refractive powering eye is more than required. The light rays are focussed in front of retina.

Hypermetropia is a condition where total refractive power is less than required. The light rays are focussed behind the retina.

Astigmatism is the difference of refractive power between two principal axis.

3. b Correction according to the age is as follows:

40 years :: +1 D
43 years :: +1.25 D
45 years :: +1.50 D
48 years :: +1.75 D
50 years :: + 2 D
55 years :: +2.25 D
60 years :: +2.5 D

4. d Age wise prescription of glasses is only applicable for presbyopia, not astigmatism.

5. a Simple myopic astigmatism is :: one axis with no number, i.e., emmetropic and the other axis is myopic. With the rule astigmatism is when the vertical curvature is more than horizontal curvature. –2D cyl at 180 means the power of –2 is at 90 degrees (Axis is always mentioned opposite).

6. d Patient should not look in the light, as it will cause pupillary constriction.

7. c The severe bradycardia is due to oculocardiac reflex, and if it starts we should immediately stop the surgery.

To prevent oculocardiac reflex, we take two measures before squint surgery:

1. We give RETROBULBAR INJECTION of lignocaine (instead of peribulbar injection).
2. We give Atropine injection that acts on the heart.

8. d There is pupillary sparing in diabetic third nerve palsy.

9. a Yoke muscles are contralateral synergist. The two muscles working in dextroversion are RLR AND LMR, and vice versa.

10. c The minimal angle of resolution is calculated by reversing the acuity value. E.g. if it's 6/60, it will be 60/6 = 10 this is for the margin of the letter. For the whole letter, we multiply by 5. Hence answer is 50 minutes (Minutes is the unit of the angle, smaller than degree).

IMAGE-BASED QUESTIONS

1. The diagnosis is:

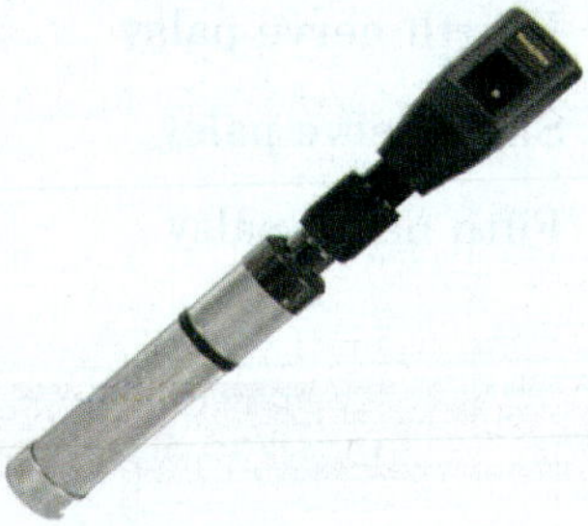

A. Direct ophthalmoscope
B. Indirect ophthalmoscope
C. Retinoscope
D. Distant direct ophthalmoscope

2. The investigation is:

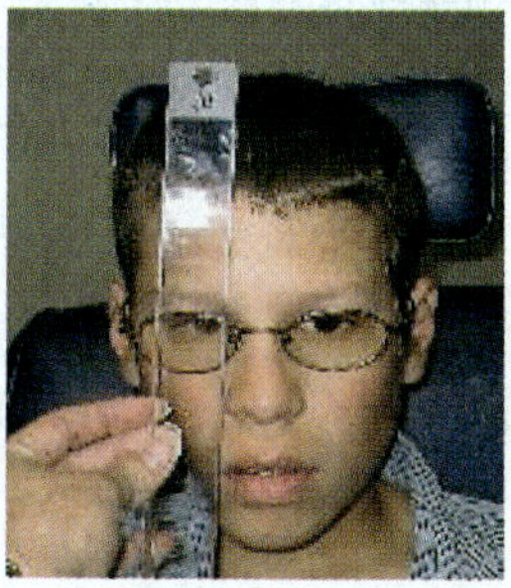

A. Hirschberg test
B. Krimskys test
C. Maddox-rod test
D. Maddox-wing test

3. The following instrument is used for:

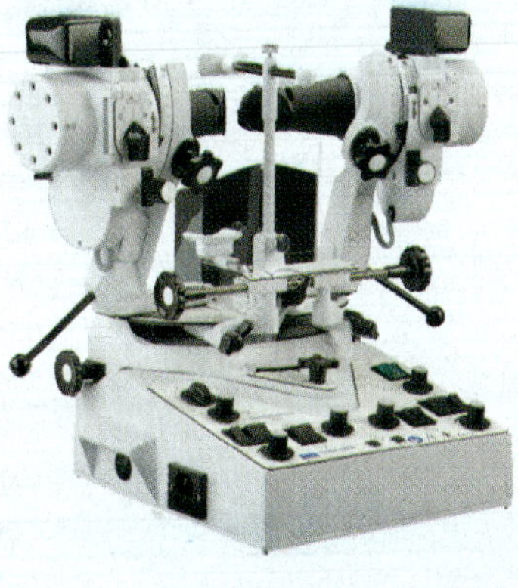

A. To measure the amount of squint
B. To check the grades of binocular single vision
C. Convergence exercises
D. All of the above

4. The diagnosis is:

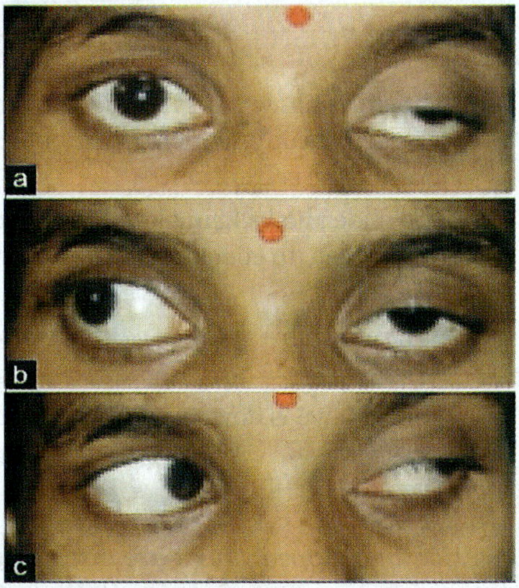

A. Third nerve palsy
B. Fourth nerve palsy
C. Sixth nerve palsy
D. Fifth nerve palsy

5. The diagnosis is:

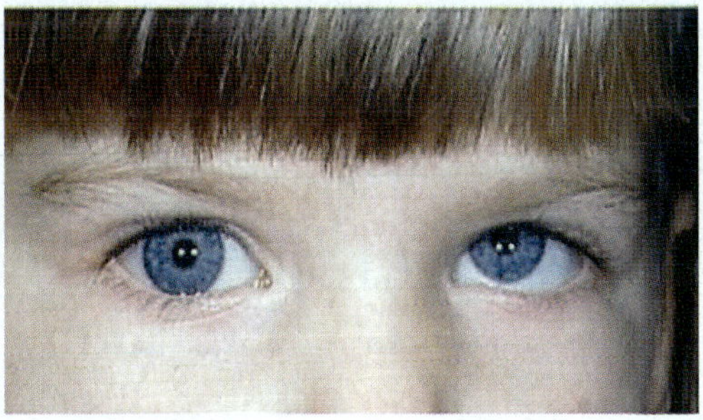

A. Third nerve palsy
B. Fourth nerve palsy
C. Sixth nerve palsy
D. Fifth nerve palsy

6. The diagnosis is:

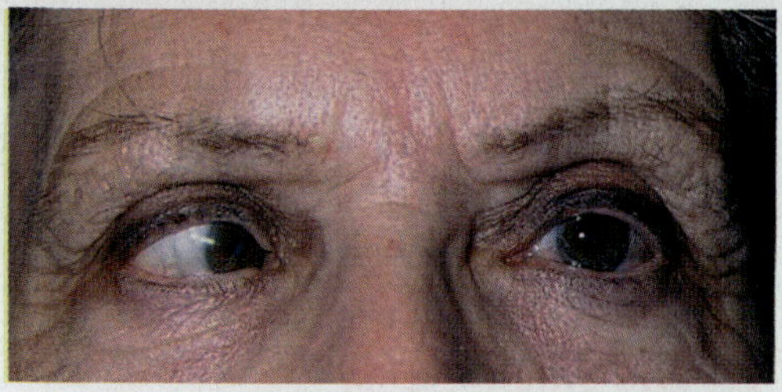

A. Third nerve palsy

B. Fourth nerve palsy

C. Sixth nerve palsy

D. Fifth nerve palsy

ANSWERS OF IMAGE-BASED QUESTIONS

1. c The slide shows a streak retinoscope for retinoscopy, which is an objective method of refraction.
2. b The slide shows krimskys test or prism reflex test, to measure the amount of squint.
3. d Synaptophore is also called amblyoscope.
4. a The left eye is down and out in primary position, with defective adduction, hence the diagnosis is third nerve palsy.
5. b The left eye is hypertropic and slightly adducted, hence the most probable diagnosis is fourth nerve palsy.
6. c The adducted position of the right eye suggests sixth nerve palsy.

GUIDANCE

Position and Appearances are irrelevant. The important thing is to carry out our personal duty, our commitment, no matter what anyone else may say. This is a life of true victory, a life of unsurpassed nobility and fulfillment.

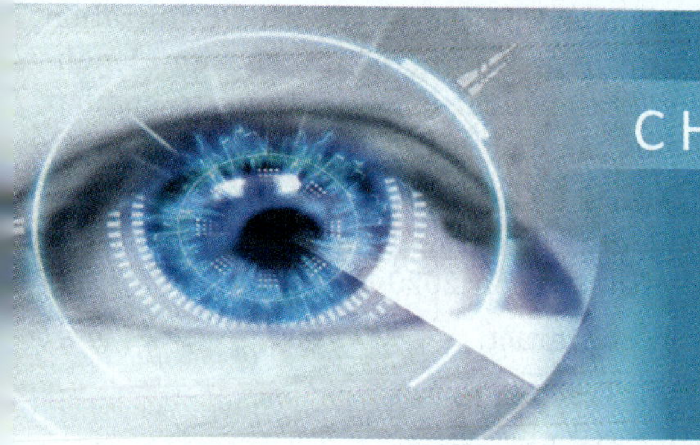

CHAPTER 14 Community Ophthalmology

WORLD: MAGNITUDE OF GLOBAL BLINDNESS

The estimated number of people visually impaired in the world is 285 million, 39 million blind and 246 million having low vision; 65% of people visually impaired and 82% of all blind are 50 years and older.

INDIA

- According to National Survey of Blindness (2001–02): Prevalence of blindness with vision of less 6/60 is 1.1%. In people of more than 50 years of age it is 8.5%.
- **Blindness with vision of less than 3/60 is 0.56%.**
- **Principal cause of blindness in India is cataract responsible for 62.6% of all cases.**
- In 1996 WHO survey, the prevalence of blindness in India was 0.7% (VA less than 3/60). And the most common cause of blindness in India—Cataract (81%).
- With 7.8 million people in India, while 45 million are visually challenged, the country accounts for 20% of the 39 million blind population across the globe.
- It is estimated that prevalence of childhood blindness in India is 0.8/1000 children in <16 years age group, implying a total of 300,000 blind children in our country.

MAGNITUDE OF BLINDNESS IN INDIA

The projected number of blind persons in India would increase to 24.1 million in 2010 and 31.6 million in 2020 (Sagar Borker–2011). As per National Programme for Control of Blindness (NPCN), the prevalence of blindness in India was 1.1% in 2001–02 and 1% in 2006–07.

RECENT CHANGE

The definition of Blindness under the National Programme for Control of Blindness (NPCB) is hereby modified in line with WHO definition: "Presenting distance visually acuity less than 3/60 (20/400) in the better, eye and limitation of field of vision to be less than 10 degrees."

CAUSES OF BLINDNESS IN INDIA

Govt. of India 1992	Percent Blindness
Cataract	81%
Refractive error	7%
Corneal opacity	3%
Glaucoma	2%
Trachoma and associated Infections	0.2%
Vitamin A deficiency	0.04%

NPCB 2001–2002

Cataract	62.6%
Refractive error	19.7%
Corneal opacity	0.9%
Glaucoma	5.8%
Posterior segment disorders	4.7%

- Percentage of surgeries with IOL implantation have increased from 20% in 1997–98 to 83% in 2003–04.
- The WHO-NPCB (National Programme for Control of Blindness) Survey (1986–89) has shown that there is a backlog of over 22 million blind eyes/12 million blind people in India. The survey has also brought out that 80.1% of these people are blind on account of cataract. Refractive errors, glaucoma, trachoma and central corneal opacities account for the rest of the blind population.

  Based on high prevalence level the states of Maharashtra, U.P., Orissa, Rajasthan, A.P., J & K and Tamilnadu were selected to be covered under the project. These seven states had the highest prevalence of blindness in the country.

Among these, U.P. has the highest prevalence followed by M.P. and Maharashtra.

VISION 2020— "THE RIGHT TO SIGHT"

- 135 million people in the world have low vision (According to the recent data).
- In general, 3/4th of world's blindness is avoidable (preventable or curable).
- Cataract is the main cause of blindness.
- Despite the best of efforts during last fifty years, the burden of blindness in the world is increasing, and the global burden of blindness can double by the year 2020. Hence vision 2020 is the common agenda launched by World Health Organization and a task force of international non-governmental organizations to combat this mammoth problem.
- The five conditions that have been identified as immediate global priorities within vision 2020 are:

1. Cataract.
2. Trachoma.
3. Onchocerciasis.
4. Childhood blindness.
5. Refractive errors and low vision.

- **The founder members of vision 2020 include:**

a. World Health Organization.
b. International Agency for the Prevention of Blindness.
c. Christoffel–Blind Mission.
d. Helen-Keler Worldwide.
e. Sight Savers International.
f. ORBIS International.

There are numerous other supporting members.

INDIAN SCENARIO

- India was the first country to launch the National Programme for Control of Blindness in 1976.
- Vision 2020 – "The Right to Sight" was launched in India at a meeting in Goa on October 10–13, 2001.
- **The target diseases for vision–2020 in India include:**

a. Cataract.
b. Childhood blindness.
c. Refractive errors and low visions.
d. Corneal blindness.
e. Diabetic retinopathy.

f. Glaucoma.

g. Trachoma (focal).

SCHOOL VISION SCREENING PROGRAMME

1. This programme uses school teachers as the initial screening personnel for identification of refractive errors in school children.
2. The programme covers only middle schools.
3. One teacher is selected from each school. The teachers are then trained in one day training sessions.
4. Abnormal vision in children is detected by using specially designed "E" card which has optotypes corresponding to 6/9 line of the Snellen's chart. All children who cannot see the 6/9 optotype with either eye are referred to the PMOA (Paramedical Ophthalmic Assistants) at the upgraded PHC (Primary Health Center) or CHC (Community Health Center) for refraction.
5. Children who need spectacles are then sent to local optician with whom the DBCS (District Blindness Control Society) has made arrangements for provision of good quality spectacles at a reasonable cost.

NPCB–National Programme for Control of Blindness was launched as a 100% centrally sponsored scheme in 1976.

GOALS

A. To reduce prevalence of blindness from 1.4 to 0.3% by 2000 AD.

B. To provide comprehensive eye care facilities for primary, secondary and tertiary levels of eye health care.

The ultimate goal of NPCB is to provide permanent infrastructure and is being done in three tier system, i.e.

1. *Peripheral sector for primary eye care:* At PHC and Subcenter levels. It is done for conditions like acute conjunctivitis, ophthalmia neonatorum, trachoma, xerophthalmia and superficial foreign body.
2. *Intermediate sector for secondary eye care:* Development of diagnostic and treatment facilities at district and sub-divisional levels under charge of an eye specialist. The conditions managed are cataract, entropion, ocular trauma and glaucoma.
3. *Central level for tertiary eye care:* Eye department of state medical colleges and establishing RIO (Regional Institutes of Ophthalmology). Major surgeries like penetrating keratoplasty and retinal detachment surgeries are done here.

CATEGORIES OF VISUAL IMPAIRMENT

WHO	VA		NPCB
	Max < than	Minimum equal to	
Normal Vision	–	6/18	Normal Vision
Low Vision	6/18	6/60	Low Vision
Low Vision	6/60	3/60	**Economic Blindness**
Blindness	3/60	1/60	Social Blindness
Blindness	1/60	PL+	Manifest Blindness
Blindness	PL-	PL–	Absolute Blindness

NEET DRILL

1. Most common cause of blindness in India is cataract.
2. Second most common cause of blindness in India is refractive errors.
3. Most common cause of blindness in the world is cataract.
4. Most common cause of blindness in developed countries is glaucoma.
5. Most common cause of childhood blindness is vitamin A deficiency.
6. Most common cause of ocular morbidity in India is: Refractive errors.
7. Highest prevalence of blindness in India is in Uttar Pradesh.
8. Best corrected vision in the better eye of less than 6/60 is termed Economic blindness.
9. The cut off vision in school screening programme is < 6/9.
10. The prevalence of blindness in India (BCVA of <3/60) in the better eye, is 0.56%.
11. The incidence of cataract in India is 62.6%.
12. SAFE strategy is used to control trachoma in the community. It stands for Surgery, Antibiotics, Facial hygiene and Environmental cleanliness.
13. *Blindness:* It is defined as best corrected visual acuity in the better eye of less than 3/60 OR visual field of less than 10 degree.
14. *Legal Blindness:* Best corrected visual acuity (BCVA) in the better eye of less than 3/60 is the legal blindness.
15. Recently in April 2017, NPCB has changed its definition of blindness as: Best corrected visual acuity in better eye of less than 3/60 or visual field of less than 10 degrees in the better eye.

MULTIPLE CHOICE QUESTIONS

1. SAFE strategy is recommended for control of:

A. Trachoma
B. Glaucoma
C. Diabetes mellitus
D. Cataract

2. The most common cause of low vision in India is:

A. Uncorrected refractive errors
B. Cataract
C. Glaucoma
D. Squint

3. Most common cause of blindness in India:

A. Trachoma
B. Vitamin-A deficiency
C. Cataract
D. Myopia

4. All are common causes of childhood blindness except:

A. Malnutrition
B. Glaucoma
C. Ophthalmia neonatorum
D. Congenital dacryocystitis

5. Under the National Programme for Control of Blindness in India, medical colleges are classified as eye care center of:

A. Primary level
B. Secondary level
C. Tertiary level
D. Intermediate level

6. Taking the definition of blindness as visual acuity less than 3/60 in the better eye, the number of blind persons per 100,000 population in India (according to older data) is estimated to be:

A. 500 B. 700

C. 1000 D. 1500

7. All of the following are given global prominence in the vision 2020 goals, except:

A. Refractive errors

B. Cataract

C. Trachoma

D. Glaucoma

8. For the field diagnosis of trachoma, the WHO recommends that follicular and intense trachoma inflammation should be assessed in:

A. Women aged 15–45 years

B. Population of 10 to 28 years range

C. Children aged 0–10 years

D. Population above 25 years of age irrespective of sex

9. The eye condition for which the World Bank assistance was provided to the National Programme for Control of Blindness (1994–2001) is:

A. Cataract

B. Refractive errors

C. Trachoma

D. Vitamin A deficiency

10. Under the School Eye Screening Programme in India, the initial vision screening of school children is done by:

A. School teachers

B. Primary level health workers

C. Eye specialists

D. Medical officers

11. Which is the most common cause of ocular morbidity in community?

A. Cataract

B. Refractive error

C. Ocular injury

D. Vitamin A deficiency

12. According to the National Programme for Control of Blindness (NPCB) Survey (1986–89), the highest prevalence of blindness in India is in:

A. J & K B. Orissa

C. Bihar D. U.P.

13. A 46-year-old female presented at the eye OPD in a hospital. Her vision in the right eye was 6/60 and left eye was 3/60. Under the National Programme for Control of Blindness, she will be classified as:

A. Socially blind

B. Low vision

C. Economically blind

D. Normal vision

14. The visual acuity used as cut off for differentiating normal from abnormal children in the School Vision Screening Programme in India is:

A. 6/6 B. 6/9

C. 6/12 D. 6/60

15. WHO criteria for blindness is visual acuity of less than:

A. 1/60 B. 6/60

C. 6/18 D. 3/60

16. Mass treatment with azithromycin is indicated if prevalence of trachoma follicles (TF) in 1–9 years population is more than:

A. 10% B. 8%

C. 6% D. 4%

17. What is the recommended ophthalmologist : population ratio in India according to vision 2020?

A. 1:5,000,000 B. 1:1,00,000

C. 1:50,000 D. 1:10,000

18. According to vision 2020 the recommendation for secondary care services including cataract surgery is:

A. 1 service centre for 5000 population

B. 1 service centre for 50,000 population

C. 1 service centre for 5,00,000 population

D. 1 service centre for 5,000,000 population

19. In a district hospital in India, an ophthalmologist is expected to perform which of the following surgeries most commonly?

A. Phacoemulsification

B. Dacryocystectomy

C. Bilamellar tarsal rotation

D. Trabeculectomy

20. Visual acuity of 6/60 is classified as:

A. Low vision

B. Normal vision

C. Blindness

D. Visual morbidity

ANSWER AND EXPLANATION

1. a	2. a	3. c	4. d	5. c	6. b	7. d	8. c	9. a	10. a
11. b	12. d	13. b	14. b	15. d	16. a	17. c	18. c	19. a	20. a

20. Best corrected visual acuity in the better eye of less than 6/60 is called economic blindness.

GUIDANCE

Pioneering takes steady dedicated efforts, it is advancing surely one step at a time.

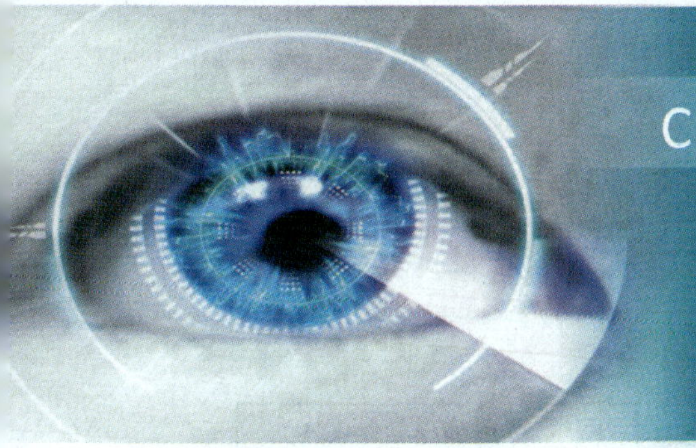

CHAPTER 15

Embryology

DEVELOPMENT OF EYE

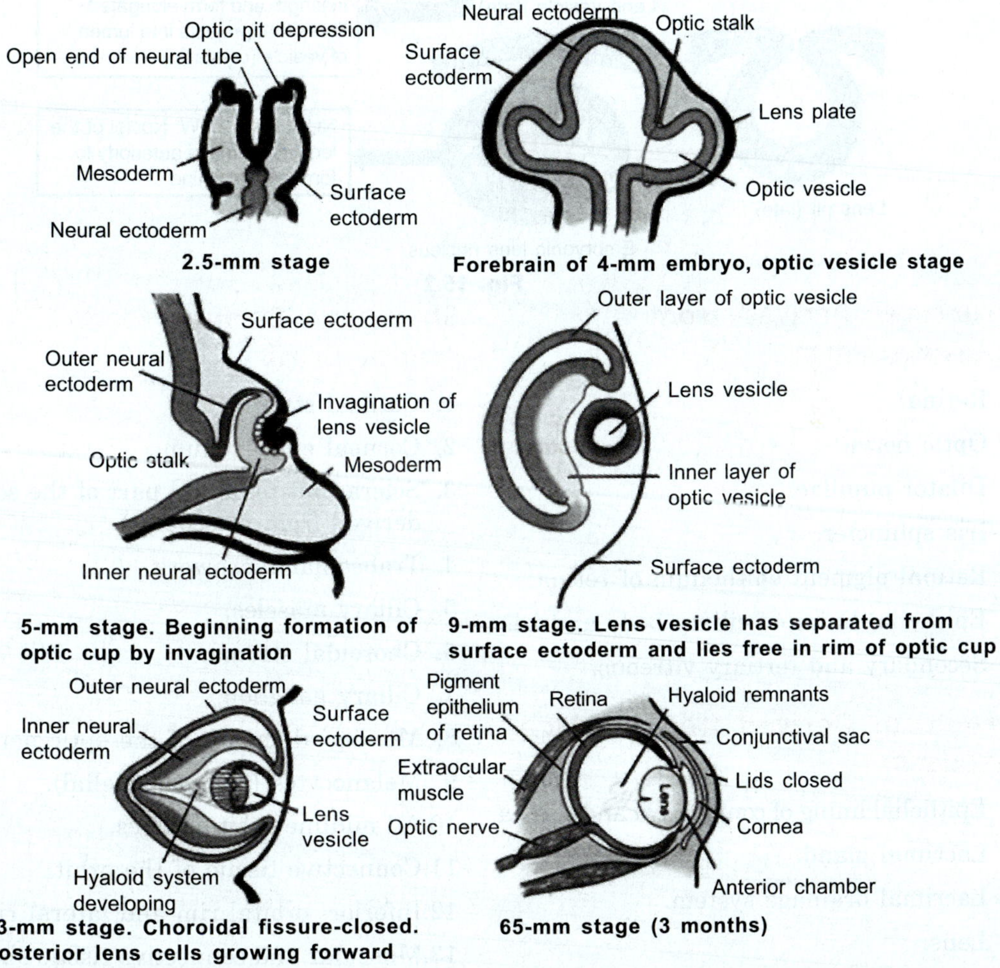

2.5-mm stage

Forebrain of 4-mm embryo, optic vesicle stage

5-mm stage. Beginning formation of optic cup by invagination

9-mm stage. Lens vesicle has separated from surface ectoderm and lies free in rim of optic cup

13-mm stage. Choroidal fissure-closed. Posterior lens cells growing forward

65-mm stage (3 months)

Fig. 15.1

DEVELOPMENT OF LENS

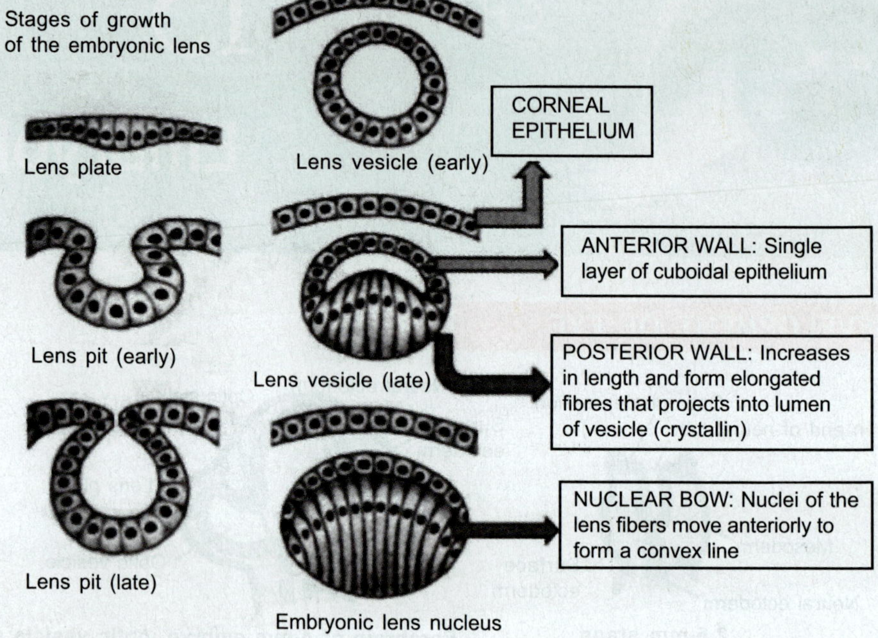

Fig. 15.2

Structures Derived from Neuroectoderm

1. Retina.
2. Optic nerve.
3. Dilator pupillae.
4. Iris sphincter.
5. Retinal pigment epithelium of retina.
6. Epithelial lining of ciliary body and iris.
7. Secondary and tertiary vitreous.

Structures Derived from Surface Ectoderm

1. Epithelial lining of conjunctiva and cornea.
2. Lacrimal gland.
3. Lacrimal drainage system.
4. Lens.
5. Skin and cilia of lids and caruncle.

Structures Derived from Cranial Neural Crest

1. Corneal stroma.
2. Corneal endothelium.
3. Sclera (but temporal part of the sclera is derived from mesoderm).
4. Trabecular meshwork.
5. Ciliary muscles.
6. Choroidal stroma.
7. Ciliary ganglion.
8. Meningeal sheath of the optic nerve.
9. Melanocytes (uveal/epithelial).
10. All midline orbital bones.
11. Connective tissue of the orbit.
12. Inferior orbital rim and lateral rim.
13. Muscular and connective tissue sheath of all orbital and ocular vessels.

Structures Derived from Mesoderm (Paraxial)

1. Fibres of extraocular muscles.
2. Endothelial lining of all orbital and ocular blood vessels.
3. Temporal portion of sclera.
4. Primary vitreous.

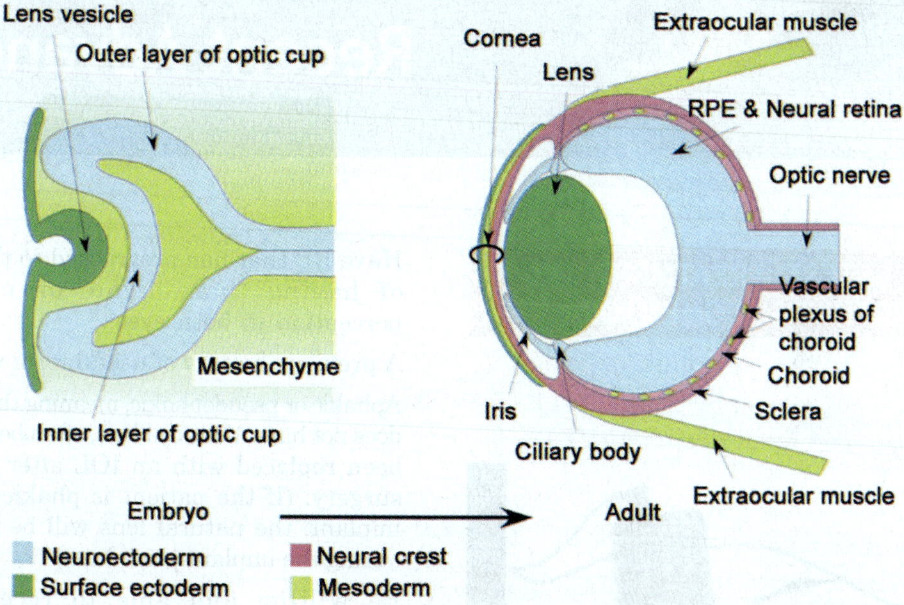

Fig. 15.3

GUIDANCE

NEVER BE SHAKEN, no matter what happens or what others may say. Never be flustered, never lose confidence. This is the way we should strive to live our lives. Being able to do so is a sign of genuine character.

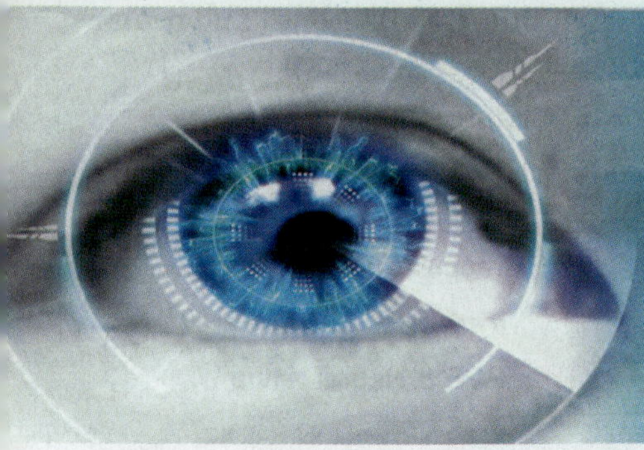

CHAPTER 16

Recent Advances

A. LATEST TREATMENT OF RETINITIS PIGMENTOSA

Argus II

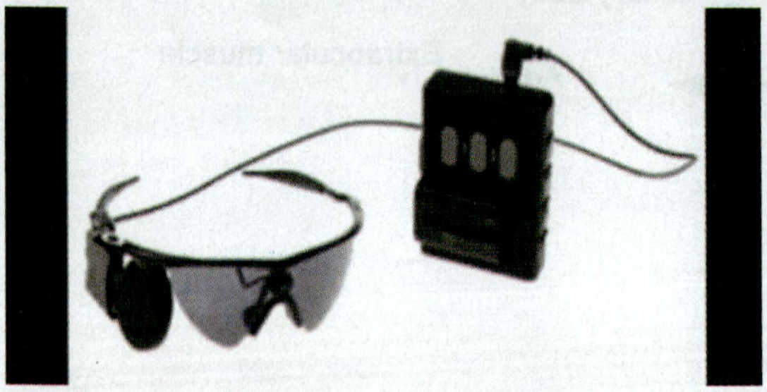

Fig. 16.1

The Argus® II Retinal Prosthesis System ("Argus II") is also known as the bionic **eye** or the retinal **implant**. It is intended to provide electrical stimulation of the retina to induce visual perception in blind individuals. It is indicated for use in patients with severe to profound retinitis pigmentosa.

Prerequisites

The implant is currently approved and intended for use in patients with severe to profound retinitis pigmentosa who meet the following criteria:

- Age 25 years or older.
- Have RP that has progressed to the point of having "bare light" or no light perception in both eyes.
- A previous history of useful form vision.
- Aphakic or pseudophakic, meaning the patient does not have a natural lens, often because it's been replaced with an IOL after cataract surgery. (If the patient is phakic prior to implant, the natural lens will be removed during the implant procedure.)
- Be willing and able to receive the recommended post-implant clinical follow-up, device fitting, and visual rehabilitation.

The Argus implant's primary external element is a digital camera mounted on eyeglass frames, which obtains images of the user's surroundings; signals from the camera are transmitted wirelessly to a computerized image processor. The processor is in turn connected by cables to the implant itself, which is surgically implanted on the surface of the person's retina and tacked into place. The implant consists of 60 electrodes, each 200 microns in diameter.

Surgical Procedure

The implantation procedure takes several hours, with the person receiving the implant under general anaesthesia. The surgeon removes the vitreous humor and any membranes on the retina where the implant will be placed. The implant is attached to the surface of the retina with a tack. The cables connecting the implant to the processor are run through the pars plana, a region near where the iris and sclera touch.

Side Effects

Among the thirty subjects in the clinical trial, there were nine serious adverse events recorded, including lower than normal intraocular pressure, erosion of the conjunctiva, reopening of the surgical wound, inflammation inside the eye, and retinal detachments. There is also a risk of bacterial infection from the implanted cables that connect the implant to the signal processor.

B. PTERYGIUM

The main challenge to successful surgical treatment of pterygium is recurrence. Autografting is a better option for preventing recurrence compared to Mitomycin C. A modification of the autografting procedure is P.E.R.F.E.C.T. Surgery.

We use a large incision to remove the pterygium, creating a large area of bare sclera and is then covered with a larger graft. This leads to very low recurrence rate of around 0.1%.

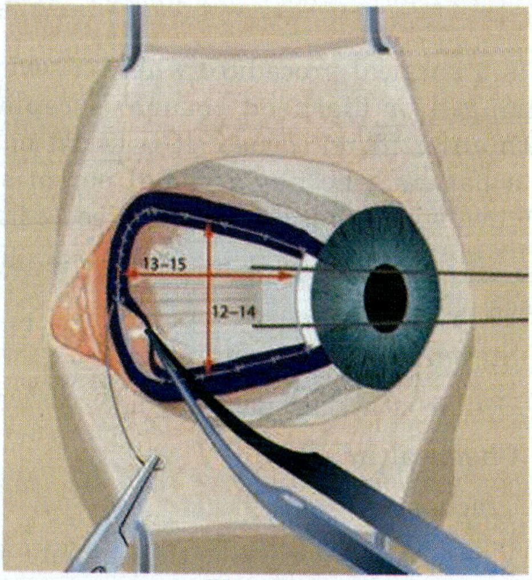

Fig. 16.2

C. FEMTOSECOND LASERS

Femtosecond laser is a focussed infrared laser, with a wavelength of 1053 nm that uses ultrafast pulses with duration of 100 fs (100 into 10^{-15} seconds) it is a solid state Nd Glass laser which operates on the principle of **photoionisation** (photodisruption), i.e., laser induced optical breakdown, this plasma of free electrons and ionised molecules rapidly expand and collapse and create microcavitation bubbles. An acoustic shock wave is produced which separates and incises the target tissue. In comparison to Nd:YAG the microcavitation bubbles produced are much smaller allowing for minimal collateral damage. In this process the collateral damage seen is 106 times less than the Nd:YAG laser which makes it ideal for use in corneal surgeries due to precision and safety. The latest femtolasers have a higher laser firing speed of as much as 500 KHz as compared to 6 KHz in the first femtosecond laser machine.

Applications

1. **Flapless refractive surgery:** It is known as ReLEx Smile (refractive lenticule extraction), Smile is: Small Incision Lenticule Extraction. We use femtosecond laser for all steps of keratomileusis procedure. A refractive lenticule is cut within the stroma, the lenticule is then extracted from the cornea, using a small incision to provide refractive correction. No excimer laser is needed and no flap is created.
2. **Femtolasers assisted cataract surgery (FLACS):** It has four applications in cataract surgery:
   - A. Corneal wound construction.
   - B. Anterior capsulotomy.
   - C. Lens fragmentation.

D. Arcuate keratotomy (AK) to address corneal astigmatism.

3. **Femto-LASIK:** Flap is created by the femtolaser and the rest of the procedure is through Excimer laser.

Other Applications

1. **Intrasomal corneal ring segment implantation:** It is used to treat post-operative LASIK complications like corneal ecstasies, pellucid marginal degeneration, and keratoconus. These rings are inserted in intrasomal channels which is created by femtolaser.
2. **Astigmatic keratotomy:** The use of femtolaser, assures higher precision, stability and more accuracy of the length and depth of the cuts.
3. **Presbyopia treatment:** Femtolasers are also used for creation of Intrasomal pockets to insert biocompatible Intra-corneal inlays for the treatment of presbyopia.
4. **Penetrating and lamellar keratoplasty:** It offers precise, repeatable parameters of diameter and depth in donor and host.

D. ANTI-VEGF AGENTS

Vascular endothelial growth factors (VEGF) are the major factors responsible for the neovascularisation. Anti-VEGF drugs block the VEGF molecules and decreases neovascularisation by decreasing the leakage and swelling of the retina.

These are:

1. Avastin: Bevacizumab.
2. Lucentis: Ranibizumab.
3. Macugen: Pegaptanib sodium.

Indications:

1. Wet ARMD.
2. Severe diabetic macular edema.
3. Severe Proliferative Diabetic Retinopathy.
4. CME (Cystoid Macular Edema) due to CRVO, i.e., central retinal vein occlusion.
5. Vitreous Haemorrhage due to DR or vascular block.

These agents are also indicated in:

1. ROP.
2. Pathological myopia.
3. Coats' disease.
4. Neovascular glaucoma.
5. Postoperatively after trabeculectomy.

The latest anti-VEGF is AFLIBERCEPT (VEGF-TRAP-EYE). In short mentioned as VTE.

E. PHACONIT

It is a minimal incision cataract surgery (MICS), with incision length of 0.9 mm. Phacoemulsification is done with a phaco probe that is without the silicone sleeve. A Rollable IOL is implanted after phaconit. These are ultrathin IOLs which are rolled inside the eye. They are made up of hydrophilic acrylic material.

F. KERATOPROSTHESIS

It is a surgical procedure where a severely damaged or diseased cornea is replaced with an artificial cornea. It is a last option in a patient who has a visual potential in the eye with severely compromised cornea.

Indications: Bilateral blindness in severe cases of:

1. Stevens-Johnson syndrome.
2. Ocular cicatrical pemphigoid.
3. Chemical injury.
4. Trachoma.
5. Vascularised cornea with complete stem cell loss and dryness.

6. Multiple failed penetrating keratoplasty.

G. GLAUCOMA

Glaucoma represents a heterogenous group of optic neuropathies with different genetic basis. In recent years impressive progress has been made on molecular genetics. Genes identified as responsible for glaucoma are:

1. Myocillin.
2. Optineurin.
3. CYP1B1.
4. TIGR.

H. LAMELLAR KERATOPLASTY

This is of two types:

a. **DALK, i.e., Deep Anterior Lamellar Keratoplasty:**

   In this procedure the recipient's endothelial layer is retained and only the anterior part of the cornea above the descements membrane is replaced by the donor cornea. It is a useful procedure in pathologies, not involving the endothelial layer like corneal opacities, corneal ulcers and stromal corneal dystrophies. The main advantage of this procedure over the full thickness penetrating keratoplasty is that endothelial graft rejection is avoided.

b. **DSEK, i.e., Descements Stripping Endothelial Keratoplasty. Also called DLEK, i.e., Deep Lamellar Endothelial Keratoplasty:**

   In this procedure only the endothelial layer with the descements membrane is replaced. It is indicated in the pathologies involving only the endothelial layer like Fuchs endothelial dystrophy, pseudophakic bullous keratopathy, posterior polymorphous dystrophy etc. The disadvantage of this procedure is high risk of endothelial rejection and endothelial cell loss ranges from 20–25%.

I. UVEITIS

Luminate Program

This is a study from Lux Biosciences for a nonsteroidal treatment of uveitis. Named Luveniq (Lx-211) or vaclosporin, it is a next generation calcineurin inhibitor and an immunomodulator. It is the first corticosteroid sparing agent available in US for treatment of uveitis.

J. ARMD (AGE-RELATED-MACULAR-DEGENERATION)

Genes associated with this disease are:

1. **ABCR gene: This was the first gene, found to be associated with ARMD. It is also responsible for Stargardt's disease. Hence, it is actually a macular disease gene.**
2. **Complement factor H: It correlates with vision loss in ARMD.**

K. ENDONASAL DACRYOCYSTORHINOSTOMY

An endonasal DCR is carried out using a thin, flexible, fibreoptic telescope called an endoscope. This is passed up the nose and guides instruments or a laser, which is used to make a small hole into the bone of the nose. A thin small silicone tube is then threaded in this passage to maintain the patency of this fistula.

Laser Endonasal DCR

Laser is focused through the transcanalicur approach to do the osteotomy which should be 8–10 mm wide. The lasers used for this purpose are Holmium-YAG laser or CO_2 laser.

Advantages of endonasal DCR are:

a. No external scar.
b. Lacrimal pump is preserved.

c. Lacrimal sac mucosa is preserved.

d. Any concomitant intranasal pathology causing epiphora can be addressed.

L. OCRIOPLASMIN (MICROPLASMIN)

It is recombinant truncated form of human plasmin produced by recombinant DNA technology. It has a proteolytic activity against fibronectin and laminin. Hence, it is useful for dissolving the protein matrix responsible for the vitreomacular adhesions.

Indication:

Treatment of symptomatic (mild to moderate) vitreomacular adhesions.

GUIDANCE

There is no need for you to be impatient. If you can achieve something very easily right from the start, you will find no sense of fulfilment or joy. It is in making tenacious all out efforts for construction, that profound happiness lies.

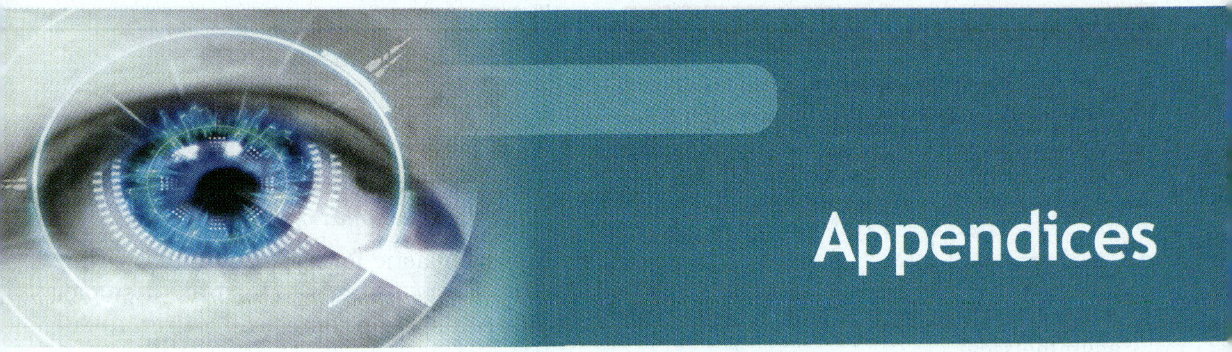

Appendices

PHACOMATOSIS

1. von Hippel-Lindau Syndrome

- Autosomal dominant.
- *Ocular Features:*
  1. 50% cases are bilateral.
  2. Multiple capillary hemangiomas of the optic nerve.
  3. Multiple capillary hemangiomas of retina.
- *Systemic Features:*
  - A. Hemangioblastoma involving cerebellum, medulla, pons or spinal cord.
  - B. Msc-lesions—Cysts of kidney, pancreas, liver, ovary and lungs.

2. Neurofibromatosis-I

Ocular Features:

1. Optic nerve glioma.
2. Other neural tumours.
3. Spheno–orbital encephalocele.
4. Eyelid plexiform neurofibromas.
5. Prominent corneal nerves.
6. Congenital ectropion uveae.
7. Congenital glaucoma (rare).
8. Choroidal hematomas.
9. Lisch nodules.

3. Neurofibromatosis-II

1. Juvenile posterior subcapsular cataract.
2. Combined hamartomas of the retina and retinal pigment epithelium.

4. Sturge-Weber Syndrome

It is a triad of:

1. Capillary hemangioma on the face called Naevus Flammeus.
2. Intracranial hemangioma.
3. Glaucoma.

5. Tuberous Sclerosis

- **Also called Bournevilles' disease or Epiloia.**
- **It is a phacomatosis with classical triad of:**
  1. Mental handicap.
  2. Epilepsy.
  3. Adenoma sebaceum.

  Ocular Features:
  - A. Retinal astrocytomas.
  - B. Hypopigmented iris spots.

MYASTHENIA GRAVIS

It is an autoimmune disorder characterized by reduction in post-synaptic acetylcholine receptors. Patients present with excessive fatiguability of ocular, bulbar and skeletal muscles.

Ocular Features:

1. *Ptosis:* Bilateral and may be asymmetrical.
2. *Diplopia:* All or any of extraocular muscles may be involved. Initially the vertical muscles are most commonly involved.
3. *Nystagmoid movements:* May be present on extreme gaze.

Investigations:

1. Tensilon test.
2. Electromyography.
3. Measurement of antibodies (to striated muscles).
4. CT or MRI of anterior mediastinum, to rule out thymoma.

Treatment:

1. *Medical*
   a. Long-acting anticholinesterase.
   b. Steroids (systemic).
   c. Cytotoxic drugs.
   d. Plasmapheresis.
2. *Thymectomy.*
3. *Strabismus surgery.*

EATON-LAMBERT SYNDROME (LEMS)

Rare Disorder

- Is a presynaptic disorder of neuromuscular junction.
- *Triad of:*
  1. Muscle weakness.
  2. Autonomic dysfunction.
  3. Hyporeflexia.
- Associated with malignancy commonly *Oat-cell carcinoma of lung.*
- Non-neoplastic form is associated with—pernicious anemia, thyroid, disease, Sjögren's syndrome and other autoimmune disorders.
- Smooth muscle, skeletal muscle and glands are involved.
- *Ocular Features:*

  Ocular features not as prominent as in myasthenia gravis.
  1. KCS.
  2. Ptosis and intermittent diplopia.
  3. Sluggishly reacting pupils.
  4. Slow saccadic velocities.

OCULAR MYOPATHIES

- Ocular myopathies are a group of rare disorders mostly sporadic or have dominant inheritance.
- *Ocular Features:*
  a. Main feature is Chronic Progressive External Ophthalmoplegia (CPEO) initially involving the upgaze.
  b. Lateral movements get involved in later stage leading to virtually fixed eyes.
  c. No Diplopia.
  d. Bilateral ptosis.
- **Three main forms are:**
  a. *Primary ocular myopathy.*
  b. *Oculopharyngeal dystrophy:* In addition to ocular feature there is weakness of pharyngeal muscles and wasting of temporalis muscle.

c. *Kearns-Sayre Syndrome:*
   1. Ocular myopathy.
   2. Pigmentary retinopathy.
   3. Heart block.

ULTRASONOGRAPHY IN EYE

- The eye scan makes use of high frequency ultrasonic waves of around 8–10 Hz.
- It is based on the principle of **"Pizeo electric effect"** where mechanical vibrations are converted into electric potentials.
- These high frequencies produce shorter wavelengths which allow good resolution of minute ocular and orbital structures. These waves can penetrate all tissues.

Modes of Display

A-scan or Time Amplitude Method: It is used for biometry, i.e., calculation of IOL power. A scan measures the axial length. Formula commonly used is **SRK-II** which is a modification of SRK-I.

B-scan or Intensity Modulation: It is used to detect lesions in orbit, eyeball, vitreous and intraocular foreign bodies.

C-scan: It is used to display soft tissues in the coronal plane of the orbit.

EMBRYOLOGICAL REMNANTS

Bergmeisters papilla: It is the hyaloid remnant on the optic disc, and presents as flake of glial tissue projecting from the optic disc.

Mittendorf dot: It is the hyaloid remnant (anterior end of hyaloid artery) on posterior lens capsule. It is associated with posterior polar cataract.

Epicapsular stars: They are remnants of pupillary membrane.

MIGRAINE

It is a familial disorder characterized by recurrent attacks of headache widely variable in intensity, frequency and duration. Attacks are commonly unilateral and associated with anorexia, nausea and vomiting.

The main types of migraine are:

a. **Common:** Headache with autonomic nervous system disturbances.

b. **Classical:** Headache with visual or auditory aura.

c. **Focal:** Headache with transient dysphagia, hemisensory symptoms or even focal weakness.

d. **Migraine sine migraine:** Episodic visual disturbances but no subsequent headache.

e. **Retinal migraine:** Acute but transient unilateral loss of vision similar to Amaurosis fugax.

f. **Ophthalmoplegic migraine:**
   - Recurrent transient III nerve palsy occurring after headache.
   - Typically starts before age of 10 years.

g. **Complicated migraine:** Failure of full recovery of focal neurological features after the migraine is over like hemisensory disturbance or partial visual field loss.

h. **Cluster headache:** Unilateral, oculotemporal, sharp, excruciating headache occurring in cluster (i.e., occurs frequently in 24 hours and then long interval of several years) in men of fourth and fifth decade. Between clusters there may be long headache-free interval for several years. It may be associated with autonomic symptoms like lacrimation, conjunctival congestion and rhinorrhoea.

OCULAR ANESTHESIA

Types

1. Surface anesthesia/Topical anesthesia.
2. Regional or Infiltration anesthesia.

Topical Anesthesia: This constitutes instillation of 4% lignocaine or 0.5–1% amethocaine into the cul-de-sac. It is commonly required for removal of corneal foreign body, gonioscopy, tonometry or syringing.

Infiltration Anesthesia/Regional Anesthesia

1. Retrobulbar block.
2. Peribulbar block.
3. Subtenon block.
4. Facial block.

Retrobulbar Block: Retrobulbar space include optic nerve, rectus muscles and tissues between them and the periorbit. It is divided into intraconal and extraconal compartment. A retrobulbar injection is any injection behind the equator of the eye in which needle lies behind the projection of the equator.

Method: Needle is introduced at the junction of middle third and lateral third of the inferior orbital margin and then directed backwards and medially towards the apex of the orbit.

Peribulbar Block:

- *Method:* Injection of 5 ml to 7 ml of local anesthetic solution in the peripheral space of the orbit (outside the muscle cone) from where it diffuses into the muscle cone and lids, leading to globe and orbicularis akinesia and anesthesia.
- *Two injections are given by 1 inch 23 G or 24 G needle:*
  a. First is through the lower lid (junction of medial 2/3rd and lateral 1/3rd).
  b. Second injection is given through upper lid (junction of medial 1/3rd and lateral 2/3rd)
- *Anesthetic solution used is:*

  2% lignocaine or xylocaine with or without adrenaline
  +
  0.5% to 0.75% bupivacaine (sensoricaine)
  +
  5IU/ml of hyaluronidase.

Subtenon Block: It constitutes the injection of the anesthetic solution (4 ml) into tenons capsule (posterior aspect) around the upper half of the eyeball and into the belly of the superior rectus muscle. It avoids the complications of peribulbar and retrobulbar injections.

Facial Block or Orbicularis Oculi Akinesia: This method is useful to block the facial nerve or its zygomatic branch to paralyse the orbicularis oculi muscle and hence prevent the squeezing of the eyelids during operation.

Methods:

1. *O'Brien's technique:* In this method 4–5 ml of the anesthetic is injected at the neck of the mandible in front of the tragus.
2. *Van-lint method:* In this method, 4 ml of the solution is injected 1 cm below and behind the lateral canthus. It is infiltrated along the superolateral and inferior orbital margin in a v-shaped manner.
3. *Atkinson block:* This method blocks the facial nerve as it passes along the zygoma. The anesthetic is injected along the inferior border of zygoma and continued along zygomatic arch towards the ear.

AUTOCLAVING

1. It is the most effective means of sterilization.
2. Steam under a pressure of 15 pounds per square inch (PSI) is used by raising the boiling point of water to 121°C. The water should preferably be distilled to prevent deposition of salts.
3. *Instrument, gowns, drapes,* dressing are routinely sterilized by autoclaving for 15 minutes.
4. *Sharp instruments*–cidex, or ethylene–oxide gas sterilization or in hot air oven.
5. *Suture materials* are usually sterilized by gamma irradiation.